PSYCHIC-NEXUS

PSYCHIC PHENOMENA IN PSYCHIATRY AND EVERYDAY LIFE

PSYCHIC-NEXUS

PSYCHIC PHENOMENA IN PSYCHIATRY AND EVERYDAY LIFE

BERTHOLD ERIC SCHWARZ, M.D.

Consultant Psychiatrist
Essex County Hospital Center,
Cedar Grove, New Jersey

VNR VAN NOSTRAND REINHOLD COMPANY
NEW YORK   CINCINNATI   ATLANTA   DALLAS   SAN FRANCISCO
LONDON   TORONTO   MELBOURNE

Van Nostrand Reinhold Company Regional Offices:
New York   Cincinnati   Atlanta   Dallas   San Francisco

Van Nostrand Reinhold Company International Offices:
London   Toronto   Melbourne

Library of Congress Catalog Card Number: 79-22701
ISBN: 0-442-25210-2

Manufactured in the United States of America

Published by Van Nostrand Reinhold Company
135 West 50th Street, New York, N.Y. 10020

Published simultaneously in Canada by Van Nostrand Reinhold Ltd.

15   14   13   12   11   10   9   8   7   6   5   4   3   2   1

Library of Congress Cataloging in Publication Data

Schwarz, Berthold Eric, 1924-
  Psychic-nexus.

  Includes index.
  1. Psychical research—Case studies.
2. Psychiatry—Cases studies. I. Title.
BF1040.S38   616.8'9'09   79-22701
ISBN 0-442-25210-2

For Lisa Thyra and Eric Rolf

Preface

In recent years there has been a reawakening of widespread interest in psychic phenomena. Psychiatrists, psychologists, biologists, physicists, and countless others have contributed to the subject. Although mention is often made of the role of emotional factors in psi, much of this is only in passing, and then these observations are frequently made by those who have not devoted their professional careers to the study of the mind, the brain, the interface, and the unconscious. Despite superb observations on the possible role of emotions in psi by parapsychologists and others, there is still a relative paucity of material by psychiatrists. As a psychiatrist, I hope that by presenting numerous examples of psychic-dynamics as experienced and interpreted in my own practice, personal life, and researches, that the reader can get an idea of how psi actually works, how frequently it occurs, how it is operative in the psychopathology of everyday life, the psychodynamics of various neurotic, psychotic and psychosomatic mechanisms, and from study of these examples, how the reader can develop his own techniques of an awareness for psi.

If the behaviorial scientist has more than a casual interest in psi or better yet, a flair for it, it is safe to predict that with study and practice he will be able to develop his abilities and that he will be swamped with psychic material. Should he so desire, by collecting possible psychic data involving himself and his family, he might be better poised to further explore this fascinating subject, seemingly without boundaries, and overlapping almost all of the scientific disciplines, waiting, yes begging, for serious attention and study for the possible benefit of mankind.

I am grateful to many of my patients and friends who knowingly or otherwise participated in these studies and who, whether they knew it or not, taught me most of what I know. One does not stand alone and it is also acknowledged that the numerous previously published psychiatric studies are gold mines of observations that are invaluable to the serious student of psychic dynamics. My thanks also go to my hardworking secretaries through the years and in particular Miss Vilma E. Semsey, who has always been willing and helpful in the typing and retyping of this material.

Many of the studies included had been previously edited by my friend, the late Mrs. Joan W. Jesurun, a master of the English language and a lady of impeccable taste and superb character. Much of what appears might have been lost for ever in the journals or left ensconsed in my files had it not been for the encouragement and kindness of my friend Martin Ebon, who suggested that I consider collecting my papers on psi and arranging them into book form. Thus, I thank all these good people for their indispensable help. They are not responsible for any errors or lack of judgement which are completely unintentional and for which I alone can answer.

My plan, from a narrow viewpoint is to be of help to my colleagues in psychiatry, and particularly to the younger ones in their training and researches, and from a broader perspective, to widen the horizons and inflame the curiosity of all potential readers who might have an interest in the subject, no matter what their particular backgrounds, or point of view. New ideas are often born of controversy. Controversy, unlike dogma, which is strangling, can become the zest of life and a motivating force.

BERTHOLD ERIC SCHWARZ

Acknowledgments

When the possible psychic examples were abridged in their original publication, new examples were substituted and the chapters revised. Hopefully then, there is no duplication of illustrative cases, unless only in passing, and then to make a point. Appreciation is given to the following organizations who permitted the reprinting of articles in total or in part:

Corrective Psychiatry and the Journal of Social Therapy for Psychodynamic Experiments in Telepathy, Vol. 9 (No. 4): 169–218, 1963; Built-in Controls and Postulates for the Telepathic Event, Vol. 12 (No. 2):64–82, March 1966; and The Telepathic Hypothesis and Genius: A Note on Thomas Alva Edison, Vol. 13 (No. 1):7–19, January 1967.

The International Journal of Parapsychology for Telepathic Events in a Child Between 1 and 3½ Years of Age, Vol. III (No. 4):5–52, 1961.

The Journal of the American Geriatric Society, Inc., for Possible Geriatric Telepathy, Vol. XXI (No. 5):216–223, May 1973.

The Journal of the American Society of Psychosomatic Dentistry and Medicine, for Telepathy and Pseudotelekinesis in Psychotherapy, Vol. 15 (No. 4):144–154, 1968; Precognition and Psychic Nexus, Part I: Vol. 18 (No. 2): 52–59, 1971; Part II: Vol. 18 (No. 3):83–93, 1971; Possible Human-Animal Paranormal Events, Vol. 20 (No. 2):39–53, 1973; Psi and the Life Cycle, Part I: Vol. 21 (No. 2):64–69, 1974; Part II: Vol. 21 (No. 3):98–105, 1974; Part III: Vol. 21 (No. 4):135–142, 1974; Part IV: Vol. 22 (No. 1):23–28, 1975; Part V: Vol. 22 (No. 2):57–63, 1975; Part VI: Vol. 22 (No. 3):91–99, 1975; Part VII: Vol. 22 (No. 4)129–133, 1975. UFO Contactee Stella Lansing: Possible Medical Implications of her Motion Picture Experiments, Vol. 23 (No. 2):60–68, 1976.

The Journal of the Medical Society of New Jersey for Possible Telesomatic Reactions, Vol. 64 (No. 11):600–603, November 1967.

Medical Times for Clinical Studies on Telesomatic Reactions, Vol. 101 (No. 2):71–84, December 1973.

Psychiatric Quarterly for Ordeals by Serpents, Fire and Strychnine, Vol. 34:405–429, July 1960.

Psychoanalytic Review for Synchronicity and Telepathy, Vol. 56 (No. 1):44–56, 1969, and Telepathic Humoresque, Vol. 61 (No. 4):591–606, 1974–75. Reprinted through the courtesy of the Editors and the publisher, National Psychological Association for Psychoanalysis, Inc., New York, New York.

Samiksa (Journal of the Indian Psycho-Analytical Society, Calcutta, India), for Death of a Parapsychologist, Possible Terminal Telepathy with Nandor Fodor, Vol. 21 (No. 1):1–14, 1967.

Introduction

It is my purpose to present to psychiatrists in particular, and to as wide an audience of intelligent laymen as possible, some of my findings in psychic research. For many readers this will be their first contact with such data, since most of the material has been published only in specialty medical journals of limited circulation. In the rare instances where examples were used more than once, new examples have been chosen to minimize or eliminate duplication.

The techniques I have used are similar to those employed in a variety of earlier published psychiatric studies, many of which were done in collaboration with other physicians during my Fellowship at the Mayo Foundation. Although the examples and psi episodes presented here pertain mainly to clinical investigations of gifted mediums (paragnosts), psi in the physician-patient relationship and in the parent-child situation, they also include an account of a field trip to the Holiness sect in eastern Kentucky where some of the devotees test their faith by the spectacular Ordeals by Serpents, Fire, and Strychnine. Also presented are some psychodynamic drawing experiments for psi; and later experiments of the UFO-psi interface, involving possible thoughtography or the appearance of UFO-like artifacts on motion picture films.

In many instances there is theoretical and clinical application not only to the practice of psychiatry, but to all the behavioral sciences, as well as broader implications for medicine. For example, the psi-induced psychosomatic states or telesomatic reactions cover a variety of conditions and might explain the precipitation, aggravation, or relief of many illnesses which without the psi hypothesis would be shrouded in obscurity. The subject matter I have chosen is not a compendium of all my published works on psi as, for example, laboratory studies of Henry Gross's dowsing[176] using the electroencephalogram, psychogalvanic reflex and electromyogram, seed-germination studies of Romano's ray,[175] a possible mitogenetic effect, and numerous papers on the UFO-psi interface published in medical journals and *Flying Sau-*

cer Review; nor does my selection include articles on basic and clinical psychiatric research projects.

Although I have memories of unusual coincidences and happenings in my childhood, this body of data is, obviously, not subject to critical scrutiny. The earliest major psi event in my life occurred in 1945 when I was on leave from the Navy in World War II. I was returning to my home when I became suddenly and progressively gripped with the horrible certainty that my younger brother Eric had been killed in action in General Patton's III Army in Germany. I couldn't shake off this thought, and as I approached my home I recognized a few cars parked in the street that belonged to family and friends. As I walked up to the door it was no surprise to learn that my premonition was all too true.

Undoubtedly this perception came from the awful news that my parents had received earlier in the evening. As I later learned, they were prepared for this grim event because some weeks earlier while all alone in Montclair, New Jersey, my mother had, presumably telepathically, perceived my brother's death and had told my father at that time.

Naturally these events jolted me and made me curious about how common such things might be, and how they work. I wondered if they might be just the tip of an iceberg or some rare and vestigial event, or if psi could encompass many less spectacular and terrible events and really be a part of everyday life. This grim experience involving my brother and mother and later myself whetted my interest in psi. I had an opportunity to further peruse many excellent volumes and journals on this subject at Baker Library in Dartmouth College. One of the books that caught my attention was about Henry Gross, the Maine dowser, by the well-known author, Kenneth Roberts.[176] Later it was my good fortune to return to Dartmouth Medical School and intern at Mary Hitchcock Memorial Hospital. While there I renewed my friendship with Herb West, Professor of Comparative Literature, who was a good friend of Kenneth Roberts. Although I never met Roberts, we corresponded about Henry Gross, and I was becoming ever more curious. For example, how could Henry Gross dowse a map of Bermuda while he was in the state of Maine and locate water—an otherwise nearly impossible finding? Was this dowsing talent related to psychic ability? If so, I wondered how this isolated psychic event would apply to Henry Gross and his family.

These questions were postponed for several years which I spent in a Fellowship in Psychiatry at the Mayo Foundation. However, while I was there, two unusual events kept my interest alive. First, I had a Phi Beta Kappa physician-patient who had earlier attempted suicide and who was admitted to the closed-ward hospital service. It developed that much of his emotional trouble was influenced by his psychic mother. The chain of spectacular psychic episodes, many of which involved his mother and himself, were noted. Through correspondence with his mother, I followed his life to his death in another state years later, from a brain tumor as proven by post-mortem. This case was published in my *Psychic-Dynamics*,[176] which also included studies on Henry Gross, and an account of a highly respected citizen and gifted psychic in my hometown, a Mrs. Krystal (pseudonym).

The second psychic situation that piqued my curiosity while in Minnesota involved a woman patient with intractable migraine. In our psychotherapeutic sessions there appeared to be many episodes of thought transference. These odd occurrences interested me intensely, and I discussed them with my supervisor, Adelaide M. Johnson, M.D. My chief concern, then as now, was therapeutic—prima non nocere—and the ethical question was: What was best for the patient? Any research interest in psi had to meet that condition or accept a secondary role. As will be seen in many clinical examples, psi is a process: when the stage is properly set, it just takes over. Psi might be akin to what some call possession. However, this "possession" is not due to an "alien" presence for which there is little evidence, but actually comes from the depths of the unconscious mind, where intuitive psychic flashes have undergone incubation and filtration by various mental mechanisms and defenses. Like the manifest content of dreams possession often seems to the uninitiated patient to be apart from himself; yet with free associations and analysis dreams lose much of their mystery and take on deeper, more complex meanings. Few subjects so tax the physician's need to try to be, at all times, both responsive and responsible.

There were always "coincidences" or odd happenings that aroused my interest. When I finished my training in psychiatry and returned to Montclair, New Jersey, in 1955, I intended to look into these matters and see if there could be anything to them. Fate intervened on the side of these goals. Earlier, Dr. Victor Johnson, Director of the Mayo Foundation, had advised me to affiliate with a medical school and continue my various researches and teaching. Therefore, when I was back in New Jersey, I wrote to Dean Clarence Brown, of the then newly founded Seton Hall College of Medicine in Jersey City. After a long wait, Dr. Brown wrote that the Department of Psychiatry was just on the drawing board and that he would write me when they were better organized. Never having heard from him, and knowing that he died in the interim, my medical school teaching career was aborted. However, this backhandedly fortuitous event gave me freedom to pursue these earlier questions. Shortly afterward I met Miss Gertrude O. Tubby, who had formerly been secretary of the American Society of Psychical Research, who lived in Montclair, and who possessed a magnificent library on psychic phenomena. Miss Tubby had an encyclopedic mind and could recall many experiences going back to nearly the turn of the century. Some involved such great mediums as Mrs. Leonore Piper, as well as her boss James H. Hyslop, also William James, Franklin Prince, Sir William Barret, Sir William Crooks, and other pioneers.

Through Miss Tubby I met a fellow townsman, Les Egbert, an engaging, successful businessman. Les, who was quite gifted in psi (see the chapter Precognition and Psychic Nexus), was fascinated with the possibility of using Henry Gross's dowsing skills for oil exploration on land that he owned in eastern Kentucky. Previously I had driven to Maine, met Henry Gross, and spent several hours with him and his family. My psychiatric interviews tended to confirm Kenneth Roberts' report on Gross, if not Roberts' interpretation. Beyond that, I learned enough to have ignited areas Roberts did not touch upon, and which pertained to psi. These fortunate events of meeting Les Egbert and Henry Gross within a short span of time dovetailed, and we subsequently made several trips to Kentucky where I could study Henry in the field, as well as additional studies undertaken in my office in Montclair.

While in the Appalachian part of eastern Kentucky with Henry Gross, Les Egbert, and others, I, by happenstance, heard about the Holiness sect and possible extraordinary psychosomatic phenomena involving the "Saints" and their apparent immunity to being bitten by rattlesnakes and copperheads, and relative protection from the effects of fire applied to their bodies or from the ingestion of strychnine. Most of my interviews with the Saints and Holiness church services were taped and filmed.

If psi was part of a continuum that seemingly involved all aspects of one's life, the quickening pace of my investigations had the effect of a psychic merry-go-round. While I was immersed in my practice and the studies of Henry Gross, my friend and classmate from Navy days at Dartmouth, Dr. Roy Swenson, kept importuning me about Jacques Romano, a man who was quite remarkable in reading thoughts. Romano, who was youthful appearing though then in his early 90s, could seemingly exert considerable control over his telepathic abilities, and he also possessed the ability to emanate a cool breeze-like sensation from his body. He was known to presidents, kings, popes, and people in all walks of life from before the turn of the century. The study of Romano then became a new salient in my psychic researches. Romano was cooperative, cheerful, full of fun, and had no ideologies, or, as he put it, "isms or spasms." He was a delightful man who could when "turned on" produce a variety of telepathic phenomena. These studies were conducted in my home and office, as well as in the field, including a radiology laboratory, and on patients at a nearby psychiatric hospital. The telepathic stunts with healthy people were as successful as with the patients who had various mental conditions as well as known brain lesions from lobotomy, tumors, etc.

While these studies were taking place, I was actively involved in psychiatric practice and raising a family. I was grateful that I never received a post at a medical school. Besides, what medical school in those days would ever tolerate such heretical research? While busy with Jacques Romano and Henry Gross, I also met Mrs. Krystal, a beautiful, elderly, remarkable patrician who was most imposing in her physical appearance and skilled in her psychic gifts. As a physician, I was particularly interested in her because of the possible tie-in between psi and her diabetes, unconscious life, family reactions, interpersonal relationships, and other significant events. It was possible to follow her abilities and conduct some psychic experiments as in the case of Jacques Romano, and later with the famous telepathist Joseph Dunninger—until the very end.

My material on Dunninger consisted of hundreds of tape cassettes and other data collected over several years. Some of this was ultra-sensitive and involved living people; therefore, in accordance with Dunninger's wishes, it was consigned to the time capsule. Some of his experiences and opinions, however, derived from his more than 50-year career in show business, will be found in the examples. With Dunninger, as with other gifted paragnosts, the best examples were always spontaneous, unplanned, and tended to catch us off guard.

Needless to say, my filing cabinets soon bulged with typed reports and tapes of many other paragnosts, spectacular physician-patient psi examples, investigations of alleged haunted houses, etc. I also kept envelopes on telepathic death experiences, examples of alleged precognition, telekinesis, human paranormal events, and alleged UFO-psychic episodes, etc. Since many of these encounters involved myself, this constituted a clinical control between myself and the paragnosts, and the patients. The data from the latter became the bulk of my material later, and cut across all diagnostic categories. The depth of knowledge about any given patient—which included reports from other physicians as well as contacts through the years with other members of the patient's families, their neighbors and friends—provided a richer understanding of the variables. Consequently, the best examples for psi were from the histories of patients and from what happened in my sessions with them, and even outside the sessions. In many instances, including studies of paragnosts Henry Gross, Jacques Romano, Mrs. Krystal, Joseph Dunninger, and others, I was fortunate to have copious collateral material obtained from other members of the family, including siblings, wives, husbands, children, and grandchildren. In most cases the psi episodes were written down as they were taking place and in many cases were dictated and transcribed shortly afterward.

Fortunately, because of the influence of Romano's lively demonstrations where "you have to see it to believe it," I gained confidence not only in considering the psi hypothesis but in using it. I was not ashamed, therefore, to record even the trivial from these early days, for as much could be learned from these as from a spectacular episode. Many things considered "coincidences" seemed to evaporate when the same types of coincidences as described in *Built-in Controls* happened again and again.

The sheer bulk of the presumed psi data indicated that psi could be "learned" and would occur under certain conditions, and that psi was clinically repeatable. Also, certain patterns of possible personality correlates began to emerge. I was encouraged by reading the works of such giants as Professor W. H. C. Tenhaeff[214-216] of the Parapsychological Institute of the University of Utrecht, and the psychiatric-psychoanalytic studies of psi as collected in George Devereux's *Anthology*.[21] I was particularly impressed by the researches of the psi-psychoanalytic quadrumvirate: Jan Ehrenwald,[36-43] Jule Eisenbud,[44-59] Nandor Fodor,[64-80] and Joost Meerloo.[124-129] I found that by studying their works with great care and rereading their articles, psi was not only an interesting subject, but my awareness for such episodes could be greatly increased. At one point in my experience, the potential ability for psi awareness was analogous to the difference between hearing "Twinkle, Twinkle, Little Star" and a virtuoso's performance of Mozart's Concerto for piano and orchestra, No. 22 in E Flat Major, K.482. These psychiatric methods of studying psi and collecting data were different in style and content from the more widely known laboratory and mostly statistical experiments in parapsychology.

Ehrenwald has often pointed out that there is no need to apologize for the criteria for psi in the clinical setting. It is second to nothing. Anecdotal material should not be disqualified out of hand as not scientific because it is not readily measurable by mathematical formulas. It behooves the mathematician and computer expert to become thoroughly familiar with psi as it is happening in the clinical situation and to devise methods that are statistically sound and yet satisfy the frustrating vagaries of psi.

Psi, as it happens in life, and as my records seem to indicate, does not appear to be an anomaly but a nearly everyday, on-going process, involving many complexities between two or more people, but possibly also many other factors, and comprising at its heart a psychic nexus.

My wife and I have seen Romano perform his enigmatic feats so many times that on occasion we have actually done the same. But perhaps due to unconscious resistance, we would recoil from the events and seldom try to repeat them because of the shock of what had happened. Nevertheless, these happenings were quite applicable in our own relationship as well as in relationships with friends, family, and others. Because of the particular chronology and type of material in the Romano studies, we started keeping records from the very first, of possible telepathic communications with our infant daughter Lisa and, later, our son Eric and ourselves.

Awareness for psi was like the story, "The Emperor's New Clothes." There it was, but because of various resistances, as cogently described by Eisenbud[50] and Meerloo,[128] these events were dissociated from, or consciously passed off as coincidences. Only by keeping records at the time or immediately after the events occurred, and then studying the data first hand were these events seemingly furthered, or perhaps a psychoneural mechanism for psi was conditioned.

In the meantime, it was evident from numerous examples that my mother was telepathic with me, my wife, and our children. This ability persisted in a spectacular manner to the end when she died of a brain tumor. The same telepathic intuitiveness was true also of my father, who in addition to being a successful physician, pursued several other careers. In one of them, his accomplishments were outstanding to say the least. As I look back on it, I suppose that in great measure his "hobby" was really an excellent outlet for his unconscious psychic abilities, or as he used to say "savvy." The difference between my mother and father, however, was that my father's attitude was more conventional, and even deprecatory, in regard to psychic abilities, whereas my mother took it for granted and made no fuss about it. Father had no *awareness* for what to me was so obvious in our numerous exchanges, which were similar to the examples recorded here. His ability, like my mother's, continued to the moment of his death.

People have frequently asked how one develops a talent for psi. I believe the answer is that most people have this latent ability but some are more aware of it than others. It is largely a matter of undoing unconscious resistance. Also, just as some people are musical prodigies and others are tone-deaf, so it is with the psi faculty. There might, therefore, be a hereditary predisposition. Moreover, a culturally favorable environment appears to be helpful. If the parents don't pooh pooh and denigrate any budding psychic ability in their children or, for that matter, the presumed psi exchanges between themselves, the phenomena are accepted for what they are: facts of life, and not suppressed and later repressed by ridicule or the like. Also, the talent of awareness for psi is hinted at by many who show keen interest in the subject, read everything they can get on it, and share their personal possible psi experiences with those who are also gifted or intrigued by the subject. These traits indicate a subliminal awareness of their own latent psi capabilities. Yet psi is elusive, for like the dream, it is disguised with various mental mechanisms and is often consigned to forbidden territory or throttled by various pejoratives like superstition, game playing, or plain rubbish. Most people are unaware of the existence of psi or of its psychodynamic meaning unless they have an intuitive talent for it or are working in a psychotherapeutic situation where psi encounters can be deciphered, made conscious, and translated into often highly charged, meaningful and enriching interpersonal events.

By keeping a record of all psi examples, including the so-called trivial ones, that go on in everyday life, success seems to breed success. If one is really interested and digs into the literature and reviews his own examples, he will be able to further cultivate his talents and understand how, as Professor Tenhaeff has shown, psi takes certain specific directions: viz., the paragnost discovers himself in his consultants. It is particularly valuable to keep these records over a long period of time. It cannot be stressed enough that the psychic function blasts the time-space barriers and is seldom the same when it is confined to the laboratory where telepathy, clairvoyance, and precognition are aseptically separated, often stripped of emotional valence, and reduced to ciphers.

Psi can be a bucking bronco. You cannot tell which direction it will take and what surprises await you. In life, as seen in a clinical situation, these variegated aspects of psi are often intermingled or occur in rapid-fire volleys that pierce the time-space barrier, shooting back into the past, as well as staying with the present and on occasion leaping into the future.

Psi has no boundaries. The definitive laboratory experiments for psi have yet to be devised. For, to paraphrase Santayana's comment on history: those who never resolved some of their early life conflicts (do not understand their personal history) are doomed to repeat them. The ceaseless bombardment of psi experiences all too often only enmeshes them in a push-pull situation—whetting the appetite yet frustrating the experients and dooming them to more of the same—usually when they least expect it. By seeking his own identity in the lives of his consultants, the paragnost—or most of those with psi talent whether aware of it or not—rediscovers through psi examples in his current life what he was sensitized to as a child and which are recycled throughout his life. This truth also holds for the psychiatrist's awareness of psi with his patients—the creative potential of psi in psychotherapy—in the countertransference.

This process is illustrated in many of the papers in this volume, and in particular the early parent-child episodes, extending into later geriatric events. An excellent clinical control is provided by one person being party to many of the recorded events and also by keeping records over a long period of time, or in many cases, over a lifetime. Through more than 20 years of practice in Montclair, for example, I have had excellent corroboration or elucidation of situations that I recorded earlier. An example: a patient once was referred to me with a chief complaint of depression and marital discord; however, it appeared that underneath her symptoms were a host of apparent poltergeists, or haunting effects, stemming from the sudden tragic death of her two sons. Her account seemed to hang together, and by grappling with the possibility of psi—the "unreal" reality—she received much relief from her melancholy. Years later, a different physician referred a patient who had been the girl friend of one of the deceased young men. This young woman, though unaware of my earlier consultation with the mother of the deceased, gave a history which corroborated, coincided, and supplemented the early events. The young woman was also involved in the hauntings, filled out the picture, and made the psychopathology even more complex and intriguing. In neither consultations were the referring physicians previously aware of the psychic factors intertwined in their patients' problems. These are not isolated examples.

Here is another, more personal example showing the desirability of keeping track of psi over a lifetime. Recently I saw Claudia (pseudonym) in emergency consultation. Her husband had died several weeks previously, and her mourning was complicated by depression and physical complaints. The main feature of her case however was that for six consecutive nights prior to her husband's unanticipated death she dreamed of her deceased mother. The mother appeared sadly shaking her head while my (B.E.S.) parents, who were in real life physician and nurse when Claudia was my baby-sitter as a child, were standing by as if to prepare her for some grim event. On the morning of Claudia's husband's death, she, for no other reason than her dreams, became upset and refused to go to work. She even asked her husband, who insisted that he was healthy, if he would phone her employer and make an excuse for her absence, which he refused to do. When he dropped dead that night, Claudia immediately thought of her recurrent dreams. Obviously they could have indicated a subliminal awareness on her part of some of the changes in her husband's health. On the other hand, the specific features of her dreams and her own interpretation makes one wonder about the psi hypothesis: (1) whether she was picking up her husband's concern over symptoms he didn't tell her about, and was not aware of himself; or, (2) perhaps her clairvoyant knowledge of his deteriorating condition, or (3) possibly an element of possible precognition. It is of interest that although I had seen Claudia only two or three times in about 50 years since she had been my baby-sitter, I had a possible telepathic death dream of her mother, and as far as I know the only dream of "Pani" (Polish for lady) in my life. Pani was my parents' cleaning woman when I was a child and Claudia was our baby-sitter. My dream was confirmed when Claudia phoned on one of the rare occasions through all these years to tell me her sad news. Claudia was always very fond of my parents, who were good to her mother and to her.

It seems evident, then, that by keeping track of events over a lifetime when studying psi—as it happens in nature and not as arbitrarily confined in a laboratory—its ubiquitous and enigmatic time dimension is seen in truer perspective. I suspect that many so-called failures in laboratory experiments, which are conventionally designed, would not be failures at all if the so-called spontaneous and extraneous developments that take place and catch everyone off guard were taken into account. Even a footnote or comment in an appendix concerning such fortuitous events could be most revealing. It is almost as reprehensible to exclude such unexpected but equally valid data as it is to falsify results. Psi has a mind of its own and like the bucking bronco will not be fenced in.

Another instructive example showing some of these complexities, and possibly telepathy and synchronicity, springs to mind. In October, 1966, when Professor Tenhaeff's star paragnost and psychic crime sleuth, Gerard Croiset,[146] first came to America, he stayed at my house. In the interim he made a quick trip to Colombia, South America, reputedly through the intercession of the Queen of Holland and upon the importunities of the Colombian Amabassador. Croiset's help was sought in a grisly murder case. When Croiset returned to the United States, he told us his opinion through a Dutch interpreter, Mrs. Cora Matteson. At the time, the newspapers ballyhooed his trip but also implied that he had failed to solve the murder. However, I remember that he told Mrs. Matteson his impressions and that he said it would be inadvisable to publicly proclaim his findings since he wished innocent people as well as himself to stay alive.

On January 6, 1971, I received a packet from Croiset sent from Holland, which contained photocopies of letters and newspaper clippings detailing his role in solving the case. But from the synchronistic point of view the story is not over. In July, 1975, my wife and I were invited to a birthday party for Galen B. Hall, my friend and personal attorney, who later became senior counsel to the International Association for Psychotronic Research. One of Mr. Hall's party guests was his son's former college roommate, a young Colombian who flew up to New Jersey for the party. He knew nothing about Mr. Hall's relationship to me nor his interest in psychotronics. However, the Colombian correctly described how some Dutch psychic had successfully solved a hideous murder in his family. Mr. Hall and I were amused at the coincidence. But the story has a final twist; for during the period June 27–July 2, 1977, while Mr. Hall was at the psychotronics convention in Tokyo, by chance he finally met Gerard Croiset. Croiset recalled the details of this extraordinary case which seemed to be forever popping up before all our eyes. Croiset penned me a note and that's where matters rest until something happens next.

Another question frequently asked is, if one possesses psychic talent, can it be helpful? In my opinion, the answer is yes, and no, depending on how it is used. For many, psi can be helpful in expanding awareness and in fine-tuning relationships to others and the environment—possibly including different forms of life such as animals and inanimate matter, as in telekinetic examples. For some who might have a tenuous hold on reality to begin with, psi can cause serious emotional problems, and the obvious advice is for such people to leave the subject alone. As is often the case in such pathology, however, such people seldom follow this advice. It is stressed again that the psychic continuum extends over a lifetime and might even extend backward and forward in time. It often involves people beyond the dyadic relationship and can possibly enmesh countless other persons, presumably known to one another. It can also be speculated that psi can engulf and bind persons unknown to one another. The sorting out and explication of these mechanisms —the hypothesized psychological, neuroanatomical, and physiological factors—is a worthwhile challenge. Psi indicates our true mammalian state of interdependency, embracing and extending from telepathic and clairvoyant contacts to telekinetic, telesomatic, and precognitive reactions.

Telepathy, as in the reported examples, might help give us a better perspective of ourselves. The examples indicate the fatuity of being pompous or taking ourselves too seriously. After all, we are all human; and nothing is more revealing, if not devastating, at times, than to have young children or our peers blurt out the naked truth about ourselves—telepathic foot-in-mouth disease—and show us precisely how we are and not how we might prefer to think we are. Telepathy teaches us, if nothing else, to avoid extremes of dogmatism and to be amenable to new ideas and different ways of approaching problems, rather than to be bogged down in stereotyped thinking.

Telepathy, and psi in general, seems to be related to creativity, and it can pierce rigid, prissy preconceptions. For example, I remember how one renowned parapsychologist once solemnly shook his head and commented that Henry Gross couldn't possibly be a good dowser because of his fondness for Kentucky bourbon. It seemed to me that this most estimable savan was missing the boat and that the question might better have been posed: what role did alcohol have in influencing Henry's dowsing either positively or negatively? His dowsing results spoke for themselves. It is for the scientist to understand the mechanism and not to prejudge character. As another example of this inflexible, if not destructive, attitude to psi, I recall how another distinguished scholar once commented that she was quite skeptical of the number of telepathic parent-child episodes my wife and I recorded. My unexpressed rejoinder, which my wife later concurred in privately, was that if the scholar wasn't so cocksure of herself and stayed home with her children occasionally instead of consigning their rearing to maids, she might have noticed similar episodes too.

As Romano demonstrated, telepathy is related to the ability to improvise. Life itself is always changing and is in a state of flux. It is these fleeting, ambient, plastic percepts on the periphery of consciousness that are transmitted, either pictographically, ideationally, or otherwise, and then synthesized and integrated completely or partially, or left to meld in the unconscious mind. It is there that they ferment and remain ready to influence future behavior, physiological reactions, or be precipitated anew when appropriately stimulated, in their original form or in various condensations. New ideas and concepts arise out of hitherto untried combinations of older ones: viz., sometimes discarded or stored thoughts, memories, behavioral reaction patterns, etc. This truth has implications for studies in psychotherapy, education, maturation, creativity, and the like.

Although the reported studies that follow are clinical and qualitative, they might have, hopefully, some value to the parapsychologist who engages in laboratory experiments because they will illuminate some of the complexities and vagaries of the indispensable, unconscious processes that comprise the anlage to the psychic faculty. As an illustration, I had a physicist professor-patient years ago who, prior to his treatment for depression and alcoholism, had never experienced any conscious interest or awareness for psi. In the course of our psychotherapeutic sessions there occurred many spectacular psychic fireworks, including his once picking up the time of Croiset's unanticipated arrival in the United States. When appropriate, some of these episodes were interpreted, and he gradually started noticing more and more of these events in his daily living. As a matter of fact, because of this new awareness he even sought out a formal statistical testing of his abilities in a leading parapsychological laboratory. One of the leading researchers in the field later told me that Professor X got the best score he had ever seen. However, the researcher missed the main point: (1) my patient's psi talent, which was hitherto latent, was awakened and developed in psychotherapy, and (2) this new awareness for psi was related to his unconscious life and the various stresses that he was learning to cope with. Recently, when I saw this patient for a recheck (12 years after our initial sessions), he was doing well and volunteered the comment that when he gets his telepathic hunches he listens to them because they are helpful and correct a great deal of the time. He has become skilled in interpreting his highly individualized personal psi symbols. He felt that because of this his life had become more meaningful, and this contributed to his success both as a teacher and in his private life. I have several physician friends who are familiar with the tenor of these investigations and who have developed their own psi abilities and awareness to extents comparable to my physicist-patient. These are realizable potentials and not occasional, singular, freakish experiences or coincidences.

In this way, then, it is hoped that the many illustrations of possible psi will encourage those who have latent psi talents themselves and care to develop them as well as those who will discover their own faculties and put them to good use. Some young people might find the psi hypothesis to be of value in their lives, enabling them to press forward to startling new discoveries. Some others might be residents in psychiatric training where knowledge of psi might have immediate research value and possible practical application.

In conclusion, this volume has been prepared as I felt it should be and as events happened and are happening—not as others who are not psychiatrists or who are not familiar with psychic-dynamics and psychopathology think it ought to be. Having traveled the long and sometimes lonely road of these researches and preparing oft-rejected and unwanted manuscripts for medical journals, I will not turn back at this time nor compromise and write a popular work on how-to-master-psi in 10 easy lessons. This might falsely simplify matters which do not have ready answers. I do not know of any shortcuts. Nevertheless, for those who are interested, the psi examples offered in this book might serve as a springboard for the development of their own personal psi talent as it exists and always has, I would suppose, in their own lives and families. It is hoped that this new generation and some who are yet to be born will come forth with new ideas and daring experiments and interpretations. Let them seek to present their material in scientific journals rather than diluting its value by rushing into print for a lay audience, where the reports are often flawed with numerous loopholes and other fatal weaknesses.

Psi is too important to be ignored by academe any longer.

Contents

A study of some provocative psychosomatic phenomena observed in some of the members and "Saints" of the Free Pentecostal Holiness Church in the mountainous rural areas of Eastern Kentucky.

Telepathic drawing experiments are described, using one agent and one or more percipients and single-agent percipient drawings and volleys of two to seven consecutive drawings. Attention is given to the prerequisite subjective mental states of the participants and to the experimental design, extrinsic and intrinsic controls, psychodynamics and interpretation of the data.

Freud's thesis that telepathy may be a form of archaic communication suggests that such contacts might well be traced between parents and children. A record of 91 apparent telepathic phenomena in a child-parent relationship is presented.

In later life, when impairment of hearing and sight, social isolation, loneliness, increased dependency, brain syndrome or other illnesses are prevalent, persons may be unusually sensitive to telepathy. Several examples are presented of possible paranormal exchanges in older persons and also data from the life of Joseph Dunninger and from psychiatric practice.

5.   Possible Telesomatic Reactions   113

The possible telepathic mediation of psychosomatic or "telesomatic" reactions are explored. In the two papers that comprise this chapter, fourteen examples of various conditions are offered.

Part II: Psychiatric Examples of Psychic-Dynamics   127

6.   Built-in Controls and Postulates for the Telepathic Event   129

A specific type of uniqueness, that of built-in controls, in which a spontaneous telepathic event will recur in an almost predictable manner when the spontaneous constellation of the psychodynamic forces for patient and physician are similar, is illustrated by a patient in psychotherapy who telepathically perceived an apparition or its equivalent at five disparate times. In the second example, concerning a patient with a chronic brain syndrome and advanced physical-mental decrepitude, a volley of apparent telepathic communications between patient and physician took place according to hypothetical telepathic postulates.

7.   Telepathy and Pseudotelekinesis in Psychotherapy   144

Data are presented about a patient in psychotherapy who had many telepathic experiences including a telepathic death dream; possible precognition of death and telekinesis; the unexpected apparition of a recently deceased neighbor; and a possible New Jersey-Hawaii patient-physician telepathic hallucination. Details are given concerning the psychic dynamic and associated factors underlying the patient's sudden recognition of four faces on a tile at the time that a specific experiment of thoughtography and telekinesis was contemplated by her physician.

8.   Precognition and Psychic Nexus   153

Presentation of the precognitive dream without the allied psychic nexus would strip it of much of its strength and present an incomplete picture. If an enlarged, more psychodynamically oriented technique were applied to the study of seemingly isolated proscopic events, precognition might be more commonly recognized.

Synchronicity is defined and related to telepathy. Four illustrations are given of how synchronicity and telepathy may happen in life. Understanding of synchronicity and telepathy can give wider dimensions to psychotherapy and show the unique interdependence of people and events.

The telepathic hypothesis offers intriguing insights into the understanding of genius. Even a limited study of Thomas Alva Edison points toward highly suggestive evidence for this point of view.

A series of possible telepathic dreams and episodes connected with the unexpected death of Dr. Nandor Fodor is explored and studied to see what telepathic overflow effect might have occurred between the writer, a psychiatrist, and his patients from the time Dr. Fodor first appeared in a dream to the time that the details of his final illness and death were learned.

Examples of spontaneously occurring paranormal events between man and beasts are presented. The link between man and his pets, and sometimes between man and exotic wild animals, is explored and speculations are offered about possible similar interactions noted from ancient times as a source of world-wide, greatly embellished legends, myths and superstitions of dragons, monsters, witches, cats, etc.

The role of telepathy is explored in (1) humorous situations with early parent-child episodes, (2) physician-patient psychotherapeutic relationships, and (3) strictly personal anecdotes obtained from patients and the writer's personal life. A deeper exploration of the subject of telepathy and humor might yield many clues about this relatively neglected but important means of human communication.

Part III: Psi and the Life Cycle   227

14.   The Seven Ages of Man: A Potpourri of Psi   229

Although at times the psychic nexus might seem more complex than the plot of an Italian opera, it is quite simple when each segment of the concatenation of spontaneous events is analyzed and finally linked together to form this larger whole. The psychic nexus is a zigzagging path that cuts across time and space and involves many people. Twenty-six cases are presented: roughly divided according to Shakespeare's seven ages of man.

15.   UFO Contactee Stella Lansing: Possible Medical Implications of her Motion Picture Experiments   267

Intensive study of the Stella Lansing effect on motion picture films, in addition to probing the fascinating mysteries of UFOs, might offer new investigative techniques and open up practical, clinically related areas of interest to psychosomatic medicine.

16.   Postscript: Possible "Impossibilities."   281

Part I: WIDTH AND BREADTH OF PSYCHIC DIMENSIONS

1
Ordeal by Serpents, Fire and Strychnine
A Study of Some Provocative Psychosomatic Phenomena

The Free Pentacostal Holiness Church[14,179,170] is a religious sect* located in the mountainous, rural regions of eastern Kentucky, Tennessee, and parts of Virginia and North Carolina. The basic tenets of the beliefs of this sect conform to fundamentalist, literal interpretations of the Bible. The members, who are mostly farmers and coal miners, are descendants of the early English and Scots-Irish colonists, and have straitlaced Calvinist backgrounds and traditions. Their speech is provincial and includes many words and expressions that Shakespeare used and that are found in the King James version of the Bible. Few have had formal education extending beyond elementary school. They are hardy people, who come from large families, and whose life histories illustrate a fierce struggle with the ravages of nature, disease and often extreme difficulties of earning a living. Their mountain culture is a patriarchy. The men work, hunt, and frequently go on their evangelical missions, while the women stay in the background and keep busy in their homes with cooking, cleaning, and attending to the needs of their large families. Many of the "Saints"** had childhoods in which one or both of their parents, siblings or other relatives died of disease, or in mining accidents, or in "shooting matches." Not a few have, or have had, pulmonary tuberculosis. Some of the leading saints had crimes of violence, bootlegging, whoremongering, and other "sins" in their backgrounds before they were "saved."

---

*Subsequently referred to as Holiness in this book.
**"Saints" is a term used to denote those consecrated church members who have extraordinary faith and gifts. In some respects they may be considered to be "ministers."

3

Most of the members do not attend motion pictures, and they abstain from alcohol, coffee, tea, tobacco, drugs and even soda pop. They battle temptation and sin with the certain knowledge of an approaching judgment day, the imminent second coming of the Messiah, and the end of the world. The realities of Satan, of sin, and of the vivid fire and brimstone of Hell strike terror in their hearts. Their faith tolerates no adultery, delinquency, lying or other forms of "backsliding." A member dedicates his whole life to "the living faith." Such are the rigors of this faith, however, that it is the exception when a member has all or even part of his family—his spouse, children, parents or siblings—as fellow-worshippers. Although the Holiness brethren attempt to convert and save souls, they use persuasion, rather than the "shooting-match approach."

It is customary for them to attend church at least two nights a week, and frequently every night. Interpreting various Biblical passages as direct commands of God, the Holiness members severely test their faith and identification with Biblical personages through "miracles," or ordeals by serpents, fire, and strychnine.[92,100,222] In this way, it can be conjectured, their previous impulses to "sin" are suppressed and repressed, while at the same time the grim threats and realities of everyday living are denied and mastered. By these highly symbolic ordeals, there is also a triumph over feelings of helplessness, and the fierce struggle with nature and the often calloused, persecuting, cognitive outside world. The successful ordeal, spectacularly dramatized before their peers and before "unbelievers," becomes an acceptable outlet and a substitute for what was often past violent, antisocial behavior. The ordeals constitute narrow escapes from torture and death. The proof and expiations afforded by the "miracles" justify the faith that there will be rewards in Heaven for the suffering and for sacrifices on earth. With the intense concentration of all their individual and collective energies epitomized in the ordeals, the Holiness people see themselves as "the [true] children of God"; and the great threat of life, bodily death, is transposed into an eternal spiritual existence. The constant repetition of this theme in their revivals protects them from doubt ("backsliding"), but, like an obsessive mechanism, it generates further need for the reassurance and propitiation of their ambivalently loved and feared Father. As an ancient religious practice of great affective force, the ordeals might then portray in microcosm all the vicissitudes of man's relationship to his fellow-man and his mystical awe of the infinite macrocosm. Other intermittent phenomena claimed by various members of Holiness have been the power of prophecy, clairvoyance, prolonged fasting and, in the knowledge of one saint, the levitation of "a bearded [backwoods] patriarch."

The report is based on four field-trip studies during 1959 of several Holiness churches and comprises first-hand observation of the various charismatic phenomena occurring during the services. The investigative techniques also included, when feasible and indicated, the use of a tape recorder, photoflash and motion picture cameras, a stopwatch, and chemical analysis of different specimens. There were psychiatric examinations of six of the saints of the church. In none of the saints who were examined was there any evidence of current neurotic, psychotic, or psychosomatic reactions, or of pathologic dissociative behavior. In general, the individual psychopathology of Holiness people was not markedly different from that of people in other sects. It is of interest that—unlike typical mystics who, in the words of one authority, "have been women, unmarried or experienced in an abnormal sex life"—the Holiness saints, by the size of their families, appear to be very active and sexually potent. However, this report is not particularly concerned with any specific details of psychopathology in individual members and reserves any further dynamic formulations for future communications.

Through the catharsis of testifying before a congregation, without the inhibiting mediation of a preacher between God and themselves, the Holiness people act out their conflicts with the often-tragic realities of their lives. The particular dissociated states of ecstasy and exaltation that occurred concomitantly with the phenomena of the ordeals were apparently necessary accompaniments. These states might be viewed as violent upheavals of the unconscious, with totally unabashed shame. At these times, all affects and imagerial contents are forthrightly displayed. The Bible comes to life. In contrast to this overwhelming display of emotion during services, however, the Holiness members express few fantasies in their everyday living. Even in their dreams, which are seldom recalled, the manifest content is reported to be about "church services, handling serpents, fire" and the like.

A typical revival meeting begins at 7:30 P.M. and lasts 3 hours or longer. It takes place in a church, which is usually a simple, square wooden frame building, or may be a concrete-block house. A meeting may even be in a private home. The churches are situated along rural roads, high in the mountains or deep in the hollows, and sometimes are accessible only by a rocky creek-bed road. Inside they are clean and are furnished with plain wooden pews and an altar. In the middle of the room is an iron coal stove. The walls have inscribed on them various Biblical passages and religious mottoes like "Jesus Saves," "Jesus Never Fails," and "Give Me My Flowers While I Live." Often there may also be a large funeral-parlor calendar with a picture of Jesus admonishing the congregation to "Go to Church," a crucifix, similar to that associated with Roman Catholic churches, and sometimes photographs of Holiness saints holding rattlesnakes and copperheads. The services are attended by 15 to 125 people. The men are clean-shaven and neatly dressed in colored pants or blue denim overalls and shirts. They sit on one side of the church and the women on the other. The women use no cosmetics, jewelry or artificial beauty contrivances. Most of them wear brightly colored cotton calico or gingham dresses. At a large service, there are usually one or two women breast-feeding their babies. The congregation is about evenly divided between the sexes and has members of all ages.

When the brothers and sisters* arrive, they go among the congregation and onlookers to greet fellow-members cordially. At times the saints, who are always males, hug and kiss each other with the greeting, "How are you, Honey?" The service starts with a stirring mountain hymn that is frequently original with the Holiness Church. Everyone sings at the top of his voice—to the accompaniment of one to four guitars, clashing cymbals and tambourines. This singing is followed by prayer. The members kneel down and, in a loud, chaotic, pandemonium of voices, individually thank God for His mercy and favors, and beseech His help for healing and for the ordeals of faith that will shortly follow. Then different members preach and testify; they confess their sins and repent; they recite their personal life experiences and compare them to their fellows' experiences and to appropriate parts of the Bible. They gradually or suddenly go into frenetic states depending on "the power of the Lord in moving [on them]." Their exaltation superficially resembles mania. At these times, they shout, scream, cry, sing, jerk, jump, twitch, whistle, hoot, gesture, sway, swoon, tremble, strut, goosestep, stamp, and incoherently "speak in new tongues" (Mark 16:17, Acts 2:1–13). The glossolalia sounds like: "ma-ma-ma-ma-ma."

When in deep dissociated trances, the members appear as if they are intoxicated, and their facies are very similar to those seen with reactions induced by mescaline and LSD 25.[198] They describe the depersonalization phenomena as: "I feel high in the spirits" . . . "happiness in the bones" . . . "a shield has come down over me" . . . "I've got conviction" . . . "I lose sight of the whole world" . . . "I can't tell if my head and face are all together" and "I can't stand under the power of God." At the apparent climax of the ecstasy, but only when "the Lord moves [them]," the worshippers impulsively turn to the screened, flat, wooden boxes containing the venomous serpents and take them out for handling. Occasionally, the "coal oil" torches or carbide lamps are ignited and the flames applied to their bodies. In rare instances the most faithful of the saints will open a bottle of strychnine, dissolve some in a glass of water and drink it.

In their comments on unsuccessful ordeals by unbelievers, the saints agreed that the "faith" would hold only when the members obeyed the inner command or impulse. In many respects, this is not unlike the apparent prerequisite for a successful telepathic experiment, with which the writer is acquainted. Success in that case seemed to depend on transmitting only when

*"Brothers and sisters" refer to the Holiness-baptized male and female members of the congregation, who participate in some of the ordeals.

the agent genuinely felt in the mood, and then using his presumably autonomous or autochthonous affect-laden ideas or complexes.[174] In both instances, then (the ordeals and telepathic experiments), critical cognition was in abeyance, or was secondary to the immediate emotional constellation.

If a member of the congregation claims he is ill or knows of someone who is ailing (it once happened that an infant was present who had a congenital deformity), the members gather around the afflicted, anoint with olive oil, "lay on" their hands and loudly pray for divine intercession and healing. During the healing rights, both because of their rigid moral code and their vulnerability to persecution, the brothers and sisters carefully refrain from the laying on of hands below the shoulders of any member of the opposite sex. In their vivid descriptions and testimonials the Holiness people claim to have cured diseases that physicians had diagnosed as hopeless: cases of what might have been tuberculosis, carcinomatosis, breast tumors, "skin cancer of the jaw," acute adenitis, poliomyelitis, other forms of paralysis, "sleeping sickness," and convulsive disorders. In a study of one of the saints, it appeared that he had a history that seemed to be compatible with a clinical diagnosis of a coronary occlusion, with either two recurrent attacks, and/or bouts of acute congestive failure. He reported that, while in the hospital and in severe distress, he was visited by members of his congregation who prayed for him. Following this moving experience, he immediately resumed his excessively exuberant physical devotions and usual form of life without any apparent untoward effect, but, on the contrary, with subjective (and objective?) improvement. Because of the enigmatic, spectacular nature of some of the ordeals, and the fervor of a faith seldom seen nowadays in perhaps more sophisticated urban circles, some of the Holiness "cures" might be profitably studied from the psychosomatic viewpoint. Although rare, there are some well-documented cases in the medical literature of spontaneous resolution of various forms of proved malignancy.[56] If one, could actually find any similar cases among the Holiness people, an intensive psychiatric study might reveal another connection between the emotions and anatomical body changes.

ORDEAL BY SERPENTS

Following the Biblical injunction of Jesus "to take up serpents" (Mark 16:18, Luke 10:19), and Paul's experience of shaking off a viper "fastened on his hand" (Acts 28:3), the Holiness members handle venomous rattlesnakes and copperheads that are caught in the surrounding mountains and fields by "unbelieving sinner boys" or by saints who inspiringly trudge these regions, put their bare hands in the rock dens, and pull the serpents out. If not bitten, and if able to handle the snakes, the worshippers then gain "victory" (over the Devil). During the actual ceremonies one to four poisonous snakes are held in the hands, around the neck, on the head, or close to the lips of the members (see Figure 1-1). Although the women also handle serpents, this ordeal is performed for the most part by the men. The snakes crawl around their hosts and are seemingly adapted to the rhythmical swaying and chanting of, "Thank you Jesus, thank you Jesus, Gloree, Gloree, Bless him Lord, bless him." Some of the serpents are gently molded into different positions by the saints. The serpents maintain these particular, and sometimes, bizarre attitudes for variable periods, and appear to be cataplectic. One brother held a rattlesnake (approximately four feet in length) in the mid-trunk region; as he stamped around the congregation, shouting his praises to the Lord, the reptile hung limply, seemingly cataplectic (see Figure 1-2), and showed no response until the worshipper paused and became silent for a few seconds. Invariably on these occasions, the serpent would start to wiggle, writhe, and then ominously rattle. It should be noted that the rattlesnakes seldom rattled when being handled during the ceremonies, but they frequently made a collective racket when their cages were disturbed. Although the author personally observed more than 200 instances of serpent handling, he has not witnessed a bite.

Many of the saints have been bitten, however. Two, in particular, claim to have been bitten more than 50 times, and two others, more than 30 times each. One claims to have handled serpents more than 2000 times in his career without once being bitten. When a Holiness member is bitten, medical treatment is refused. The saints use no definitive treatment and rely solely on their "faith in the Lord" for a cure.

Four saints studied knew, among them, of only 18 Holiness people who had died of snake bites in 31 years. They cited examples of men and women in their 70's and 80's who survived bites. Although there are instances of children, as young as four years of age, handling the serpents at the services, and also other instances where infants inadvertently handled serpents in private homes, no member of the Holiness Church knew of any case when a child was bitten. A saint asserted that when a person is bitten there is a free flow of blood and intense swelling and pain. From their combined experiences, the saints believe that the mortality and morbidity does not depend on the site of the bite since they have been bitten on the faces, necks, hands and lower extremities without any significant difference in the final outcome. However, some of the brothers and former members of the faith were observed to have snake-bite complications of auto-amputation of digits and parts of hands.

Three brothers, who, in their collective lifetime experiences, have been bitten more than 100 times, and, on some occasions, two to three times almost simultaneously, concluded: "A rattlesnake bite gives numbness, difficulty in

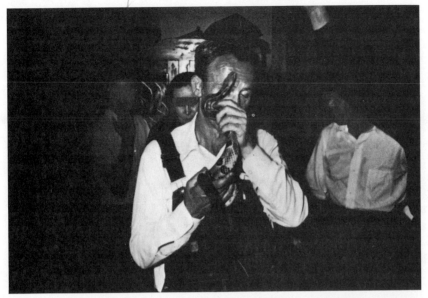

Figure 1-1. A Holiness saint with "victory" over a rattlesnake.

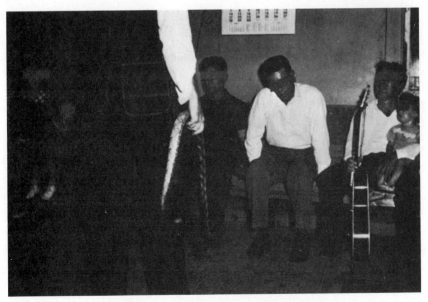

Figure 1-2. A brother, in exaltation, and his apparently cataplectic rattlesnake.

walking, talking, weakness and a 'drunken-like' feeling, like having a shot for a tooth-pulling. A copperhead bite doesn't have these effects but feels like fire and there is much more swelling. The poison makes you hot and the blood thin. You [can] bleed to death." In the cases of these three saints, there were apparently never any sequelae. It was difficult to ascertain how frequently bites occurred through the years, the species of snakes involved, the sizes or estimated ages of the snakes, how many members subsequently received medical treatment, and the final outcome.

When a bitten member suffers complications or dies, it is because "he didn't have enough faith." As an example of the relationship between their beliefs, their faith and the ultimate results of handling serpents, many persons told how one famous saint successfully handled serpents for 30 years until he believed a sister's prophecy of his own approaching death from a snakebite. As prophesied, he was bitten and died. Although the history could not be verified in all the salient details, it was stated that this saint had received similar bites throughout his career without any fear of dire results or any lasting complications.

Discussion

What is it that might account for the apparent ability to avoid being bitten when in such intimate contact with these dangerous reptiles? In some way, it might be related to the magnitude of dissociation or trance. Indirect evidence in support of this supposition is the fact that those who have been bitten the least number of times appear to be very gentle and kind people who handle the serpents only "when the Lord really moves on us; this is not for show. God won't let 'em open their mouth. The snake would dart at me but hit can't open hit's mouth." The saint who was alleged to have handled serpents more than 2000 times without being bitten was a particularly kind and gentle individual. On the other hand, those who have been bitten many times are, perhaps, not so cautious and gentle in handling the serpents. Some frequently handle snakes in their homes or in church without "the command of the Lord," or the deep dissociative state. One brother who once handled 26 serpents at the same time was, of course, more likely to be bitten, and he was bitten. Nevertheless, he suffered no complications. The particular minister who was never bitten in 2000 experiences said that he quaked in terror on seeing or handling harmless garter snakes or black snakes when he was not in a trance.

Many of the snakes appear to react in a fashion analogous to other animals observed in various states of hypnosis (Totstell-reflex), that is, from a light drowsy-like state to complete cataplexy.[199,213] The saints reported one unusual and enigmatic situation where it was alleged that two sisters frequently handled rattlesnakes that died (of fright?) during the ordeal. It is plausible then to conjecture that the rhythmic stimulation to the serpent, combined with its possible terror during the experience, might produce, in the snake, reactions varying from relative inertia and drowsiness to cataplexy and even death.

Practical considerations in the evaluation of the treatment of snake bites in medical practice might make it worth while to determine the mortality and morbidity of untreated rattlesnake and copperhead bites in the Holiness members. For instance, from some of the historical data of members incurring repeated and even multiple simultaneous snake bites—and where no tourniquets, cruciate incisions, antisera, transfusions and the like were used —questions might be raised about current therapy and the pathophysiology of snake bites.[122,143] However, this should not be construed to mean that current established therapeutic procedures should be abandoned or radically modified. After further investigation and documentation of untreated snake bites in Holiness members, however, might there be some value in doing careful immunologic studies? Possibly Holiness donor-blood or some of its derivatives (globulin fraction?) could be studied for possible use in the therapy of those envenomed people who are sensitive to hyperimmune horse protein or directly allergic to the venom itself. Perhaps performing such suggested studies on Holiness blood would yield results different from similar tests reported by Parrish and Pollard.[143] In the case of the Holiness people, some of the saints have been bitten many more times, much more frequently, and more often have had multiple bites than the subjects reported by these two authors. Furthermore, since most of Parrish and Pollard's severly envenomed cases had received large amounts of antivenom, the active immunity in this group might be expected to be lower than that in the Holiness group—if the factor of immunity is involved in the Holiness group. The material presented would seem to point to the importance of the bitten saints, attitudes and "faith." In any event, these potential by-products of this investigation are of secondary importance, compared to the fact that human beings in states of exaltation can generally handle poisonous snakes without being bitten, and that, most frequently, when bitten, they do not die. The real question that should be asked is how? Or why?

ORDEAL BY FIRE

In the ancient history of many Western peoples, the ordeal by fire plays a prominent role. In medieval Europe, the Christian clergy officiated at ordeals, which included boiling water and oil, red-hot iron and burning logs, to determine the guilt or innocence of people. The legal term, *judicium ferri,* was derived from these particular rites, and the still prevalent custom of taking an oath in court can be ascribed to related ordeals. Eventually, the fire ordeal became so dangerously prevalent that the church outlawed it in the Fourth Lateran Council in 1215. Nevertheless, the rites persisted. In 1725, for instance, during the bloody French Reformation, it was reported that "a convolutionary called 'La Salamandre' remained suspended for nine minutes over a fiery brazier, clad only in a sheet, which remained intact in the flames."[14] At approximately this time in America, the French missionaries reported that the Indians of the St. Lawrence River region and Great Lakes had various fire ordeals, including successful handling of hot coals and stones, plunging their arms into boiling water, and walking through fire.[91] In many similar forms, the fire ordeal was widespread in other cultures and parts of the world for centuries, and exists today or did very recently in Ceylon, the Fiji Islands, Hawaii, and India. [57,117,123,92,100,222] In the 1860's, the famous medium, D. D. Home,[16,103,117] is alleged to have handled hot coals many times and once "kneeled down, placed his face right among the burning coals and moved it about as though bathing in water." Another more recent event occurred in New York City some years ago when a Hindu mystic, Kuda Bux, was reported to have safely walked over charcoal that was measured to be burning at 1220° Fahrenheit.[130,156]

This part of the present study concerns the first-hand observation of 13 members of the Holiness sect and their experiences with fire handling. They base their ordeal on various parts of the Bible (Isaiah 43:2, Daniel 3:25), and, as with the serpents, they usually take to the fire at a climactic point in the revival. At such times a rag wick placed in a milk bottle or tomato juice jar full of "coal oil"* is ignited. The flames are orange-yellow and shoot 8 to 24 inches high. The worshippers slowly move their outstretched open hands and fingers over the midpoint of the flames for times ranging from 3 to 5 seconds or even longer. (See Figure 1–3.) Frequently, one turns the burning torch horizontally and puts the proximal flame to the palm of his hand for 5 seconds or longer. On three occasions, two of the saints put their exposed toes and the soles of their feet directly in the flames for 5 to 15 seconds. As noted with the fingers, the flames were observed to pass through the interdigital spaces. In one instance, the most faithful saint smeared fuel oil over hands and feet, and then proceeded to hold them in the midst of the flames for more than 10 seconds. Although there was some thick white smoke, the fuel oil on the skin did not burn. (See Figure 1–4.) The saint then cupped the palm of his hand and tried to ignite the little pool of fuel oil in it with the blazing torch, but it only flickered a few times. As controls, an iron poker and a wooden dowel, that had fuel oil sprinkled on the surfaces, quickly burst into flames when in contact with the torch. On 13 occasions,

*Kerosene.

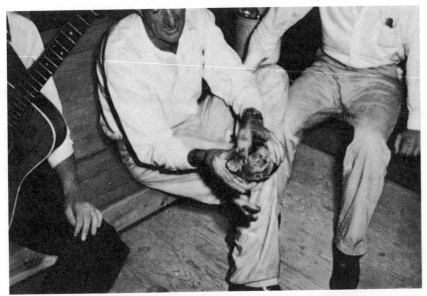

Figure 1–3. A Holiness saint with his thumb in a "coal oil" torch flame.

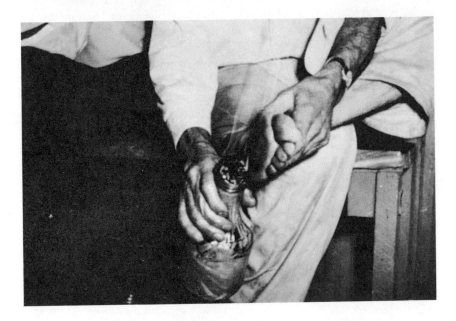

Figure 1–4. A Holiness saint with his foot in a "fuel oil" torch flame. His hands and foot glisten from the previous immersion with "fuel oil." Also note dense white smoke at base of flame and sole.

5 different women moved the midpoint of the torch flame backward and forward directly under their elbows, forearms and upper arms for a few seconds —or longer. One of the women had chronic blotchy erythema of the exposed parts of her body (actinic dermatitis), and she claimed that this condition developed every spring and persisted throughout the summer until fall. There was no change in her condition, locally or diffusely, before or after the ordeal. Once a sister handed the flaming torch to an old man sitting in the back of the church. Apparently moved by the fervor of the services, he acquired an immunity for the first time, applying the flames to his hand without burning. On three occasions, three different women held the blaze to their chests, so that the flames were in intimate contact with their cotton dresses, exposed necks, faces and hair. This lasted for longer than a few seconds. Twice, at separate times, one of the "most faithful of the saints" slowly moved the palmar and lateral aspects of one hand and the fifth finger in the midpoint and tip of an acetylene flame (produced by the reaction of calcium carbide and water in a miner's headlamp). He did this for more than four seconds, and then repeated the procedure, using the other hand. Later that same evening, he alternately applied each hand again to the acetylene flame for slightly longer periods. Once this saint, when in a relatively calm mood, turned to a coal fire of an hour's duration, picked up a flaming "stone coal" the size of a hen's egg and held it in the palms of his hands for 65 seconds while he walked among the congregation. As a control, the author could not touch a piece of burning charcoal for less than one second without developing a painful blister.

In all these fire ordeals, except one, there were, apparently, no evidences of painful reactions; and there was no erythema, blistering, charring, singeing, suggestive odor of a burn, or gross change in sweat production. Just once, when a brother handled the torch, there was a slight singeing and an associated odor, where some hair on the dorsal distal forearm burned. In no instance though, was there ever any evidence that clothes had been either scorched or burned. Although some of the men had calluses on their palms and soles, others, including "the most faithful saint" did not. The women, of course, had no calluses on their forearms, arms, necks or faces. In no case, was any change found before or after the fire ordeal, upon examining the affected body parts for superficial touch, pain and temperature sensitivity, or astereognosis. On the occasion when the most faithful saint immersed his oil-soaked hands and feet in the flames, he washed his hands shortly before the ordeal. As a control, the author could not keep his own hand closer than 3 cms to the "coal oil" torch flame at its base for longer than one or two seconds without pain or the danger of getting burned. Other control attempts, under ordinary circumstances and simulating the ordeal, were impossible to complete, because of almost instantaneous pain and the risk of incurring severe burns.

Careful history-taking of these people revealed no discrepancies in their accounts of the fire ordeal, and brought forth more interesting and suggestive data. For instance, "the most faithful saint" inaugurated his gift 26 years ago by rushing to the hearth, balancing—with his hands—red-hot logs on his shoulders, and walking around the congregation without any ill effects to his person or clothes. Another minister* is alleged to have jumped up on a red-hot iron stove, to have sat on it, and to have put his exposed feet and legs among the glowing coals while he delivered his sermon. A third saint has a reputation for putting his head and neck in a red-hot stove for "many seconds or a few minutes." However, no observer claimed to have actually timed this. The same man is also reported to have had a welder's acetylene torch applied to his outstretched upper arm for many seconds, and also later to his forehead, against which was placed a piece of paper which instantantously disintegrated. In neither case was there any burn to his skin or shirt.

The fire ordeal has been undertaken by male and female worshippers from 7 to 80 years of age. It is alleged to be a not uncommon practice to hand red-hot coals among the congregation during winter service ("it feels like velvet") and for "the young girls to hug the red-hot stovepipes and pass around a hot [glass] lamp chimney." Also, on occasion, the fire immunity has been seemingly conferred by the saints on newly converted spectators at the services.

An interesting story was provided by one brother who reported applying the "coal oil" torch flame to the palm of his hand for several seconds with complete immunity until he noticed that a piece of wick was breaking off. This trivial incident was enough to cause him to awaken from his trance and engender anxiety. At this point, he suffered a very discrete and localized blistering burn. The surrounding area that had previously been in contact with the flames during the trance and had been of no apparent concern to him showed no burn.

In a like manner, a sister who had, during previous ordeals, frequently handled a hot glass chimney, developed blistering burns when one evening while at church, the electric power failed, and in a reflex action, she grabbed the brightly burning kerosene lantern that was hanging on the wall. She was not entranced at that particular moment. The fact can, therefore, be noted that when Holiness members are not entranced, they, like everyone else, suffer burns, are afraid of poisonous snakes, and possibly are more frequently bitten by them.

---

*Or "saint." They are ordained in their own church.

Various brothers and sisters emphasized their accounts by telling how "sinner people" when intoxicated with alcohol, or disbelieving what they saw, attempted to duplicate the feats, suffered bad burns of the skin, hair or clothes. As an example, a scoffing brother of the most faithful saint, held his finger for a fraction of a second in the acetylene flame and rapidly developed blisters in the exposed area. There have been reports in the literature[57,130,156] of similar experiences where those "without the faith," or not in complete trance, have been severely burned. Some of these people were ministers of sects other than those of the fire-handlers, who tried to prove the trials fraudulent. They apparently considered them to be superstition or heresy, or perhaps felt the need to expose as hoaxes something that differed from, or threatened, their own convictions. However, it can be surmised that there was a close connection between their not being in receptive, dissociative states (their lack of "faith") and their suffering serious burns.

Discussion

It appears to be fact that some people in a state of religious ecstasy and faith can have varying degrees of immunity to burns on their body and their clothing. However, what explanation for these phenomena, if any, can be offered? It should be frankly admitted that careful critical studies ought to be undertaken, so that the collateral historical data can be scrutinized, and the observed data can be further explored and measured. The problems in a study of this kind are manifold. One must establish rapport, obtain cooperation, and then adjust to quick-moving, ever-changing conditions. The fire ordeal studied here is part of a church service, and there is much compulsive and excessive motor activity. In addition to these factors, there is the problem of measuring flame temperatures, distance from flame, time of exposure, the particular part or parts involved, the effects of movement on such a part, and at all times, the apparently fundamental relationship to the underlying and varying degrees of ecstasy or dissociation.

Despite the many drawbacks of the present field-trip observations, which are admittedly not comparable to well-controlled laboratory investigations where the data are accurately measured[17,55,102,134,135,136,204] there still exists the fact of varying degrees of fire immunity and no satisfactory explanation. In this regard, for those who would insist upon strict laboratory controls during the fire ordeal, one should recall the previously noted example of the man who, while in a trance, became aware that the burning wick was breaking and thus came out of his trance and suffered a burn, when moments before this, flames had licked his hand without effect. Similarly, interjecting the body of an overzealous experimental interference (with its necessary demands for frequent and strict controls and checks) may sabotage the trance, taint the results, lead to false conclusions, and expose the participants (and the observer?) to serious bodily harm.

The patent freedom from pain in the fire ordeal is not unusual when consideration is given to the related conditions of spectacular hypnotic anesthesias[231] and the categorial emotional aspects of pain perception.[4,114] Although no striking chemical changes have been associated, to date, with hypnotic anesthesias, such anesthesias are incontestable facts, and, similarly, the religious dissociations might also have no readily indentifiable chemical changes. Hypnotic anesthesia has been studied with scalp electro-encephalography, and, in one instance, with depth electrography, but in neither case has there been a clear-cut major electrophysiological change in comparison to control states.[200] Even though the formidable technical obstacles could be overcome, it would then be reasonable, by analogy, not to anticipate any gross electrographic changes during the fire ordeal.

The fact that there is absence of pain does not explain the immunity to burning, but it also does not necessarily mean that the two phenomena are unrelated. Evidence in favor of some neural factors, however, is provided by experiments where blistering has been produced during the hypnotic trance[225] and by some studies by Sevitt[204] on guinea pigs, which led him to conclude that: "burns [that] just produced a definite increase in capillary permeability in the intact skin, failed to affect the capillaries of the denervated skin." He also noted the observation that transection of the spinal cord decreased inflammatory edema and degree of hemoconcentration after burning. In any event, it is difficult to see how these rather scanty data could be transposed and sufficiently magnified to account for the high immunity to burning in the fire ordeals.

Kolb[114] has shown how the presence, absence or degree of pain is closely related to meaningful past life experiences, current attitudes, symbolic values and whatever conscious and/or unconscious significance the pain-associated situation or body part might have for the patient. In a comparable way, it can be supposed that the success of the fire ordeal depends on the worshipper's experiences, beliefs and particular body image. The Holiness worshippers are compelled to apply the flames to the bodily parts when and where "the Lord moves on them." Since, from suckling infancy and childhood, many of the Holiness people have witnessed or heard about such ordeals from relatives and friends, it is reasonable to suppose that in their minds there can be no question about the reality of such phenomena, or for that matter, other "miracles" mentioned in the Bible. "It is a matter of having enough faith and living the right kind of life." To the worshippers, it is the unbelievers or "sinner boys" who are strange and illogical; they act "rationally," and of course do not really expect fire immunity, and are subsequently burned. Therefore, for the believer, success, freedom from pain, and complete immunity to the fire are anticipated; and the results conform to this projected body image.

The effects which, in more ordinary situations, would be expected to occur do not result. Thus, there are: (1) the lack of effect of the flame on the skin during the trance (when, seconds after, a localized burn resulted when the individual came out of the trance); (2) the lack of burn when the flame was applied to the forehead (while a piece of paper interposed between the flame and forehead disintegrated in the fire); and (3) the failure of "coal oil," smeared on the hands and foot of the believer, to ignite when the torch was applied (while similar "coal oil" smeared on a poker and wooden dowel burst into flame in similar circumstances).

A Holiness member's faith has the strength of an incorruptible obsession. As an example of this, and of indifference to worldly matters, one saint (perhaps wisely?) refused much material wealth for "going on the stage with his wife and baby" (to perform the fire ordeal). The members are always careful to refrain from doing anything which would compromise their convictions and jeopardize their exaltation and gifts. For instance, it is reported that one member successfully handled fire until he returned from military service and tried to resume his ordeals, when he was badly burned. "He lost faith in the service; didn't live the right kind of a life." Those who participate in the most unusual feats must keep at them compulsively so as not to develop fear and lose ability. Being totally immersed in his faith means that a member is ready to leave his job, family and personal comforts at almost any time that the "Lord moves" (him) and go to evangelistic revival meetings, bedside prayers for healing, and so forth.

Although the believers' attitudes toward strangers varied between wholehearted acceptance and cooperation to suspiciousness and withdrawal, these disparate factors never seemed to alter their exaltations significantly or change the frequency, content or magnitude of the phenomena from one meeting to another. When in exaltation, they are in another world, and, as freqently noted with mescaline and LSD 25 reactions, they are relatively unresponsive to the distracting external stimuli of their immediate environments.

Another possible concomitant to the trance might be an increased efficiency of circulatory cooling mechanisms. However, this would not seem to be a plausible explanation because the "believers" were in varying degrees of excitement (increased cardiac output). Some were relatively tranquil on occasion. If circulatory factors were important, there would have to be an enormous increase in cooling ability to protect what were often large areas of the involved skin from the direct local effects of the flames on epidermis, corium and subcutaneous tissues. Furthermore, these tissues should respond locally to the flames and in a great measure be independent of the circulatory factors. Clinically, it should be noted that in several instances the fingers and toes, which are particularly vulnerable to serious burns[55], were unduly exposed to flames.

The hypothesis first put forward by Albertus Magnus[222]—that the fire-handler's skin is protected locally from fire with a "recipe"—would not be relevant, because, as far as the author knows, there is no such preparation; and, in one instance, to forestall this criticism, a saint washed his hands before the ordeal, and the results were the same.

Since none of the "believers" took any drugs, the ingestion of drugs for protection cannot be considered possible. Humoral mechanisms are unlikely, because nothing has been isolated as yet which affords any significant protection against burns. If the procedure could be carried out without ruining the trance, it would, of course, be of interest to analyze, chemically and/or biologically, blood specimens obtained from Holiness people while in resting control states and while in states of religious exaltation, before and shortly after their fire ordeals—to see if any protection could be discovered for animals or humans undergoing experimental burns. Although the states of exaltation sometimes superficially resemble pathologic frenetic conditions, it should be pointed out that manic patients and agitated schizophrenics can develop bad burns, even though in some instances they appear to be, like Holiness people, subjectively free of pain. The suggested explanations of immunity from burns are, therefore, all inadequate, because in the literature, in histories given by the Holiness members, and in some instances that were confirmed by direct observations by the author, the apparent immunity to burning is even extended to other people watching the services and to clothing. "Brother [Smith] put hot coals in his shirt." In one reported case of 70 years ago, Crookes[16] tested, in his laboratory, a fine cambric handkerchief that the medium D. D. Home had folded around a piece of red charcoal, then fanned to white heat with his breath without damaging the handkerchief. Crookes concluded that the handkerchief "had not undergone the slightest chemical preparation which could have rendered it fire-proof."

It was unfortunately impossible to measure in each instance the time of exposure and distances between the source of heat and bodily part in the examples reported from the Holiness sect. Nevertheless, in many of these phenomena, common sense and the reported experimental data (where lesser thermal stresses were imposed with resultant tissue injury) would indicate that the temperatures of the flames that were used (coal oil, acetylene, burning coal; and also the history of alleged contacts with red-hot and white-hot iron) were high enough so that the exposures witnessed should have sufficed to produce serious burns. The questions—why these people are not burned on their bodies and what are their projected body images when in their exalted states—remain a mystery for future probing.

ORDEAL BY STRYCHNINE

Mark 16:18 says ". . . and if they drink any deadly thing it shall in no wise hurt them." With this scriptural verse as a command, some of the saints undergo the ordeal by strychnine. This particular poison is most commonly consumed because of its ready availability, known toxicity, and widespread use as a rodenticide. However, it is also reported that "believers" have swallowed lye without any complications. The ordeal by poison is rare, and the ingestion of strychnine is believed to be the severest trial of faith. This event usually occurs at the acme of a service, and in the two observed instances it occurred in men 52 and 69 years of age. Their estimated weights, were respectively, 68 and 75 kilograms, and it was three hours since they had eaten. Immediately before the ordeal one of the saints alternately got up and sat down in his pew, trembled, cried and laughed. He discussed his one-and-one-half-inch-thick walnut coffin, funeral plans and experiences with "boogery" ("playing with the Devil") until he felt "the power of the Lord descend" upon him. While he was "hollering" and raving, the younger saint, who had just finished his ordeals with the flaming torch, copperhead, and blazing stone coal, paced the floor, puffed, whistled, and exhorted his brother minister to do what the Lord commanded. Suddenly, after the tumultuous "Resurrection Hymn" the older saint took out his pocket knife, pushed down the seal on a new bottle of strychnine sulfate, opened the cap, and transferred an amount of the poison on the knife blade to a glass of water. He stirred it and within 12 seconds took two to three swallows and then passed the glass to his friend, who rapidly imbibed an apparently equal amount.* "In my stomach it feels like cold water, you can sprinkle it on my tongue and it tastes better than honey." Between them, the two saints drank slightly more than 80 ml or a total of 34.4 mg of strychnine sulfate.** Both

---

*The total quantity taken by the two saints was estimated by measuring the column of strychnine sulfate solution in a slightly conical glass tumbler, then aspirating into a syringe an aliquot part which still remained in the glass.

**The qualitative and quantitative analyses of some of the portion remaining from the orally ingested aqueous solution, of suspected pure strychnine sulfate, were performed by William J. Lane, development chemist, analytical laboratory, Schering Corporation. "The total sample [of alleged strychnine sulfate] remaining in the vial was found to be 3.53 grams indicating that approximately 220 mg. had been removed if the label is assumed to be correct. A 1 mg portion of the powder was ground thoroughly into 300 mg of dried potassium bromide and a pellet was pressed from it and examined by infrared using a Beckman IR 5. A similar treatment was afforded a known standard sample of strychnine sulphate. The resulting spectra were identical in all respects. The submitted sample also gave positive tests for strychnine sulphate as outlined in N. F. X[139] and the British Pharmacopoeia 1953.[9] These tests indicate that the material in question is strychnine sulphate. Aqueous solutions of a standard strychnine sulphate were prepared containing 1, 2, 3, 4, and 5 mg per 100 ml respectively. These samples were examined on a Cary recording spectrophotometer from 200 to 400 mu. The resulting curves were all of the same shape and Beer's law was obeyed when optical density was plotted against concentration. This relationship is the basis of the quantitative analysis of the submitted aqueous solutions.

ministers immediately returned to their preaching, jumping, handclapping and singing. Eight minutes later, the younger saint kindly permitted a blood specimen to be taken for analysis, and 26 minutes later he produced a urine specimen. However, to this date, conditions have not made it possible to analyze these specimens. At no time after drinking the strychnine were there any twitches, convulsions or other signs and symptoms.

Of all the Holiness people that were observed, only four gave histories of undergoing the strychnine ordeal. The saint who was alleged to have put his head into the red-hot iron stove, with live coals, claimed to have taken strychnine four to five times in his life, and "I feel the Lord—a cool feeling go down on my neck. I once took half a bottle of it."* In no reported instances, were there ever any complications. In order to emphasize the danger of the strychnine ordeal, the preachers tell how ministers of other denominations have sprinkled some of the Holiness strychnine solution taken by the saints on meat for a dog who died while convulsing shortly after biting into it, or have told how a cat was similarly killed.

Discussion

The strychnine ordeal is an unusual feat, since strychnine[22,207] is readily absorbed from the stomach and intestine. In amounts varying between 5 and 20 mg it can produce convulsions in 15 to 45 minutes that could be fatal. The ordinarily fatal dose by the oral route varies between 60 and 90 mg. Furthermore, it is a characteristic of strychnine to make the subject who ingests it more responsive to various sensory stimuli (as lights, claps, pain, and so forth) which can precipitate convulsions. In sharp contrast to habituating drugs like the barbiturates, the repeated use of strychnine does not lead to tolerance, but on the contrary to an increase in nervous system susceptibility and effects.

It should be stated that the exact dose of strychnine sulfate that was orally taken by each saint was unknown. However, at best, if the total imbibed solution was evenly divided, then each should have had at least 17 mg. If it were not drunk in aliquot parts, one should have had a dose of more than 17

Two aliquots were taken from the submitted solutions and were diluted to 100 ml. volume with water. The solutions were examined using a Cary recording spectrophotometer between 200 and 400 mu. The resulting curves were identical in shape to curves of similar concentration of standard strychnine sulphate solutions. Calculations showed that there were slight differences in the strengths of the examined solutions but that they were of the same general magnitude, being 0.46 mg/ml and 0.41 mg/ml respectively, the average of these results being the reported value of 0.435 mg/ml. The aqueous solutions gave positive tests for strychnine sulphate as outlined in N. F. X and the British Pharmacopoeia 1953. The shape of the above ultraviolet curves also substantiates these identities."
*Strychnine Sulphate, Merck, used by the Holiness saints is dispensed as 3.75 grams per bottle.

mg and the other a lesser amount. However, whether each saint received approximately 17 mg or one saint more, such an amount, by way of the method and times of administration might have been sufficient to produce convulsive, other toxic, and/or possibly, even lethal effects.

The data in an isolated and unique situation like this are too scant upon which to make generalizations. It should also be stated that the dosages employed, although presumably in toxic amounts, might have been insufficient to produce convulsive effects. The dangerous nature of this ordeal naturally precludes any thought of experimentation by using human beings. However, as in the ordeals by serpents and fire, these unusual reactions are fact; and they occur not infrequently. Therefore, it should be possible to study this ordeal further, and gather information which might elucidate the influence of the exaltation on the possibly changed absorption, detoxification, and/or metabolism of strychnine. It can be supposed that the apparent immunity to convulsions and other sequelae is related to these altered factors. Yet, like the ordeals by serpents and fire, the very nature of the strychnine trial makes it most difficult to study and obtain specimens without subjecting the participants to more serious hazards. It is noteworthy that the turbulent church services themselves provided a very intense and variegated form of sensory stimulation, which, in this respect, should have been an additional risk. As in the cases of failure to be bitten by the poisonous snakes or to suffer burns, perhaps the exaltation in this case was an important reason why no convulsions ensued. The only remotely similar situation the author could recall was where, in one instance at least, a blind faith in a scientific opinion (exaltation?) might have accounted for an extraordinary protection against serious effects, illness and possible death. That was at the turn of the last century when von Pettenkofer, in an attempt to disprove Koch's thesis that a cholera culture was highly poisonous, swallowed "virulent choleric culture from Gaffky's laboratory along with Emmerich, Stricker, Metchnikof, Ferran and other pupils."[89] As in cases of suicides, homicides, and accidental deaths from strychnine, laboratory workers and others have become seriously ill and died as a result of the accidental ingestion of the comma bacillus. Perhaps then, exaltation—through its concomitant physiological changes—can act as a potent protective mechanism against the dangerous effects of strychnine, or, by analogy, some other poison.

Any minimal traces of data in this regard might throw some light on how the emotions can, in some instances, affect the thresholds of nervous-tissue irritability and discharge, and, for example, how convulsive-seizure thresholds can be influenced by prevailing affects. For instance, clinicians have long been aware of the fact that some seizures in epileptic patients can be precipitated by significant emotional experiences, whether happy, unhappy, conscious or unconscious. Some support for this opinion is provided by the observation of a seizure occurring in a 46-year-old catatonic woman during depth electrography and a structured interview.[98] The patient (with her family members) was thoroughly studied via the collaborative technique and with concomitant scalp electroencephalography and depth electrography. This observation was unique, because the patient had had no spontaneous convulsive seizures for more than 40 years before the structured interview.

In contrast to this catatonic woman, or to epileptic patients who can have convulsions when surprised or overwhelmed with anxiety, the worshippers in the strychnine ordeal are aware of their experience and, from their previous trials and faith, have some understanding about what they expect will happen. By the gradual build-up of exaltation, they have time for mastering their anxiety and for apparently (internally) bracing themselves against any untoward effects. They dissociate from the threat of certain death by invoking the "power of the Lord" and then acting out the possible counterphobic defense of ingesting the strychnine. Other tangential support for this hypothesis might be provided by the common clinical observation that some patients, in different degrees of excitation, can show wide variations from time to time in the dosages of intravenously administered, short-acting barbiturates necessary to induce sleep.

Further support for this thesis may be provided by patients who, in undergoing pentylenetetrazol (metrazol) activation of an electroencephalographic focal discharge, show variations from time to time in the amount of drug necessary to precipitate a focal convulsion. In both of these situations, then, the factors of previous experience and attitudes might be instrumental in mastering the anxiety and, secondarily, in affecting various neural thresholds. If the biochemical changes associated with the affective state responsible for the altered convulsive-seizure thresholds in the strychnine ordeal could be better defined or identified, there might be some clues here for the pathophysiology of convulsive disorders.

SUMMARY

Some of the cultural and psychodynamic background factors for the members of the Free Pentacostal Holiness Church are described. Particular attention is devoted to the relationship between their states of exaltation that occur during the religious services and the more than 200 observed instances of successful manipulation of poisonous rattlesnakes and copperheads. Also, the salient details are given of the many instances where several different worshippers, during ecstasy, handled "fuel oil" torches, acetylene flames, and flaming coal without having either thermal injury to either their bodies or clothing. As a final psychosomatic phenomenon, the ordeal by poison is described, where two ministers, in exaltation, ingested presumed toxic doses of strychnine sulfate solution, without any harmful effects. These observed data are related to additional material obtained in histories from Holiness people, reported similar data in the literature and some hypotheses toward the understanding of these phenomena. From the study of these ordeals by serpents, fire and strychnine, some possible practical applications to various fields of medicine are mentioned.

ACKNOWLEDGMENT

The author, who is of a nonsectarian Protestant background, hopes this report has been fair and factual, and he thanks the many ministers, brothers and sisters of the Holiness Church whose kindness, help and desire to show the medical world "the workings of the Lord" made these studies possible.

The author also wishes to note that, through the generosity and skill of Dr. Kenneth A. Hawkins, Mr. Wilbur S. Felker, and Mr. William J. Lane of Schering Corporation, Bloomfield, N. J., it was possible to obtain laboratory analyses of the specimens in the strychnine ordeal.

2
Psychodynamic Experiments in Telepathy*

PART I–INTRODUCTION

Since the time of Franz Anton Mesmer[150] a number of physicians have remarked on paranormal, psychic phenomena. One of the first contributions made from the psychodynamic standpoint was Stekel's monograph[209] on the telepathic dream. He noted the influence of strong emotions, such as love, jealousy, and anxiety, on the occurrence of telepathy in the agent-percipient relationship. Shortly after Stekel, Freud[81] made a brilliant contribution to psychic research by stating that if telepathy were a fact, then what telepathically transpired between agent and percipient should conform to the principles of the unconscious: the psi phenomena should exhibit distortions of perception caused by the unconscious which would be similar to those occurring in dreams and in the psychopathology of everyday life.

Eventually the application of the psychoanalytic method unmasked a wider reservoir of hitherto unrecognized psi phenomena in ordinary life. Many psychiatrists, psychoanalysts, and parapsychologists since Freud have written of their personal and clinical experiences with telepathy (e.g., [21,37,64,203,214]). Although specific psychodynamic formulations seem to vary among investigators, there is general agreement that when telepathy occurs during therapy it is most frequently the outcome of an unconscious, emotionally charged process having libidinal or interpersonal significance for both patient and physician. In recent years special emphasis has been attached to the details of the psychoanalytic transference-countertransference relationship. It has been surmised that the existence of countertransference is one reason why more complete reports of telepathic events in therapy are

---

*Dedicated to the memory of Reverend Timothy V. A. Kennedy, M.D., who encouraged the author's research into the relationship between psychic phenomena and the human mind.

not published; Eisenbud,[44] for example, has frankly stated his reluctance to go into detail lest he be too revealing.

Although among modern researches some very significant contributions have come from the work of Dr. J. B. Rhine and his associates at Duke University,[151] there appears to be a certain gap in quality and meaning between the results of laboratory experiments and the spontaneously occurring telepathic events of clinical practice which evidently represent subtle, unconscious factors. For this reason it seemed desirable to the author to devise experiments whose method and interpretation would be based, in so far as possible, on psychodynamic principles.

None of the experiments reported herein was coercive, preplanned, or otherwise consciously reflected upon. A general rule was adopted of avoiding any method of random selection of targets, since it was felt that such would dampen spontaneity and substitute an enforced or too cognitive approach. It was thought that random methods of choosing the subject of a drawing could not conform to the agent—precipient emotional nuances of the moment and might lose the subtle, unconscious factors most responsible for transmission. It was considered that the results would be more analogous to the many incidental reports in the clinical literature, and thus that it would be well worth the risk of an impure telepathic experiment by using psi in a more natural and casual as well as a more purposeful manner. The admitted weaknesses of having no absolute control would, it was hoped, be counterbalanced by the gains induced by more favorable and natural emotional circumstances. The questions of intrinsic controls will be touched on later.

In some respects the experiments described in this study resemble earlier studies in the transmission of drawn images reported by Myers,[137] Warcollier,[229] Sinclair,[205] and Carington.[12] However, for the most part those pioneer studies were too descriptive, elaborately statistical, and cognitive, and were sometimes mystical.

The experiments reported herein were undertaken only after an intensive study of telepathic experiences noted personally in everyday life and in psychoanalytic therapy. These experiences were similar to many described in the literature. The agent (B.E.S.) attempted to cultivate a passive, anxiety-free, subjective state that he had learned from a prolonged first-hand psychiatric investigation of a 95-year-old telepathist, Jacques Romano. In working with this subject, who seemingly could exercise some degree of control over his psi abilities, it was well observed that when agent-percipient transference (positive or negative) was achieved the agent could occasionally transmit a first fleeting thought or impression that occurred to him. It further appeared that when these first impressions—which were the agent's autonomous, or autochthonous, ideas—were uncritically and passively accepted by the agent himself, they were most likely to be successfully transmitted to the percipient.

PART II—PROCEDURE

Concerning the physical health of the participants, it can be stated that all were without symptoms of impairment other than occasional head colds or episodes of la grippe, which had no discernible effects on the perceptions. The effects of various drugs on telepathic function were not studied; the rare use of acetylsalicylic acid and heavy consumption of coffee seemed to make no difference.

In all experiments, except when specifically noted to the contrary, the agent was in one room and the percipient in another room far removed, so that no communication was possible other than through an intercom apparatus. For example, when all the double windows (regular and storm) and the doors were closed and the agent, seated at his desk in his office on the first floor, shouted a name, letter, or digit, it was impossible for the percipient, at her desk in the electroencephalography laboratory on the second floor, to hear the message or any other oral sound.

The percipient's station is directly over the kitchen, which in turn is adjacent to the agent's desk. The kitchen is separated from the agent's office by outside shrubbery, a wall 9 inches thick, a built-in bookcase 11 inches deep, and 4 feet 8 inches high and filled with journals, a loose cotton-padded satin-brocade wall cover, steel kitchen cabinets 1 to 2 feet in depth and holding china and pots and pans, and a formica-like material 1/8 inch thick covering the wall. The ceiling of the agent's office is 11 feet high and 14 inches thick. Together with the floor of the room above, it consists of 12 by 2 inch beams, two oak floors, and plaster. The floor of the percipient's room is covered with a padded carpet. The agent's desk area is under the ceiling that forms part of the outside copper roof for this section of the house. The area of ceiling-floor overlap for the agent's and percipient's rooms is 2 1/2 by 13 feet. That particular floor area of the percipient's room is completely taken up with an electroencephalographic apparatus, patient's chair, portable (folding) bed, and photic stimulator.

The percipient was an acquaintance and subsequent patient of the agent, and there was no overt anxiety during the experiments. On occasion the agent and the percipient were many miles distant from each other. The experiments were conducted under ordinary lighting conditions at any time of the day or night. No attempt was made to eliminate extraneous noise (e.g., telephone, doorbells) or other kinds of distraction. The environment usually was familiar to both agent and percipient. When the agent was in a mood to experiment, and it was a feasible time, he would ask over the intercom,

"May I send you a picture?" After the percipient said "Yes," all communication through the intercom between agent and percipient was discontinued. When the percipient had finished making her drawings, she would call through the intercom, "All right." At no other time during the experiment was the intercom apparatus open between agent and percipient.

One picture was sent or a volley of several pictures in rapid succession, depending upon the particular nuances of the moment and the feelings of the agent and the percipient. The single drawings were usually jotted down by both participants in a matter of seconds and the volleys of drawings seldom lasted more than a few minutes.

The agent's drawings were quite crude, whereas the percipient's were more expert and artistic. Although both agent and percipient usually made drawings of what they visualized in their minds' eye, neither exerted himself concerning this, and often words were written in addition. The agent believes his auditory imagery is better than his visual, whereas the reverse is applicable to the percipient. At no time during the transmission were the thoughts of either agent or percipient ever spoken.

One or several drawings might be made during a day, or again nothing for several days. The agent made his choice of target after becoming as passive as possible and then graphing the first "thought" or impression that arose— sometimes a clock before him, sometimes an object outside of his actual vision. The preliminary instructions to the percipient were, "Put down anything that comes into your mind or any associations that you get." The agent then began asking the percipient over the intercom, "May I send you a picture?" This was rapidly repeated for as many times as the agent felt like it. A separate piece of paper was used by the agent and the percipient for each drawing and association. A lead pencil was employed most of the time, a red pencil occasionally.

Although one person was used as the percipient for most of the experiments, four others were used on various occasions. Sometimes three percipients and one agent were used simultaneously. All these persons were friends of the agent and, again, no tenseness or anxiousness obtained. In the latter instance (agent-percipient transaction) additional rooms were used. As previously, the agent was stationed on the first floor and the percipient, 4, at the electroencephalographic laboratory on the second floor. Percipient 3 was stationed in the sitting room on the second floor, and another participant, the agent's wife, I, in the dinette area of the kitchen on the first floor. None of the participants knew of the wife's uninvited intrusion in the experiments and she, on her own initiative, made drawings which she timed by the kitchen clock. The wife knew about the experiments but her timing was determined on an unconscious basis. Percipient 3's station in the sitting room is

66 feet from the electroencephalographic laboratory as measured via the hallway. The more direct route between the electroencephalographic laboratory and the sitting room, 58 feet, is obstructed by the interposition of four walls, one brick chimney, and numerous doors. The door to the sitting room has soundproof insulation. Thus, again, it was not possible to communicate verbally between the areas involved in the experiment.

The preliminary instructions were the same as with two people except that the first percipient, 4, pressed a bell button, rather than called through the intercom, to signal the second percipient, 3, to draw his picture and write his associations. When the experiments were completed, all pictures were compared and charted. Usually this was done immediately after completing the experiment, but sometimes hours or a day later. In more than one-half of the experiments, accurate facsimiles were made of the drawings, which are given as Figures 2–12–2–21. The remaining drawings are described in Tables 2–1 and 2–2 on pages 53–57.

PART III—RESULTS

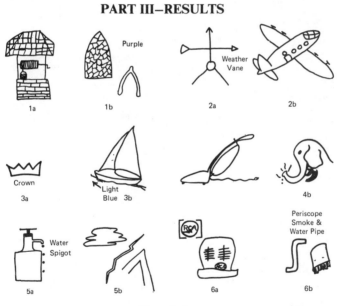

Figure 2–1.

Figure 2–1. The brick well and shingled roof, *1a,* is perceived as a mosaic church window and a wishbone, *1b.* The weathervane, *2a,* is perceived as an airplane, *2b,* of a similar shape. The crown, *3a,* is represented by a sailboat, *3b,* with the words "light blue" pointing to the waves. This crown was a trademark observed on a box with light-blue-to-aqua stripes on it; perhaps the corrugations of the crown suggest the waves of water (see *Figures 2, 5a and 5b*). The vacuum cleaner, *4a*, might be symbolically related to the elephant with his trunk and water spray, *4b*. The water spigot in *5a* is symbolically represented by the cloud, the flash of lightning, and the right-angled pipe, *5b*. The drawing of the microphone, *6a*, was accompanied by the following sentence: "I focus via tubular vision, yet I perceive the arrow." The agent peered through his curled fingers and hand which formed a tube. His attention was arrested by the arrowlike dash in the RCA trademark. His percept is represented as a square mail sack turned upside down with letters (communication) protruding and a tubular structure called "periscope, snake, or waterpipe," *6b*. If a mirror is held up to his latter structure, it resembles the flash of lightning in the RCA trademark (see the little figure, upper left, *6a*) which originally was being observed but was not drawn.

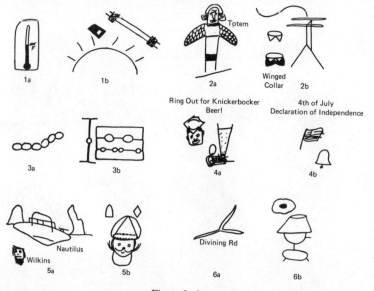

Figure 2–2.

Figure 2–2. The thermometer at 100° F, *1a*, is received as the sun a meter, and a long tubular structure, *1b*. The winged totem pole, *2a*, was perceived as a winged collar and a tall television aerial with two antennae, *2b*. This might be suggestive of the wings and rather large ears on the totem. The six links of the chain, *3a*, are perceived as six links in a square area, *3b*. The three-cornered Father Knickerbocker hat, *4a*, posed a drawing problem for the agent: in making the drawing he associated to George Washington and wondered if there would be some perception of this "foreign body" thought, as well as of the jingle "Ring out for Knickerbocker beer," which he simultaneously "heard in his mind." It was responded to with the visual-auditory complex of "Fourth of July, Declaration of Independence," American flag with the stripes (bars of music), and a bell, *4b*, which approximated the theme song; it was also noted that this was one of the very few times that the percipient entered the office at the end of the experiment singing, (associated motor response). In *5a* the bearded Arctic explorer Wilkins, the submarine *Nautilus*, ocean, and icebergs were perceived as a Santa Claus. *5b:* here the serrations of the fur on Santa Claus' hat might be suggestive of waves of water (cf. Figures *2-1 3a* and *3b*). Finally, the divining rod, *6a*, is repeatedly used in forming the lamp and shade, *6b*. Although the percipient did not explain the black area, it might have pertained to the agent's association of oil discovery with a divining rod.

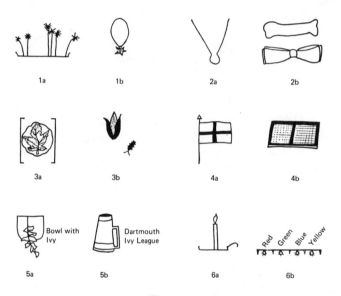

Figure 2−3.

Figure 2−3. Several stellate flowers, *1a*, are perceived as a necklace and starlike jewel, *1b*. The clip *2a*, seems to have received multiple representation in the bow tie, *2b*, and, to a lesser extent, in the bone. A bronze ashtray with a multicolored honeycombed maple leaf, *3a*, (which had been looked at but not drawn) was perceived as an ear of corn (in nature usually golden yellow) and a serrated structure resembling the corrugations of the leaf, *3b*. The Swedish flag, *4a*, becomes without any association a rectangular structure, *4b*. The bowl with ivy, *5a*, was represented as a beer mug, *5b*, with the associations, "Dartmouth Ivy League." The lighted candle, *6a*, is multiplied and improved upon in a battery of four multicolored electric lights, *6b*.

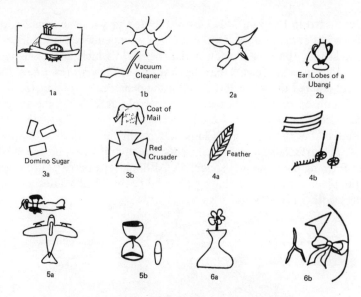

Figure 2-4.

Figure 2-4. The (bracketed) paddlewheel steamboat, *1a,* was mentally visualized while the agent reclined in a barber's chair many miles distant from the percipient, who drew a paddlewheel-like structure and a vacuum cleaner, *1b.* The bird, *2a,* might be symbolized in the vase and words "earlobes of a Ubangi," *2b;* and the percipient thought of the deformed Ubangi ears (wings); possibly the beak is suggestive of the prominent Ubangi lips. The domino sugar cubes, *3a,* might have been multiplied in the rectangles of the coat of mail or transformed into the emblem of the "Red Crusader," *3b.* The feather, *4a,* may have been divided into a pair of skis and the segmentlike tracks in the snow, *4b.* The lateral view of the biplane and dorsal view of the extended cockpit of the monoplane, *5a,* might be suggested in the hourglass and capsule, *5b.* The flower in the vase, *6a,* is not unlike the flowery bow-tie, *6b,* which could be a condensation of the shapes of both vase and flower.

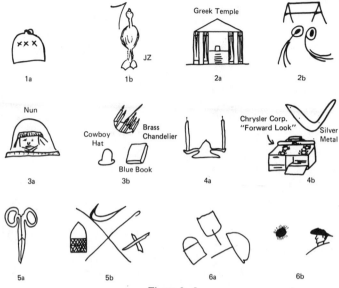

Figure 2–5.

Figure 2–5. The poison jug with "XXX" on it, *1a,* might be symbolically related to the dead duck with three symbols, (*7, J, Z*) *1b.* For the Greek temple, *2a,* the agent had the "foreign-body" association of the Trojan horse and this was drawn as a wooden carpenter's horse and filamentous designs suggestive of the carvings on the columns, *2b.* The drawing of the nun and golden rule, *3a,* shows similarities to the cowboy hat, *3b;* the brim of the hat might correspond to the ruler. The lighted candles on the brass chandelier and the blue book would not be inappropriate to the religious motif. The silver candelabra and lighted candles, *4a,* are represented by the "silver metal" auto trademark and completely lighted gas stove, *4b.* The scissors, *5a,* receive multiple representation with the two large crisscrosses and lattice window, *5b;* possibly a segment of the handles of the shears is pictured in the crescentlike image. The beach motif of shovel, pail, and umbrella, *6a,* was responded to with a bright sun and head with a sombrero, *6b.*

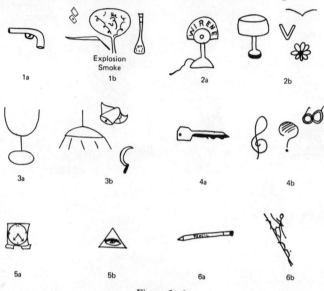

Figure 2–6.

Figure 2–6. Only once (*1a* and *1b*) in the series of experiments did the percipient agree to reverse roles with the agent. On this occasion the agent received the angular structure suggestive of the gun and the drawing of an explosion with the additional associations of "smoke or tornado." Also noted, and complementary, were playing cards and a bottle of wine. The microphone with station letters, *2a*, was perceived as a similarly shaped lamp and flower, *2b*, plus the *V* which, when doubled, would be a *W*, the first letter of the station and first fleeting thought. The symbol in *3a* is not unlike the inverted light or, in a fragmented form, the hand sickle, *3b*. The door key, *4a*, might be related to the musical clef, *4b*, that gives the key, although of another kind; the question mark and glasses vaguely resemble and duplicate the key. Drawing the clock, *5a*, was accompanied by the question "What will the effect be if I look at this object through telescoped hands?" The association was well received by the drawing of an eye looking through a triangle, *5b*. The pencil, *6a*, might have some resemblance to the straight line representing a mountain slope with a man ascending, *6b*. There are six letters in the word "pencil" and the mountain climber must contend with five stones; possibly the letters have some connection with the stones.

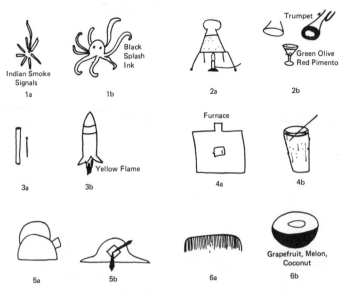

Figure 2-7.

Figure 2-7. The seven radiating sticks of an Indian campfire and black smoke with the accompanying association "Indian smoke signals" are perceived as an octopus and the words "black splash ink," *1b.* The flask on the stand and the Bunsen burner, *2a,* are perceived as the multiplied funnel-like motif of the cocktail glass and trumpet, *2b.* The bell of the horn resembles the edge of the customary wire-asbestos grill. The percipient wrote, "I saw three objects but forgot one while drawing." The cigarette and the match, *3a,* are represented with the drawing of the rocket and the words "yellow flame," *3b.* The furnace, *4a,* may be represented by an opposed image in the tall, cool, icy drink, *4b.* The kettle, *5a,* is visually suggestive of the clock and one of the hands, *5b.* The comb, *6a,* elicited the response "grapefruit, melon, or coconut," *6b.* This was not considered particularly valid until, much later in the series when the comb was again drawn (Figure 2-11: *3a* and *3b*) a similar and ludicrous response was obtained. It would be quite a feat to comb a grapefruit, melon—even a hairy coconut—or a bald head.

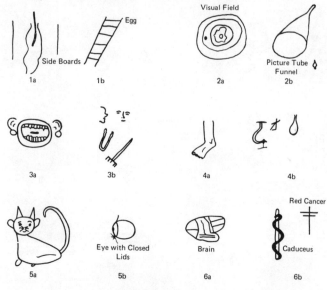

Figure 2–8.

Figure 2–8. The first drawing, *1a,* was made many miles distant from the percipient. At the time the agent had been called for consultation at the hospital but did not know what medical problem he would encounter. However, he jotted down a stomach with indwelling tube and sideboards and words which turned out to be appropriate to his patient: "ruptured aneurysm and delirium." This was responded to with a ladder (sideboards), *1b,* and the word "egg" (stomach or aneurysm as the laity might think of it). A visual field, such as that used in examining eye function, *2a,* was represented by a drawing variously described as "picture tube, funnel, glass, perfume," *2b.* The bizarre mouth, teeth, ears, and earrings, *3a,* might have some functional connection with the symbolical rake and nutcracker which can suggest biting, crushing, and grinding. The profile and frontal view of a partial face help to complete the drawing of the "faceless" mouth. The L-shaped foot, *4a,* was perceived as a hook, which is almost L-shaped also and a mirror image (see Figure 2–1: *6a* and *6b*). The strange or poorly drawn cat and whiskers, *5a,* has some similarity to the eye with closed lids, *5b;* the eyelashes correspond to the cat's whiskers. The diagram of the brain, *6a,* was accompanied with the association "EEG diagram and recent red circle marking site of brain tumor." This was perceived in the drawing of a caduceus and a cancer cross similar to that used in fund-raising emblems in cancer research with the words "red, cancer," *6b.*

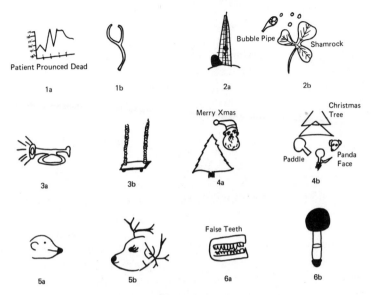

Figure 2–9.

Figure 2–9. The temperature chart, *1a,* had the accompanying statement, "Patient pronounced dead." It was drawn when the agent had attempted to make his mind a blank and then took a medical journal and opened it to an advertisement from which the drawing was made. The symbolism of the response, a stethoscope, *1b,* was accentuated later when it was volunteered that immediately after this experiment the percipient had, in fact, taken her temperature. This was not done at any other time, and there was no conscious awareness of the possible connection between her motor acting out and the experiment. The drawing of the oil well derrick, *2a,* suggested to the agent because of his concern over some investments as well as his 2-year-old daughter's shouting of the word "oil" when the agent was thinking of it (automatic motor telepathic response). Although the oil well was not eidetically perceived, perhaps the shamrock and bubble pipe, *2b,* symbolically expressed the percipient's (or agent's) ambivalence: good luck, fatuous pipe dreams, or someone "forever blowing bubbles." The blasting trumpet, *3a,* was drawn after the agent had stepped to the back of his house and was indecisive about removing his child's swing for the approaching winter. The percipient's swing, *3b,* perhaps was connected with both the agent's irritation over the swing and the slang word "swing" (music). When the percipient presented her drawing she pursed her lips, which was unusual for her and may have been a motor expression of trumpet playing. (see Figure 2–2: *4a* and *4b*). The Christmas tree and Santa Claus head, *4a,* yielded triangular structures with the words "Christmas tree," a panda face, key ring chain, and paddle, *4b,* all three could be fragments of *4a.* In the case of the peculiar mouse head, *5a,* and deer head, *5b,* there was a slight deviation from the usual order of the experiments. The percipient had asked the agent at the end of one day whether he had sent her a picture. His answer being "No" he then volunteered to draw his first impression, which was the animal resembling the mouse. The percipient then gave the agent her drawing, which had been made earlier, at 2:05 P.M. The agent was quite surprised, because it was at this approximate time that a patient, then beginning therapy, had been relating her first (and most important) dream: "I walk up an old street, a deer crosses the street, there's pandemonium. I call for my husband to shoot the deer. Just as he is about to shoot the deer, I wake up." The patient's associations to the dream were related to conflicts about accepting her role as a woman and her hostility toward the male sex. The false teeth, *6a,* is the particular impression that came to the agent's mind on a date prior to seeing a certain patient. This patient was an acutely disturbed adolescent showing marked dissociation and a possibility of acting out by running away from home and a mother she consciously hated. It seemed that her disturbance was precipitated by false teeth. The patient had been looking forward to spending a weekend with her boy friend after finishing her mid-term school examinations, but a "kick in the teeth" came when she received a long-distance telephone call from her fiancé telling her that he would have to break his date because, while playing football, his false teeth had been knocked out and he had to go to the dentist for emergency care. The patient repressed all rage and dissociated from this incident but became overtly disturbed when she received a second telephone call, this time from her mother: she was informed that mother was breaking her promise by prohibiting the patient's visit to her fiancé at a later date and insisting that she come home and take care of her younger sister instead. Shortly after this incident, the parents were unexpectedly called out of town because of a death in the family. Thus, it was apparent that the patient might have had much repressed hostility and anxiety over this symbolical castration (false teeth): breaking of boy friend's date because of false teeth, mother's broken promise concerning a date, death in family with abandonment by parents, and finally need to care for younger sister. In the experiment, the agent was surprised when, later in the day, he was told that approximately 15 minutes prior to his drawings of the false teeth his wife was "reading a Christmas short story about an aunt with false teeth, this aunt always left them around and this annoyed the children." The percipient's response to the false teeth was an aseptosyringe, *6b,* which was also called a penis and reacted to with blushing. The psychopathology seems to be compatible with this fellatio-like or oral-sadistic type of response and is also in harmony with the patient's similar character structure.

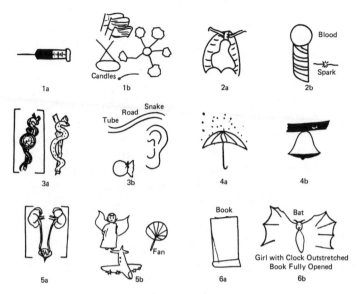

Figure 2–10.

Figure 2–10. These drawings represent experiments in which a red pencil was spontaneously used by either agent or percipient so that a red target object might be either transmitted or perceived. A syringe, *1a*, was drawn with a red pencil and reacted to in *1b* with tubular structures and needles as well as candles; the red, white, and blue stripes of the American flag are suggestive of the red syringe calibrations. The postero-anterior X-ray silhouette of the chest with (red) heart, *2a*, seems to be represented by the red and blue barber pole, *2b*, with the word "blood," as well as the two lines with a spark in the gap; the horizontal lines divided by the spark might be suggestive of the clavicles and sternoclavicular joints. The bracketed drawing of the red caduceus and seal of Hippocrates, *3a*, was looked at by the agent and then drawn without the seal. It was perceived as a tubular structure described as "tube, road, snake," a pouch turned on its side, and an ear, *3b*. It would seem that the percipient received the caduceus partially, the undrawn seal carrying a profile of Hippocrates being incompletely picked up and magnified. The umbrella and rain, *4a*, were represented as a red bell, *4b*. The bracketed drawing of the kidneys, ureters, bladder, and urethra, *5a*, had been observed in a medical journal where it was colored red. The agent wished to transmit this over several miles, so he telephoned the percipient to suggest an experiment at a later time that evening. The percipient's father, who had never met the agent, answered. Almost his first words were of her history of pyelitis in babyhood. However, the percipient not being home, the agent let the matter rest, and the experiment was performed at a later date under the usual conditions. At that time the pictures of an angel, airplane, and fan were drawn, *5b*. Perhaps the paired wings and lateral lines of the trunk are suggestive of the kidneys and ureters; the fan is quite reminiscent of the bladder. As to the airplane it might be an addition to what was not drawn but possibly unconsciously thought of by the agent: the airplane is a common symbol of the genitals and as such would not be inappropriate to the percipient's psychopathology. By drawing the plane she made a more complete sketch of the genito-urinary tract. The next target was the book *Sexual Deviations* randomly opened to a chapter on vampirism, *6a*. This was reacted to with a (red) drawing of a bat and the words "girl with a cloak outstretched . . . book fully opened." In this instance, as in the previous one (Figure 2–10: *5a, 5b*) the use of red may have had some erotic significance.

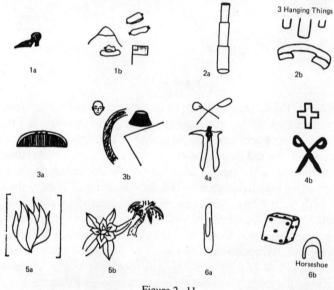

Figure 2–11.

Figure 2–11. The agent's drawings *1a, 3a,* and *5a* were in red and the percipient's drawings *2b, 4b* and *6b* were in red. The red shoe, *1a* may be related to the red, white, and blue American flag and the hot dog, *1b;* the latter response was consistent with the percipient's frequent use of colloquialisms; "my dogs are burning and killing me." The telescope, *2a,* was partially received as "three hanging things" and audio-visually received as a French telephone, *2b*. The response to the red comb, *3a,* of a bald-headed man, a semilunar darkened structure (head of hair?), and a lampshade may have a humorous connotation and seems to have some similarity to the response to the comb obtained in Figures 2–7: *6a* and *6b*. The right angle is suggestive of the perpendicular teeth of the comb. The picture of the bald-headed man evoked a smile from the agent because he immediately thought of it as a likeness of one of his father's closest (and only completely bald-headed) friends, E. J. W. The percipient, of course, knew nothing of E. J. W. However, the surprise came a short time later when the agent's mother telephoned to say that she had just heard of E. J. W.'s sudden and unexpected death. This was a shock, since E. J. W. had been in apparently excellent health. Since the times of the percipient's drawing and the agent's mother's learning of the death approximately coincided, this particular drawing experiment may represent a complex telepathic transaction between the percipient, the agent, and the latter's mother. The speculum and shears, *4a,* are represented by red scissors and the Red Cross medical symbol, *4b.* The bracketed drawing of a red flower-like structure, *5a,* was conjured from an advertisement and perceived by the percipient's looking around the room and noting a bedspread with a similar red flower, *5b.* The paper clip, *6a,* may have had some relationship to the horseshoe, *6b;* the clip has three horseshoes in its structure.

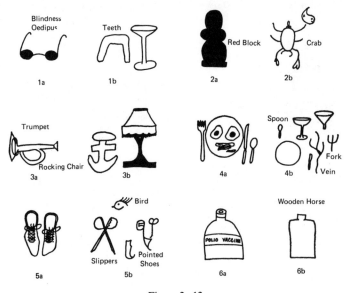

Figure 2–12.

Figure 2–12. The smoked glasses and associations "blindness and oedipus," *1a,* were suggested to the agent by a difficult problem he had with a patient affected with psychic blindness and some incestuous conflicts. The percipient drew a tooth structurally similar to the glasses and the symmetrical cocktail glass. Blindness and a tooth are symbolically related and quite suggestive of the patient's castration anxiety; in fact, the patient frequently equated blindness, tooth extraction, and castration. The drawing for *2a* was made from observing a child's red block. It was picked up many miles away as a red crab, *2b*, the body of which resembles parts of the block. The trumpet, *3a*, gave drawings of an ornate lamp and iron anchor, *3b*, which resembled the instrument. The fork, knife, spoon, plate, and bacon and eggs, *4a*, were perceived in a fragmented and disorganized order, but with all those objects, plus the added feature of a cocktail glass, *4b*. The laced slippers, *5a*, were preceived eidetically in *5b* as shears and ornate pointed shoes; the lace motif suggests the feathers from the head of a bird. The polio vaccine bottle, *6a*, was eidetically perceived as a bottle in *6b*.

The remaining single-drawing experiments are charted in Table 2–1.

VOLLEY-OF-DRAWINGS EXPERIMENTS

In the experiments now to be reported, the images were rapidly transmitted and received as "volleys" at times given at the base of each figure. However, the drawings and associations were on occasion compared much later.

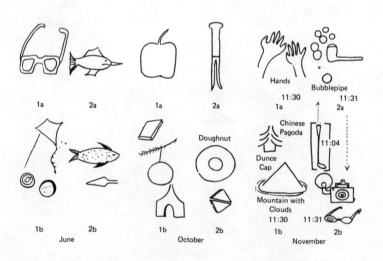

Figure 2–13.

Figure 2–13. These three two-image experiments were done in different months. In June, the percept of eyeglasses, *1a*, was suggestively received as two round cans with a line drawn from one and the bent tail of a kite approximating the other, *1b*. The immediately following drawing of a swordfish, *2a*, was eidetically perceived as a fish and a spear, *2b*. The October experiment with the drawing of a red apple *1a*, gave eidetically a red Christmas tree ornament, a book, and an archway, *1b*. The clothespin, *2a*, yielded a doughnut and sandwich, *2b;* possibly the gap between the sandwiches was suggestive of the split in the clothespin. The male-female symbolism (clothespin, doughnut) may be significant because of the recurrence of this type of response (Figure 2–9: *6a* and *6b*). In November, the outstretched hands *1a*, were copied from a drug advertisement appearing in a psychiatric journal: the effectiveness of a tranquilizer medication for organic psychoses was stressed. When drawing the hands, the agent wondered if any of his associative material pertaining nonverbally to patients with senile delirium and impaired intellect would be transmitted. Possibly this was the case, because a Chinese pagoda with radiating roofs (fingers) and "mountains with clouds" and the words "dunce cap," *1b*, were obtained. The mountain with clouds is an enlarged picture similar to the ten finger tips and nails. It might also suggest the serenity induced by tranquilizers. And the response, "dunce cap" was not inappropriate for a lay person who equated psychiatry with delirium, mental deficiency, and the like. The second picture of the volley, transmitted one minute later, consisted of a bubble pipe and nine bubbles, *2a*, which was received as a camera with flash attachment and eyeglasses. There are nine round structures in the percipient's response and the right-angle flash attachment and bulb are suggestive of the pipe and bubbles (see Figure 2–2: *3a* and *3b*). An additional surprise was afforded when the percipient produced from her pocket a drawing of a golf club—the time: 11:04. Perhaps the golf club was the real original, and the agent's bubble pipe only a spurious one.

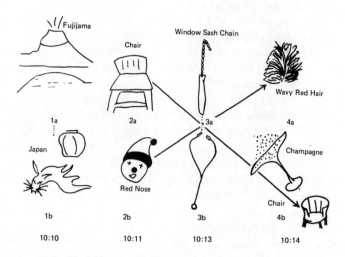

Figure 2–14.

Figure 2–14. These four images were "sent" between 10:10 and 10:15 A.M. The dragon with flames shooting from his mouth, the lantern, and the word "Japan," *1b,* are clear symbolic associative responses to the erupting volcano, "Fujiyama," *1a.* The stethoscope, *3b,* either with the diaphragm hanging from the single hose or visually inverted so that the metal ear pieces seem to form a weight suspended from the hose are suggestive of the window sash chain and weight, *3a.* Perhaps the glass of bubbling champagne, *4b,* is visually related in fragmented form to the weight motif and links of the chain, *3a.* The eidetic crisscross between the chair *2a,* and chair *4b* is apparent. The red-nosed clown, *2b,* and wavy red hair, *4a,* might be related to the agent's irritation over the telephone importunities of a wavy-haired redheaded relative of a patient (drawn without a face) then under treatment. In this instance the color red may, in addition to identifying an important aspect of the agent's associations, indicate his anger. The percipient had never met the relative in question, however, her successive associative drawings of red-nosed clown, stethoscope, and glass of champagne and chair are suggestive of an unconscious recognition of the physician's annoyance with the patient's petulant relative and of the need to relax in a comfortable chair with a glass of champagne. The bleary-eyed red-nosed clown might be an excellent crisscross complement to the (faceless) wavy red hair. The question remains whether the percipient's red-nosed clown provoked the agent's drawing of the red hair or was a response to other earlier unconscious thought processes of the agent (see Figure 2–13: November *2a* and *2b*). In such a short interval volley irritation may well have been a factor in the crisscrossing and reversal of the agent and percipient roles.

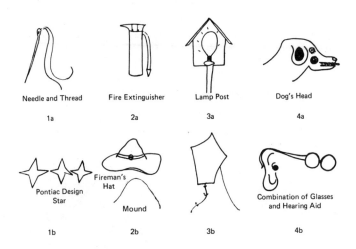

Figure 2–15.

Figure 2–15. In the needle and thread picture, *1a,* the needle point was drawn first; perhaps the multiple points of the three stars, *1b,* are related to the needle point and the stainless steel needle and the shiny chromium are certainly alike in color and even substance. The fire extinguisher, *2a,* was drawn two minutes later and was perceived as a red fireman's hat and a mound, *2b.* There was, however, an interim of several hours before the percipient reported her perception, and during that time some interesting events transpired. One hour after making this group of drawings the agent left his office to go Christmas shopping. At approximately 11:45 A.M. he bought a rather expensive fire extinguisher and a can of pine deodorant for his wife. This was extraordinary for him, since it was not his intention and these two items were hardly suitable Christmas gifts. He thought it was foolish, but on the other hand just felt compelled to buy them. While driving home he decided to give both presents at once, rather than to wrap them and wait until Christmas. He brought the gifts into the kitchen, and immediately noticed acrid fumes. His wife excitedly told him that in his absence (approximately 11:45 A.M.) there had been an electrical fire in the deep-fat fryer, which had burned a hole through the aluminum pot and stainless steel spoon. There had never been a fire in the house. This combination of a controlled experiment and some additional spontaneous telepathic events seems to raise the question of precognition, unusual coincidence, or both, and the agent's compulsive telepathic reaction (see Figure 2–13: November *2a* and *2b*). Three minutes after the drawing of the fire extinguisher, a five-cornered lantern and lamp post, *3a*, was drawn and perceived as a similarly shaped kite and tail, *3b*. The last drawing of this volley, made one minute later, was the dog's head *4a*, which was perceived as a combination of glasses and hearing aid, *4b*.

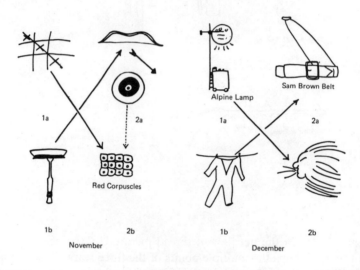

Figure 2–16.

Figure 2–16. Possibly the less striking results of this experiment can be attributed to the percipient's anxiety over scheduled surgery on a body part of psychosexual significance to herself. However, this fact was not made known to the agent until after the experiments. The tick-tack-toe drawing, *1a*, was perceived as a divided area of many squares, *2b*. In the squares are round objects, and these figures are the percipient's impression of red corpuscles. They might also be related to the drawing of a bull's-eye target, *2a*. The line drawn through the three X's of the tick-tack-toe possibly was associated with an arrow and with the bow-and-arrow-like razor, *1b*, appearing in *2a* as bow, arrow, and target. The percipient's anxiety may have accounted for this crisscross phenomenon. A crisscrossing occurs again between December's alpine lamp, *1a*, and the North Wind, *2b*, and between the X-shaped long underwear, *1b*, and the Sam Brown belt, *2a*. When the agent (correctly) drew this belt, he wondered whether there ought to be straps over each shoulder so that an X would be formed. At the conclusion of this volley of drawings the percipient was staring out the window and sobbing. Later it appeared that she was upset because of intense rage toward a male friend. She had treated him rather sadistically and his failure to respond as the percipient thought he should only produced more rage and guilt. Here, again, is the situation of rage and the crisscross phenomenon. It may be noted also that the long underwear drying on a clothesline, *1b,* is complementary to the hot, bright rays of the alpine lamp.

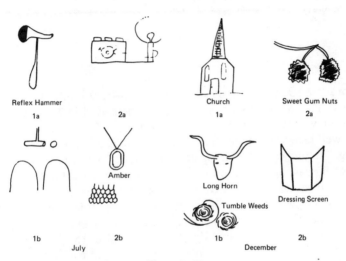

| Reflex Hammer | | Church | Sweet Gum Nuts |
| 1a | 2a | 1a | 2a |

	Amber	Long Horn	Dressing Screen
		Tumble Weeds	
1b	2b	1b	2b
July		December	

Figure 2–17.

Figure 2–17. The reflex hammer, July, *1a,* was received as a croquet mallet, ball, and wires, *1b.* Perhaps the curved wires are related to the photoflash unit attached to a camera, *2a.* The amber pendant on the chain in *2b* may have some connection with the particular amber flash bulbs the agent used and was thinking of in making the drawing of the camera and flash attachment. The December church, with a long, narrow, pointed steeple, two symmetrical windows and the central door, *1a,* is perceived as the long-horned steer with prominent eyes, *1b.* The other response of tumbleweeds, *1b,* resembles the agent's next drawing of sweet gum nuts, *2a.* While drawing these he wrote "looking out the window (at the sweet gum nuts)." Here may have been an instance of the agent's visual motor response to the percipient's image of tumbleweed, and the "looking out the window" action could have been perceived as the *2b* windowlike drawing of a "dressing screen." The actual dressing screen in the agent's office is made from three window screens. There also seems a crisscrossing of this percept with the two symmetrical church windows and door, *1a.* The experiment was successful despite the fact that it was the only time a third party was present with the agent during the actual drawing: there was no overt anxiousness.

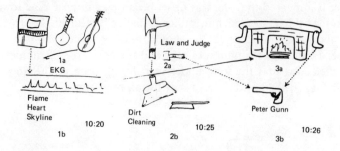

Figure 2–18.

Figure 2–18. Of the three musical instruments in *1a* only the piano keyboard with its dark keys seems to have been perceived in *1b* as the electrocardiogram with the rhythmic QRS complexes. The fasces and gavel, *2a*, are visually well related to the dustpan and broom, *2b*, and the association "law and judge" to the words "cleaning up dirt," which could be a symbolical definition of the law appropriate to a lay person. The brick fireplace, burning logs, and flames, *3a*, seem to have come from the percipient's earlier associations of "flame, heart, and skyline," *1b*, while the red brick may be related to the red heart. The fireplace flames, as drawn, are reminiscent of the New York City skyline as it appears from the agent's office. The gun and the comment "Peter Gunn" (a television detective), *3b*, could be a condensation of the stockings on the fireplace, *3a*, and the agent's preceding associations of law and judge, *2a*. (Peter Gunn refers to a television sketch in which the detective is frequently involved in law-enforcement problems).

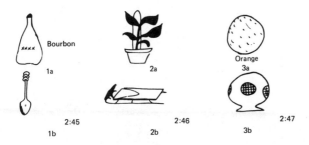

Figure 2–19.

Figure 2–19. The bourbon decanter (imagined as an ornate one), *1a,* was perceived several miles away as an ornamented silver spoon; the two drawings have some resemblance. The philodendron plant, *2a,* became a sled, *2b.* The connection, if any, seems remote, but when the sled is rotated 90 degrees counterclockwise, there is some visual affinity between it and the philodendron: the main stem of the plant is backed by a board with parallel edges, and the darkened side (front view) of the sled, in turn, is flanked by two parallel lighter lines. Turned around, the dark areas of the sled suggest the stem and leaves of the plant. The drawing of a navel orange, *3a,* which immediately followed and an interfering association of the agent's, that of a face, was picked up as a diver's helmet, *3b:* the helmet is globular like an orange, is worn on the face, and would have a face looking (appearing) through.

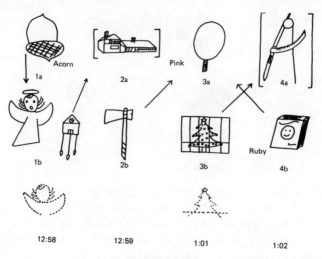

Figure 2–20.

Figure 2–20. This, one of the last volley-of-drawings experiments, is of clinical interest. The percipient participated only reluctantly and then re-fused to associate further, and the agent was most angry. The results seemed to indicate two reversals of agent-percipient roles and the crisscross phe-nomenon occurs at the end. The acorn, *1a,* apparently suggests the round angel's head, the wings shaped like a quartermoon, and the symmetrical strands of hair (crosshatching on acorn); see the dotted sketch below *1b.* However, the additional response of a pendulum clock in the shape of a house, *1b,* may have impelled the agent's going into the recesses of his desk and pulling out a postcard of a restaurant, *2a,* which he erroneously believed he was sending. The spurious response of a tomahawk (percipient's rage?) *2b,* to the restaurant again seems to have given the agent an image of a ping-pong paddle—a rather ludicrous comedown. The drawing of the Christmas tree through bars, *3b,* was perhaps too formidable a drawing test for the agent who, therefore, again reacted physically by entering his desk, this time pulling out a drawing compass. The geometric similarities are noted in the dotted sketch below. The agent's spurious compass was taken as a book with a round face on the cover and the word "ruby," *4b.* Perhaps the round face and the word "ruby" were related to the pink paddle of the preceding exper-iment, thus completing the crisscross, or they were a condensation of the disc and two arms of the compass, *4a.*

The consistency of reversal of the agent-percipient roles, in association with the crisscross phenomenon, suggests the significance of the percipient's quality of response, the reciprocating influence of anger, and the value of training or practice in one role.

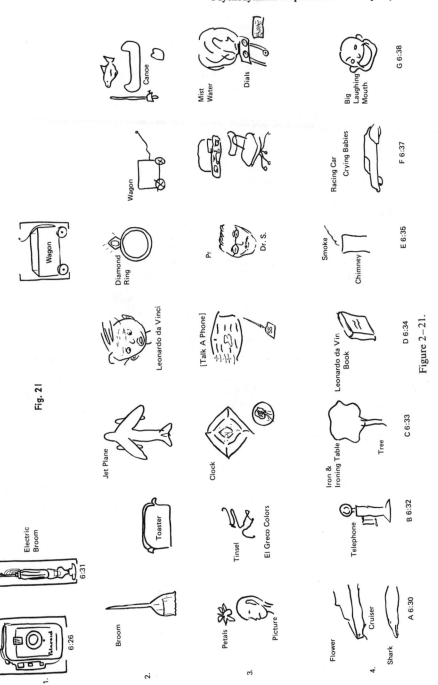

Figure 2–21.

Volley-of-drawings Experiments Four Persons

Figure 2–21. In this experiment the agent, 2, and two percipients 3, 4, were in separate and isolated rooms. An uninvited participant was the agent's wife, I, in still another isolated room and who without any warning or previous plans rather mirthfully entered the series by writing down her spontaneous and unsolicited images at the exact time of their occurrence.

Percipient 4, B. A. Ruggieri, a physician, is well-known to the agent and his wife. Percipient 3, Roman Mercier, a soldier, is the brother-in-law of Dr. Ruggieri, is only casually acquainted with the agent and his wife and was brought along by Dr. Ruggieri as a surprise to the agent. The experiment was entirely spontaneous. There had been no previous mention of experimentation when 3 was invited to participate. In short, this was the first such experiment for I, 3 and 4, Thus, a housewife, a soldier, and two physicians, none with a history of unusual psychic experiences, formed the group making 24 drawings within a period of 12 minutes.

Possibly I's Polaroid camera was a factor in 3's banal but entirely appropriate response of "picture." The broom, *2a,* inverted might resemble a tulip, a flower being the image received, *3,* and associated to, *4.* The electric broom, I, appears a good response to the agent's percept. The chromium-plated electric toaster, *2,* perhaps was a picking-up of the electric broom. The silver tinsel, *3,* again may be related to the chromium toaster or the wires of the electric broom or both, as may be the old-fashioned upright telephone, *4,* in a general way. The jet plane, *2,* apparently suggested the cruiser or shark, *4,* but perhaps it was a visual approximation to the telephone. The electric clock also seems to tie in with the broom and toaster and so does the association to an iron and ironing table, *4* (heat as well as electricity).

Possibly the Talk-A-Phone panel, *3,* connected with the telephone, participant *4.* For the first time since the beginning of the volley (the first two being the two brooms and the flower petals and flower), a very good hit was made with the World Publishing Company trademark of the tree, *3,* and an almost identically shaped tree, *4.*

TABLE 2–1.   Single Agent-Percipient Drawings.

		Comments*
1.	Apple = diamond ring	Ss
2.	Venetian glass vases in arch = arch and design	Ss
3.	Three Ballantine beer rings–bowling pins and ear	Ss
4.	Polka-dot bow-tie = nutcracker	Ss
5.	Dove = artist's easel	Ss
6.	Christmas trellis (drawn in red) = Christmas ornaments with word "red"	Ss
7.	Snifter glass = sun or egg yolk and telephone pole	Ss
8.	Mouse's head = barn, hay, cows	Highly symbolic if anything; mouse in hayloft?
9.	One-dollar bill = mallet	Head of Washington in oval, similar to mallet head.
10.	Stapler = geometric form	Ss
11.	Vase with ivy = two bridge spans and waves	Ss
12.	Pill case = sea urchin	Dots for spines = pills.
13.	Cup and saucer = fish mounted on plaque	Ss
14.	Sail boat = bell and telephone	Ss
15.	Pen knife = leather camera case	Strap of camera case poised like hinged blade.
16.	Old-fashioned locomotive = four structures like locomotive chimneys	Ss
17.	Football, helmet, and jersey with a "D" = puff, mushroom, umbrella, and D-like symbol	Ss
18.	Oil derrick and water lily = ladder plus "black and green" and rain and wagon	Ss; symbolic.
19.	Shrunken Jibaro head = whistle	Ss
20.	Carousel with horses = moth and green leaf with design	Ss
21.	French telephone = mushroom	Ss
22.	Pine tree = Doctor's sign on pine fence post	Ss
23.	Deer's head with antlers = vase	Ss
24.	Yellow sign, "Taxi" = half sliced egg and word "yellow"	Matching of color yellow.
25.	Pocket watch and seven other items = autoclave timer	Eidetic.
26.	Coat-of-arms and three other items = gold shield-shaped electric fixture	Eidetic.
27.	Electric iron = sunglasses	Ss symbolic of heat.
28.	Bermuda shorts = windmill, block "A," and canoe	Ss of shorts and windmill; symbolic.
29.	Stethoscope = geometric shape plus train	Ss

TABLE 2–1. Single Agent-Percipient Drawings. (Cont.)

30.	Lamp and cord = sliding pond and splash	Ss
31.	Lawn mower = florescent lamp	Ss when rotated.
32.	Flower = design, fish, and train with two wheels	Ss
33.	Ball, bat, and glove = 23 stick men and (thumb-shaped) cemetery, tornado (bat), and sail boat	Ss
34.	Bathing suit = geometric design	Percipient had just bought bathing suit.
35.	Camera screw = rear-view mirror with eyes	Ss
36.	Flash gun and camera = round bird bath	Ss
37.	Pitcher, flower, nurse's hat = needle and thread and pen	Ss
38.	Old-fashioned radios with two symmetric dials = two symmetric minnows, water, and bow of boat	Ss
39.	Elephant's head = slice of bread turned sideways and half moon	Ss
40.	Three capsules = diamond	After shuffling and cutting deck, correctly called the 8 of diamonds (clairvoyantly), this spontaneous experience apparently perceived, whereas the more cognitive three capsules was not.
41.	Baby's bottle and iron = iron anchor, leaf, and honeycomb	Ss
42.	Covered wagon and horse = envelope and wings, picture on a lampshade	Ss spokes of wheels similar to folds of envelope, wheels resemble orange. Cover over wagon is similar to lampshade.
43.	Moon with crater (of burnt-out volcano) = skate with red eyes and tail, turban with red stone	Color red symbolizes old volcano.
44.	Cup of coffee and doughnut = bottle of ink	Bottle of ink resembled jar that contained coffee; color of both was black.
45.	Elaborate tall brick chimney = long-necked turkey and feathers	Ss
46.	Tape recorder = tennis racket with only vertical strings	Ss circle with tangential tape.
47.	Nefertete bust = can of beer	Ss
48.	Pearl necklace and window = leopard with spots	Ss
49.	Vine = bird and many straggly lines	Ss and complementary response.
50.	Zebra = sailing ship = sailing ship	The two percipients picked up agent's fleeting thought of Viking ship which was changed to Zebra (similar to striped sails of painting that was visualized.)
51.	Harp = Tie on 45 degree angle and golf bag	Ss

TABLE 2–1.   Single Agent-Percipient Drawings. (Cont.)

52.	Plate, knife, fork, spoon = toaster and the three figures *P, 3,* and *h*	Syncretism; *3* = fork, *h* = knife, *P* = spoon.
53.	Typewriter = open book with print	Open book with print similar to typewriter keyboard or to printed pages of open book.
54.	Sailing schooner = broom	Ss
55.	Wheel and arrowhead = keyhole	Ss
56.	Insecticide spray can = long-necked turkey	Syncretism
57.	Dollar bill = canoe on water with oval seat in middle	Similar symmetry; dollar sign (*$*) resembles design on canoe? Eidetic multiplied.
58.	Peter = face of girl	Name chosen is that of male child who has many feminine physical traits.
59.	Record = axle of auto wheel, half moon and letter "B" with rows of dots	Ss
60.	Milk bottle = geometric design with five cylinders	Ss
61.	Dagger with red blade = oil derrick and tennis racket	Shaded handle of tennis racquet similar to dagger.
62.	Cacti in sun, hammer-and-sickle = skull, face with sunbonnet, letter "A," and rectangle	Skull of steer in desert thought of but not drawn—complementation.
63.	Pistol = sail boat and face of girl	Ss
64.	Turtle and feet on hot coals = spiral, shoes, heart, and shells	Spiral resembles turtle shell, heart (red) symbolic and Ss to hot coals; shoes complementary to bare feet on hot coals.
65.	Ballentine's three beer rings = bottle of beer	In composing chart could not find note for this, despite search for several minutes; set drawing on my desk; received note from percipient two days later with words "strange impression of a bottle of beer."
66.	Clock with hands set at 7:25 = circle enclosed in half a square	Ss

*Ss = structural similarity.

TABLE 2–2.   Vollies of Drawings Experiments.

Experiment number	Serial number	Time		Comments*
I	1	3:25	(*a*) Snow man = (*b*) Christmas star, Waterfall	Symbolic of winter: *1a* and *1b*.
	2	3:30	(*a*) Photos of two faces = (*b*) can opener	Crisscross geometric shape and symbolism between *2a* and *3b, 2b* and *3a*.

TABLE 2–2. Vollies of Drawings Experiments. (Cont.)

Experiment number	Serial number	Time		Comments*
	3	3:33	(a) Cartoon of skiing around tree = (b) eye (looking)	
II	1	1:08	(a) Flashlight = (b) sailor jumper and striped tie	Is lion's head, 2a, on sailor's jumper, 1b a ludicrous criss-cross? Percipient irritated.
	2	1:10	(a) Lion's head = (b) hand towel	
	3	1:11	(a) Hand saw = (b) lantern	Teeth of saw, 3a, related to towel design, 2b, and perceived geometric shapewise as lantern, 3b.
III	1	4:30	(a) Crystal ball on wooden mount = (b) flowers and Christmas tree	First experiment for this percipient; criss-cross, eidetic, and geometric shape: 1a and 2b, 1b and 2a.
	2	4:31	(a) Christmas tree (b) cartoon figure, a shmoe holding hemlock	
IV	1	12:40	(a) Black frying pan = (b) darkness and night	Second experiment for this percipient. Symbolical: 1a and 1b.
	2	12:41	(a) Desk pen = (b) food, fun, and goblet	For desk pen, 2a, agent first looked at blunt artist's pen point (goblet), but did not draw – did picture of pointed desk pen. Blunt pen point on first impression condensed with black frying pan, and association of grilling sausages (food) perceived as food, fun, and goblet, 2b.
	3	12:43	(a) Fingers and hand = (b) two packages with ribbon and bow—word "covered" (do not open)	Complementary response between 3a and 3b.
	4	12:44	(a) Sailing ship with wind blowing its flag = (b) racing car moving fast	Movement and drawing of wind, 4a and 4b.
	5	12:46	(a) Electric bulb = (b) numbers 15, 8:30, and 431	Agent thought of special 15 watt bulb needed for hall lamp; possibly the number 15, 5b, was perceived.

TABLE 2-2.   Vollies of Drawings Experiments. (Cont.)

Experiment number	Serial number	Time		Comments*
V	1	1:00	(a) Long doorkey = (b) "sounds very wavy, length, depth, hollow, empty" (to receive key)	Third experiment for this percipient, complementary response; male-female symbolism.
	2	1:01	(a) Glass ash tray = (b) clock	Geometric similarity.
	3	1:03	(a) Claw hammer = (b) keyhole, keys, and question mark	Question mark viewed horizontally similar to claw hammer. Are the keys 3b, a tardy perception of long doorkey, 1a?
VI	1	7:52	(a) Postage stamp with corrugated borders = (b) toothbrush	First experiment for this percipient. Structural similarity between corrugated borders of postage stamp, 1a, and tufts of toothbrush, 1b.
	2	7:53	(a) Silver Chalice with water = (b) large ocean liner on water	Agent's object contains water; percipient's object is contained by water.
	3	7:55	(a) Scotch Tape dispenser = (b) pipe with bubbles	Dispenser, 1a, is fragmentally perceived as complex geometric design (plaid), 3b.

*a = agent
b = percipient.

It is plausible that there was a connection between the picture of Leonardo da Vinci, who was imagined as a mad genius, and the earlier "El Greco's colors," 3, as well as the "picture," 3. A near-direct hit was scored for the fourth time with the associative response of "Leonardo da Vinci book," 4, to the drawing of the mad da Vinci. The rectangular-shaped book somewhat resembles, furthermore, a Talk-A-Phone panel and they both register language.

The agent's wife entered the experiment for the last time with a child's wagon, 1. The diamond ring was perhaps suggested through the agent's unconscious awareness of his wife's unsolicited and unexpected intrusion. If so, the drawing of the agent and the word "psychiatry," 3, were entirely appropriate: participant 3 in linking the agent's wife with her husband, also was signifying his unconscious thinking of her participation in the experiment. Further, perhaps the portrait and association "psychiatry" was a telepathic condensation of the agent's earlier mad da Vinci and participant 4's da Vinci book. The chimney and smoke, *4,* suggest the glitter (dispersions) of the diamond, *2.*

Another near direct hit, this time for all participants, is registered in *2,* the same baby's wagon of the previous intrusion of the agent's wife, in the wagon-shaped dictating equipment with two large symmetrical dials plus the chair with four wheels, and in the toy racing car and association "crying babies." This was an unusual success.

The last notion sent—canoe, fishing rod, fish, and heart, *2,* may be associated with the much earlier cruiser and shark, and the immediate *3* response of "mist and water" plus duplicated fishing rods and reel-like fragment (dials). The big laughing mouth, *4,* is shaped somewhat like the canoe; the percipient said the mouth was all he immediately saw and that the rest of the picture was filled in. The big laughing mouth might also be heard as a hearty laugh.

This interaction illustrates the complexity and the frequently fallacious use of the words "agent" and "percipient." The responses are so enmeshed that the prescribed roles are often reversed without any conscious awareness. The results of the unexpected and well-recorded participation of the agent's wife strengthen the impression that experiments are most successful when done spontaneously and with the use of material presumably chosen naturally. There was hardly any question of tenseness, self-consciousness, or other inhibitive attitudes. The responses came from the first fleeting impression or free association, or from the prevailing mood.

The remaining volleys of drawing experiments are charted in Table 2–2.

The detailed psychodynamics of the participants are unknown. Superficially, they are all healthy and asymptomatic.

PART IV–THE MAJOR PERCIPIENT

The necessity of professional secrecy and the desire to limit self-revelation preclude a detailed analysis of the two persons and their roles in the single-person experiments. Ellen, a young, rather vivacious, impulsive woman, was "interested in the occult," and after the completion of all the drawing experiments she agreed to psychiatric investigation over a period of several sessions. Although she was not a professional medium and had had no personal psychic experiences, Ellen's background may have predisposed her to some of her particular imagerial and associative responses.

Ellen's history included dissociative behavior like syncope, sleepwalking, sleeptalking, daydreaming, and the capacity for going into a deep hypnotic trance. She had intense, hostile, dependent identification with a cold, denying, and competitive mother, which may have been related to her persistent need to please, appease, and coinciliate authoritative figures. At home she was never permitted to show any hostility; her slightest legitimate protest was enough to precipitate the mother's long tirade of obscene language and abuse, alternating with days of sullen silence and refusal to communicate verbally. Besides repressing much of her resentment toward her mother,Ellen introjected all her mother's distorted values, as well as her guilt. She had her mother's many superstititions about menstruation, pregnancy, and the opposite sex. There was seldom any display of affection from the mother. As an example, Ellen never had a birthday party and was not permitted to have friends to her house lest her mother comment "you're nice to everybody except your family."

Ellen was enuretic until puberty and had had incapacitating dysmenorrhea. In addition to these characterological traits she had much psychosexual confusion. The mother encouraged, then angrily broke up, liaisons between her daughter and countless sadistic men. She even condoned a prolonged unnatural relationship with a close male relative, with the ambiguous warning that Ellen should not tell her father. Ellen had a recurrent dream of "snakes all over the floor, crawling over my legs and arms." Her relations with men were also patterned on the sadomasochistic ones she observed at home between her mother, father, and four year older brother. The men were the butts of the mother's sharp tongue and petty tyrannies. They never protested but passively accepted all the effeminating humiliations that were foisted upon them. Despite the contradictions, the marriage and family life were touted by the mother as perfect. Father and brother, together with the daughter, uncritically accepted all the unreal, warped, and many incredible values of the mother. They had blind faith in the mother's omnipotence and omniscience.

Although the father was quiet, ineffectual, and physically seductive with Ellen, he could accept her display of hostility, and when not under the mother's domination he could be capable of warmth and kindness. The older brother who was unreliable and fired from many jobs was showered with the mother's compliments and fine fantasies "for his extraordinarily bright future." At such times the daughter was scolded if she did not echo her mother's spurious praise of the brother and thus demonstrate that she was a "loyal member of such a close family." Ellen hated the favored brother and she had a guilty remorse when she treated him and other men in a cruel fashion and they did not respond by fighting back. At such times she had less pleasure from her sadism and possibly more anxiety from her increased titre of repressed hatred that then threatened to get out of control. The failure of the men to stand up to her and set limits to her hostile acts only increased her inner turmoil and confusion.

It might be conjectured that the percipient was quite suitable for these studies because of an uncritical and infantile belief in the occult. This would not be unlike her unlimited and unrealistic faith in her mother's superstitions and belief in her omnipotence. Many of her telepathic perceptions seem compatible with her unconscious life. Perhaps her intuitive empathy in ferreting out all the subtleties and variations in mood of her unstable, sadistic, and chameleonlike mother—her expertness in perceiving the wishes and values of an authoritative figure—were good practice for attempting experiments of this order. It is plausible also that her telepathic abilities were useful in helping her to conform to the mother's demands and bridging the hiatus of an often grossly impaired communication: a primitive means of adaptation and survival.

The percipient apparently had excellent eidetic ability and it might be supposed that this talent was defensively adapted to her developmental fixations from her early oral-dependent stages. Her tendency to dissociation and her great need to please might have been telepathically extended via vivid visual and associative imagery, as suggested by the experiments reported herein.

Ellen's exhibitionism and hostile seductive life experiences may have been sublimated in the experiments and have afforded her a vicarious gratification. In the close agent-percipient relationships in which the one unconscious communicated with the other there was ample opportunity for subtle interplay of libidinous forces as well as an expression of ambivalence. The permissive nature of the experiments afforded the percipient indulgence of her unsatisfied dependency strivings and the means of winning approval from an authoritative figure without there being any strings attached. She could attempt to seduce, complement, and successfully compete with an authoritative figure without the danger of being squelched as she repeatedly was in her life situation. Thus her intense, unresolved, oedipal problems and sibling rivalry could have found an outlet in the experiments. A suggestive example of the percipient's psychosexual confusion and erotization of the experiments was her reluctance to reverse roles with the agent. The only time she agreed to do so was when she drew a picture of a pistol which was well perceived as an explosion (Figure 2–6: *1a* and *1b*).

During the experiments the percipient seldom saw a connection between any of the matched drawings. In many instances the agent's stimulus was received with compulsive motor actings out besides the more usual employment of visual, auditory, and associative memory channels (Figure 2–2: *4a* and *4b;* Figure 2–9: *1a* and *1b, 3a* and *3b;* Figure 2–11: *5a* and *5b;* Figure 2–17: *1b* and *2a*). The one time that the percipient was consciously uncooperative there was an unconscious reversal of roles and the agent's motor acting out (Figure 2–20: *1b* and *2a, 3b* and *4a*).

Apparently, when a red pencil or an allusion to color was spontaneously used by either the agent or the percipient, the response might have had some hostile or erotic significance. Interestingly enough, whenever red was used it earmarked both of the matched drawings and might even have expedited the transmission (see Figure 2–8: *6a* and *6b;* Figure 2–10: *1a* and *1b, 3a* and *3b, 5a* and *5b, 6a* and *6b;* Figure 2–11: *1a* and *1b, 4a* and *4b, 5a* and *5b;* Figure 2–12: *2a* and *2b;* Figure 2–14: *2b* and *4a*).

Throughout the investigation there was neither striking improvement nor deterioration in the degree of success. Yet when either the agent or the percipient had some anxiety, or the percipient reluctantly participated in the volley-of-drawings experiments, the results did not deteriorate as much as they changed qualitatively. Further, when the percipient no longer acted as percipient, but tended to reverse roles with the agent, the quality of response took on a new, more complex meaning (Figures 2–14 to 2–20). Although there are not enough data for one to formulate a conclusion, they seem to indicate the significance of this percipient's role and her underlying sado-masochism. It should be emphasized that even when there were anxiety and hostility in the relationship the exchange of emotion was still marked.

At no time during the experimentation was the agent or the percipient ever consciously aware of the degree of success or failure in comparison with previous drawings.

PART V–GENERAL DISCUSSION

It is seen that a certain amount of psychodynamic interpretation can be useful in the analysis of telepathic phenomena, and vice versa; although, clearly, an immoderate or otherwise injudicious use of either would endanger further research–if not the participants!

As stated in the beginning of this report, the ordinary scientific methods of investigation were felt to be improper to the phenomena in question. If the customary formal controls had been employed, the subtle emotional factors hypothesized as necessary for the actual telepathic experiments might have been adversely influenced, and thus even the chances of success might have been jeopardized. To paraphrase Jung,[110] a too rigid approach that attempted to fit irrational phenomena into a preconceived pattern might upset Nature's performance by cancelling the necessary emotional values. The many connotations in the drawings and associations are witness to the manifold difficulties in establishing criteria for any quantitative analysis. It might further be supposed that the unusual spatial-temporal dimensions and infinitesimal propensities of the unconscious are of such magnitude that for this type of experiment a simple ordinary quantitative method or system of controls could not be applied without throwing the baby out with the bath water. On the other hand a qualitative inspection of the drawings and associations reveals what may be called successful telepathic transmission, albeit with frequent distortion.

It should be mentioned that there are certain controls afforded by the nature of the experiment itself: the percipient's pictures and associations are entirely analogous to those produced in other studies reported in the literature[12,137,205,229] and again, in many of the instances described, when very similar targets were used at widely varying times, the responses given were also similar to earlier percepts.

Some examples: Figure 2–2: *6a* and *6b*, and Figure 2–3: *2a* and *2b;* Figure 2–2: *5a* and *5b*, and Figure 2–9: *4a* and *4b;* Figure 2–5: *5a* and *5b*, and Figure 2–11: *4a* and *4b;* Figure 2–7: *6a* and *6b*, and Figure 2–11: *3a* and *3b.*

Further controls are afforded by the responses to the spontaneous use of the red pencil and, more particularly, by the many occasions in the volleys of drawings in which either direct or crisscross successes occurred in close order (Figures 2–13 to 20).

The drawing responses become more meaningful when they are considered as part of the total response of the human being. Although the agent selected the object, the part of the object or the derived concept that was transmitted or perceived conformed to the agent's or the percipient's particular unconscious attitudes and values. (Figure 2–1: *6a* and *6b;* Figure 2–5: *1a* and *1b;* Figure 2–9: *3a* and *3b*).

Certain characteristics of many of the percipients' drawings are suggestive of what Meerloo[124] has described as an archaic mode of communication, and what Ehrenwald[39] noted to be characteristic of the drawings of a brain-damaged patient suffering from optical agnosia and apraxia. In some ways the telepathic drawings also structurally resemble drawings of patients with apractognosia due to involvement of the parietotemporoccipital junction of the minor hemisphere.[101] As in the case of images drawn in various aphasic states, the percipient drawings often can be related to the recognition of a figure, its recall, revisualization, and association. However, as in the aphasic state, there is confusion at the most conscious level of comprehension; at this stage the response is usually incomplete and rarely understood. Many of the drawings demonstrate the substitution of simpler, more concrete, automatic and incomplete aphasia-like mechanisms.

Illustrations of some of these infantile modes of communication and related mechanisms are the following:

Symbolization and condensation: Figure 2–1: *5a* and *5b;* Figure 2–2: *1a* and *1b;* Figure 2–3: *5a* and *5b;* Figure 2–8: *3a* and *3b, 6a* and *6b.*

Multiplication, perseveration, and fragmentation: Figure 2–2: *6a* and *6b;* Figure 2–3: *2a* and *2b, 6a* and *6b;* Figure 2–4: *3a* and *3b;* Figure 2–5: *4a* and *4b;* Figure 2–10: *1a* and *1b.*

Eidetic imagery: Figure 2–2: *3a* and *3b;* Figure 2–5: *5a* and *5b,* Figure 2–9: *5a* and *5b;* Figure 2–12: *4a* and *4b, 5a* and *5b, 6a* and *6b;* Figure 2–21: I-E and 2-F, 3F and 4-F.

Visual-auditory synesthesia and use of colloquialisms: Figure 2–4: *1a* and *1b;* Figure 2–5: *1a* and *1b;* Figure 2–11: *1a* and *1b, 2a* and *2b.*

Rotation and right-left mirror reversal: Figure 2–1: *6a* and *6b;* Figure 4: *6a* and *6b;* Figure 8: *4a* and *4b;* Figure 14: *3a* and *3b;* Figure 2–19: *2a* and *2b.*

Possible precognition: Figure 2–13: *2a* and *2b;* Figure 2–15: *2a* and *2b.*

It is of interest that many of the possible telepathic drawings are, on qualitative inspection, strikingly similar to the drawings produced by Fisher's subjects in experiments on visual subliminal stimulation and the Urbantschitsch phenomenon.[58-62] In a later communication Friedman and Fisher[84] mention the similarity between parapsychological findings and their drawings, but after mention of the telepathic hypothesis they offer the opinion that "some of the results claimed for parapsychology may be based, instead, upon subliminal registration." However true this seems, one might wonder about telepathic transmission in their experiments on subliminal stimulation and thus, by inference, the necessity of designing still more subtle emotional controls that would omit the possibility of telepathic or clairvoyant leakage. Little has been said about the possibility of leakage in such experiments, although much has rightly been said about subliminally faint visual and auditory stimulation and its role in explaining alleged instances of telepathy in the psychoanalytic situation. It would seem to be entirely plausible that subliminal stimulation is closely related, too, and leads straight into extrasensory perception. The notes of Fisher and Paul[60] on factors involved in subliminal stimulation are also entirely germane to problems of telepathic communication. Such factors include "the capacity for free fantasy, the nature of the emotional relationship between subject and experimenter, and the unconscious meaning of the particular stimulus as well as the experimental situation to the subject, differences in cognitive organization and style, variations in the defensive and adaptive characteristics of the ego, the state of consciousness, etc."

Many of the drawings carry the concept of movement, action, or change.

Figure 2–1: *2a* and *2b,* and *3b* (the waves), *5a* and *5b;* Figure 2–3: *1a* (growing flowers) and *3a* and *3b* (growth).

The subjective technique of making the mind passive and then seizing on the first impression that arises, may be analogous to an atavistic mode of perceiving change and action—a protective alerting mechanism which we call a hunch or intuition. In many drawings it was frequently the "foreign-body irritation," the trivial thought intruding from the periphery of consciousness, that was successfully transmitted, rather than the more consciously determined thought.

Figure 2–1: *6a* and *6b;* Figure 2–6: *5a* and *5b;* Figure 2–8: *6a* and *6b;* Figure 2–9: *3a* and *3b;* Figure 2–10: *3a* and *3b.*

The telepathic function is probably a useful adaptive mechanism working in concert with the other modalities of perception and having the complementary function of perceiving changes, in the environment and affects of people that are significant to the percipient. There is for example, a mother's intuition about dangers to her children and mention may be made of the infant's manifold nonverbal responses to his mother and his environment.[125] In nature, animals often depend for their life on the ability to sense quickly changes in their environment, even impending earthquakes, through communication channels unknown to Man.[227]

SOME REMARKS ON ARCHAICNEURONAL MECHANISMS

It has been hypothesized that telepathy is dependent on archaic neuronal mechanisms. The hippocampus is a phylogenetically old cortical associational area that correlates olfactory, gustatory, visceral, auditory, visual, somasthetic, and sexual sensation. MacLean[121] has described how this primitive area of early myelination might be implicated in psychosomatic disease and various emotional reactions. It can be speculated that the limbic area also is involved in telepathic transmission and reception. For instance, the heteropsychic telepathic percepts in the hippocampus could be relayed to the occipital lobes where the impression could be clairvoyantly synthesized, and/or to the temporal lobes where it could be clairaudiently perceived, or to other particular nervous pathways for appropriate discharge and synthesis. As an example, relayal to hypothalamic areas could account for various psychophysiological effects. The interpretation of the percept or discharge could depend on the early conditioning experiences. In the experiments reported here the libidinous tinge of many of the drawings, the multiple distortions, and the visual-auditory and seemingly synesthetic responses suggest the reputedly manifold functions of the allocortex, which interprets experience in terms of nonverbal emotional feelings, rather than the neocortex whose functions are cold, logical, abstract cognition. Possibly, the not infrequent rotation or reversal of an image and multiplication of percept can be ascribed to this area and its ancient functions. It may further be remarked upon that earlier in Man's evolution the color red had particular alerting quality for survival, and that before steroscopic vision the eyes functioned separately.

The limbic area has been implicated in the auras and seizure discharges of psychomotor epilepsy.[121] The dejá vu attacks and automatisms are reminiscent of the minus functions[39] of sleep, hypnotic trances, effects of various hallucinogenic drugs,[142] other dissociated states, and the subjective states signified by these telepathic drawing experiments. Because of the experimental design it was not feasible to study any of the responses in these various states with the electroencephologram.* Automatisms can occur with mental diplopia or complete retrograde amnesia concerning the complex behavior exhibited during the seizures. Similarly, a telepathic event often occurs before agent or percipient is aware of what has externally taken place that is related to it, and the sequence of events leading up to the telepathic experience often cannot be remembered. As an analogous example, the countertransference situation in therapy frequently prevents recognition of the occurrence of a telepathic event because of its association with something of unpleasant personal significance to the physician; it is possible that such painful preoccupations continue to reverberate in the unconscious without being relayed to the appropriate cortical areas for synthesis and conscious comprehension.

SUMMARY

A telepathic drawing experiment using one agent and one or more percipients in single agent-percipient drawings and in volleys of two to seven consecutive drawings is described. Attention is given to the prerequisite subjective mental states of the participants and to the experimental design, extrinsic and intrinsic controls, psychodynamics and interpretation of the data. In more than 1200 drawing experiments, varying degrees of success were obtained in a great number of cases. It is postulated that telepathic perception is most commonly an unconscious process and can occur more frequently than has been supposed. The psychological and physiological significance of the reported data is discussed.

---

*In some carefully controlled studies with a few gifted sensitives and a 10-channel Medcraft electroencephalograph there were no significant changes in the recording when the eyes were closed and telepathic events occurred: the tracings are indistinguishable from normal ones.

LEGENDS

Figures   2–1—2–12 Single   agent-percipient   drawing   experiments, a = agent; b = percipient.

Figures   2–13—2–20 Volley of agent-percipient drawings experiments, a = agent; b = percipient.

Figure   2–21 Agent-percipient   transaction,   2 = agent;   3 = percipient; 4 = percipient; I = agent's wife.

3

Telepathic Events in a Child Between 1 and 3-1/2 Years of Age

Although Stekel was the first psychoanalyst to report several telepathic dreams and observe that telepathic events occurred in people bound by strong emotional ties, it was Freud who showed how telepathic events might be more common than usually recognized, if cognizance were taken of the psychodynamic mechanisms.[47] Despite Freud's discoveries that telepathic phenomena might be profitably studied and understood through psychoanalytic techniques, comparatively little experimental work based on psychodynamic principles has been reported. Freud and others hypothesized that telepathic transmission was an age-old means of communication, and that the material produced was of a purposeful, significant nature. However, this clue and the inference that telepathic events might be more readily discerned between young children and their parents received little direct attention until Burlingame's analytic observations of children and their mothers while under treatment,[10] and Ehrenwald's provocative discussions of the possible role of parent-child telepathic communications in the genesis of various behavior disorders.[38] Because of the relative paucity of such reported material, it seemed that there might be some value in studying any further observations regarding telepathic communication between children and their parents in everyday life. If such could be demonstrated, then perhaps intensive psychodynamic study of these early telepathic communications might lead to the uncovering of hitherto unexplored, but nevertheless significant factors in the genesis of various psychopathological states, like, for example, the dissociative experiences of hysteria and schizophrenia.

In an earlier investigation by the author,[174] he reported all the data in a series of over 200 agent-percipient telepathic drawing experiments, in which it seemed that telepathic communication, although at times highly disguised, was not at all infrequent and seemed to follow psychodynamic mechanisms and recognizable patterns of brain function. Furthermore, by using volleys of drawings, the agent-percipient roles were demonstrated to be more complex than their face-value definitions would indicate; and the possible telepathic contagiousness of some events was shown to extend to and act on many people not participating in the experiments and in unanticipated ways. These telepathic events seemed to follow psychodynamic laws that could not be quantitatively analyzed without the difficulties of losing much qualitatively valid data. It was conjectured that quantitative techniques and controls as understood and applied in the more normal type of experiments might, if rigidly employed here, tend to inhibit the telepathic phenomena by dampening interpersonal spontaneity and the subtle propensities of the unconscious mind.

The telepathic drawing experiment studies were undertaken while conducting a prolonged and intensive psychiatric investigation of a 95-year-old telepathist, Jacques Romano, who apparently could exercise a fair degree of control over his abilities.[181] When "reading minds" or doing telepathic phenomena with playing cards, Mr. Romano seemed to be in a trance which placed him in close contact with his own and other people's preconscious and unconscious. During many of these sessions, the author's wife watched Mr. Romano "perform" and she too learned to recognize some of the myriad subtleties of her own often quickly changing emotionally colored thought processes while concomitantly engaging in social intercourse with another person. By recognizing and being able to salvage the fleeting thoughts of her reveries and daydreams, which are repressed almost as quickly as they occur, she discovered how, while in a minor dissociative state, she could comprehend the often rapid unpalatable intrusions and instinctual reflections of herself in relation to another person and his expressed or reflected thought content. It thus became possible to learn how to register mentally many of the quickly occurring, presumably telepathic events that took place between a parent and his child, as contrasted with the usual perceptual-associational-motor (nonverbal) communications between parent and child.[201,202] With the parent's progressive experience in this technique of "mental diplopia," a nucleus of presumably telepathic material could be distinguished from the other more usual, but often no less subtle and devious, parent-child communications.

In addition to the developmental reasons previously mentioned, the child seemed a good subject to study because his vocabulary is limited and this would minimize the verbal distortions that make adult-to-adult transmission much more complex and difficult to analyse. There would also be no motive for unconscious deception. Furthermore, Burlingame's clinical observations and Ehrenwald's brilliant deductions would suggest that any work defining the recognizable frequency, content and significance of telepathic communications between a child and his parents would indicate the importance of such processes in normal development, learning and the psychopathology of health and illness.

The participants in this study include, except where noted to the contrary, the author's wife, Ardis, his daughter, Lisa, his son, Eric, and himself. The following reported, presumed telepathic incidents, occurring within the family circle, and the surrounding explanatory factors, were recorded by Lisa's parents immediately or shortly after their occurrence. The earlier telepathic events in this series often surprised the unsuspecting parents and, unfortunately, in this still exploratory stage, not as much data concerning the parents' reactions were recorded as was the case in the later events. At those times, the events were more frequent and perhaps because of the previous experiences, less startling. Lisa, of course, had become much more verbal as she grew older.

As can be noted, many of the reported events are good examples of presumed telepathy. Other events are suggestive and some very doubtful. However, all the possibly telepathic data were listed since it appeared that telepathy worked in harmony with other bodily processes and by listing all the events, questionable as well as striking, it might become easier to distinguish some fundamental pattern. It was technically feasible to record most of the recognized telepathic events because Lisa was a baby and had almost her only interpersonal contact with her parents. As Lisa progressed in her development and broadened her interpersonal contacts the reporting of all possible telepathic events became virtually impossible and thus the "sample" with the parents became more complex and dilute.

In order to understand better many of the following possible telepathic events, some pertinent developmental data should be mentioned. Ardis' pregnancy and delivery of Lisa were uneventful. Lisa was born November 24, 1956, and, aside from infrequent upper respiratory infections, her development and health have been uneventful. At seven months of age Lisa said "Mama," "Papa" and used some unintelligible jargon. At ten months she said, "Hi" in response to greetings; and at eleven months, "hot" for toast, (hot cookie) radiator, and red Christmas tree lights. Lisa once burned her hand on these lights. At that time she also noted the color "red" in magazine advertisements and red Christmas ribbons. She understood the difference between "dog" and "doll" but occasionally confused the two in her speech. She said "bow-wow" on seeing a toy dog or teddy bear and "quack-quack" on seeing a duck. At one year, she waved "bye-bye" under appropriate conditions, and also screamed when she was inadvertently put to bed without her rag doll. At one year and three weeks of age, while looking at a Christmas tree she reacted with awe and said "ah, ah." She would turn her head toward the Christmas cards on the fireplace mantle and say "See!" Another common phrase at this time was "pretty bracelet." Since these early beginnings her use of language has become progressively more complex.

Lisa might have had nightmares at eight months of age when teething. She would fall asleep for an hour, then wake up screaming. When she became oriented and saw that she was all right, she would be put back to bed and sleep without interruption. However, she did not give any verbal account at this time.

At one year five weeks of age, she had a nightmare and awoke in a trance-like state, screaming and shouting, "See! See dog!" She had been thrashing about and crying in her sleep, with her eyes closed. She held her upper extremities and fists in a hyperflexed position and appeared to be frightened. She continued to scream until awakened, then when her eyes were opened, and she was correctly oriented and comforted by her parents, tranquillity was restored. Lisa then said in response to her parents' affectionate tone of voice and caresses: "The dog is gone, bad dream, mommy and daddy are here, Lisa will be all right." [Although the author could not find in the literature dreams (verbally described) of a child as young as one year five weeks of age, it is noted that Grotjahn's psychodynamic comments on verbally reported dreams of babies were entirely applicable to this case (see Grotjahn, M.: Dream Observations In a Two-Year-Four-Months Old Baby, *Psychoanalytic Quarterly*, 7:507–513, 1938).]

Between 15 and 16 months of age, shortly after her brother Eric's birth and arrival home, Lisa had recurrent nightmares and would wake up screaming, "Baby, baby!" It was difficult to awaken her from these dreams and console her. At other times she would look inside the baby carriage, pull the covers back and shriek. Only when she was shown the baby and could see that he was all right did she immediately cease. However, her sibling rivalry and ambivalance towards her brother have been diminishingly manifested, to this day, by her occasional alternate patting and striking Eric. All other developmental factors including standing, walking, bladder and bowel training were uneventful. Lisa has no neurotic character traits.

The following is a listing of presumed telepathic events:

1. *September 13, 1958, Saturday.* While reading a new text book, I slowly drifted away mentally and thought of telephoning my friend, Floyd, and asking him if he would care to go to Luigi's Restaurant. As I silently hesitated between either reading and satisfying my intellectual appetite or gratifying my gastronomic desires by picking up the telephone and making the

necessary arrangements, Lisa interjected, "Telephone." I was far from a telephone. By her remark, Lisa catalyzed her father's basic need.

2. *October 12, 1958, Sunday.* I was talking to Ardis about buying some small plastic containers in which she could put leftover foods. Although I did not say so, I considered that the rather large containers we owned were a useful size only for the dessert, Jello. At the very second when this silent thought occurred to me, Lisa screamed "Jello, Jello!" This dessert is one of her favorites. Although she might have said this by associational processes it was an unusual response for Lisa at this age.

3. *October 20, 1958, Monday 5:00 P.M.* I walked into the kitchen feeling quite exhuberant and thought I would clown by showing Lisa a Nijinsky-like kick. However, before I could demonstrate she started to kick and do a little dance. She had never done this before. In this way, perhaps, she acted out, in motor fashion, my happy behavior that was about to emerge from its silent incubation.

4. *December 27, 1958, Saturday, 12:05 P.M.* Ardis was perplexed since our regular baby sitter was caring for her incapacitated husband, and, because of the holiday season, it was difficult to obtain a substitute baby sitter for just one night. In the past Ardis had heard the name of a woman which at this moment she was silently recalling to memory before making her telephone call. At this exact time Lisa started saying, "Mrs. Axwell, Mrs. Axwell," the name of the baby sitter. Lisa had never met this sitter, and, if her name had ever been mentioned in Lisa's presence, it must have been many months previously.

5. *December 29, 1958, Monday, 4:36 P.M.* Having used all our available liquor entertaining, Ardis was, perhaps half ruefully, thinking to herself, "Well, we will not have any more liquor with dinner." Simultaneously with this thought, Lisa started shouting, "Give me a drink of ginger ale!" Ardis almost invariably drinks ginger ale and bourbon, and at such infrequent times Lisa is given a small glass of ginger ale.

6. *January 21, 1959, Wednesday.* While playing, Lisa, out of context, said "Eric" (her brother) and "Kugel" (baby sitter) as I thought of them. There had been no previous conversation about these people.

7. *February 27, 1959, Friday, 8:30 P.M.* Ardis was in her bedroom speaking to her mother-in-law on the telephone. Lisa was in her crib in her room and the two heavy doors which separate it from Ardis' room were closed. When Ardis finished her conversation she went into Lisa's room and Lisa said, "You were talking to grandma; she's sick in bed." This was correct. Although it is conceivable that Lisa could have overheard the conversation, it should be stated that Ardis has a very soft, quiet voice, and under simulated controlled conditions it was hard to hear her voice, and impossible to under-

stand what she said on the telephone in her room from the place where Lisa's crib stood. Lisa is very attached to her grandmother.

8. *February 28, 1959, Saturday.* Ardis is thinking of cake, and Lisa shouts, "Cake." There was nothing, to my knowledge, immediately available that might have tended to provoke such a thought in Lisa's mind.

9. *March 13, 1959, Friday.* Last night I had a nightmare during which I saw a lion climb up the wall of a room and cross the attic rafters. I was trapped on the beams and defended myself by slamming a hammer down on the lion's toes. At the exact moment when I woke up, Lisa also awoke explosively, screaming and vomiting. She had no recognizable illness at the time and had had no apparent nightmares for many weeks. We went back to sleep. Shortly before I awoke a second time, at 6:40 A.M., the hypnopompic vision of the lion reappeared, and Lisa again woke up screaming. Usually Lisa would sleep through in an undisturbed state and awake at 8:00 A.M. Although Lisa gave no verbal hints about the content of her dream, it is of interest that I do not recall dreaming of a lion or other animal since my personal psychoanalysis several years ago. It may be conjectured that Lisa had a terrifying dream about an animal which I received and which awoke me twice, simultaneously with her. Lisa's Oedipal dream might have coincided with incompletely resolved problems of a similar nature in myself.

10. *March 19, 1959, Thursday, 6:00 P.M.* Lisa has been fussing and screaming for a long time. Ardis is sick in bed with the grippe. It was my unexpressed wish that Lisa go to bed much earlier than her usual time (7:30–8:00 P.M.) and without the long harangue this earlier bedtime might precipitate. At the exact moment of my thought and wish, she looked up at me and said, "Lisa very tired, wants to go to bed."

11. *March 28, 1959, Saturday.* Ardis thought, "I must have my hair fixed." Lisa blurted out these exact words in reference to herself immediately after Ardis' thought.

12. *April 12, 1959, Sunday, 1:00 A.M.* Possibly in anticipation of my approaching field trip to study ordeals by serpents, fire and strychnine, I had a dream about a great many rattlesnakes. At a particularly vivid point in the dream, Lisa woke up screaming.

13. *April 21, 1959, Tuesday.* Ardis was thinking, "Why was the white apron hung in the back vestibule?" Lisa said these words. At that particular time Ardis was in the kitchen and occupied with other matters. The apron had been hanging in the vestibule all day and no one commented until Ardis thought of it and Lisa commented.

14. *May 5, 1959, Tuesday.* Ardis thought of Mrs. Long and Lisa simultaneously said, "Mrs. Long." This woman who had been my secretary was in frequent contact with Ardis.

15. *June 13, 1959, Saturday, 12:30 P.M.* I was sitting at the kitchen table

reading a magazine article, and there was a photograph of Senator Clinton
B. Anderson and Chairman Lewis Strauss. The photograph was smudged,
and it appeared that Strauss had a moustache. I was looking at it and trying
to decide whether Mr. Strauss did or did not have a moustache. Lisa, who
was sitting at the opposite end of the table and who had no idea of what I
was looking at, suddenly laughed and called, "Moustache, Daddy! Moustache!" I have a moustache.

16. *June 14, 1959, Sunday, 12:30 P.M.* I took a can of tomato juice and
was reading the advertisement on the label for buying some beautifully
initialed drinking glasses. In my boredom and perhaps passive state, I casually imagined how monogrammed glasses would look. Lisa, who was sitting
in the high chair at the opposite corner of the room, and could not see this,
suddenly said, "New glasses, new glasses." Ardis, who was also close by
wondered about the commotion and I turned the can to show her the particular advertisement.

17. *June 23, 1959, Thursday.* Lisa's grandmother who usually telephones
before driving over to visit, happened to come to the house as a surprise.
Lisa greeted her and said, "Grandma is going to take Lisa shopping to buy a
new raincoat for Lisa." Grandmother was quite taken aback, because no one
else knew of this, Ardis was not at home, and this was the specific purpose of
Grandmother's surprise visit. Grandmother wondered how Lisa could have
guessed the secret and then remembered having once remarked that she
would buy Lisa a raincoat.

18. *July 1, 1959, Wednesday.* I was reading some particularly fine print in
a newspaper column on the Rockefeller family and their oil investments. At
this juncture, Lisa shouted, "Oil!" She had not said this word for many,
many days. However, she had formerly been aware of my previous interest
in and minor explorations for oil, and she now was very alert, attentive and
in a state of rapport with me.

19. *July 6, 1959, Monday.* It was a clear day and Ardis was riding in the
car with Lisa. While driving, Ardis was pondering whether to accept Floyd's
dinner invitation. She equivocated because of some pressing work that I had
and my reluctance to go out socially at such times. While she was thinking
about this, Lisa said, "It's raining on Uncle Floyd's house now!" Lisa correctly named Floyd and by mentioning the unpleasant connotation of "raining," she might have echoed my negative sentiments about dining out.

20. *July 8, 1959, Wednesday, 9:00 A.M.* While taking Lisa downstairs by
the hand I was thinking of "radiating" the hybrid corn. This was part of a
control in some experiments undertaken at that time. Simultaneously with
this thought, Lisa said, "Radiation, radiation." Although she had seen this
done in the past she did not understand the meaning of this word, and, aside

from my silent thought, there was no discernible reason why she should have said this.

21. *July 19, 1959, Sunday.* I drove the car with Lisa to the outdoor vegetable market. She had not been there in almost a year. While I was pulling up to the curb, she suddenly blurted out "Pumpkin." On leaving, I thought to myself, "A marvelous memory that she can say 'pumpkin' when it was many months ago, when she was so tiny, that the clerk gave her a pumpkin." While these thoughts quickly flashed through my mind, and this was more than 15 minutes since arriving at the market, Lisa again shouted, "Pumpkin, pumpkin." This might be an example of how a fleeting thought that darts through the mind might be facilitated in its telepathic transmission by the concept of arriving or leaving, the element of change or separation between people, or people and an object; or the change in anxiety threshold that one experiences in adapting or changing in his dependency states. Such is the time that a decision must be made or an affect reaction is crystallized in reference to another person or object of symbolic significance. Could this forceful reaction have accounted for Lisa's correct remembering or guessing?

22. *July 21, 1959, Tuesday, 6:00 P.M.* It was after dinner and I was taking a walk in the backyard with Lisa. While going down the hill and holding on to her hand, I noticed a few stray leaves on the ground from the pear and apple trees. The thought crossed my mind: "I wonder if the pear tree will die with these leaves coming down?" Lisa then verbally repeated the same words. When I asked her why she thought that she said, "Mommy said so." I later checked with Ardis, who said she has never commented on the pear or any other trees to Lisa. During this walk Lisa was very affectionate.

23. *July 23, 1959, Thursday, 5:45 P.M.* Ardis' eye fleetingly caught sight of a piece of chocolate frosting adhering to a bakery cake box. It was her intention to clean the box off in order to make it more presentable. This particular box was hidden behind many pots and pans and completely out of view from Lisa, who had just come into the room. Before Ardis could clean the box, Lisa, while looking out the window, on the opposite side of the room, at Dr. L's house, suddenly said, "Annie has chocolate outfit!" Annie, Dr. L's daughter, who is one year older than Lisa, was nowhere in sight. However, Lisa is fond of chocolate. Ardis is reluctant to give her chocolate and ruin her appetite for other foods. By her condensation Lisa gave the valued chocolate (outfit) to her rival, Annie.

24. *July 24, 1959, Friday, 12:33 P.M.* During this luncheon hour Ardis was thinking of having the car washed. In her complex flash-imagery, she recalled how the men wear boots and raincoats at the car wash. At the juncture of these fleeting associations of Ardis, Lisa said, "Dr. L. has raincoat and boots on." Dr. L., our friend, was not in view, and it was a clear day. Ardis had not mentioned the possibility of having the car washed. It is of

interest that Lisa would possibly condense the thoughts of raincoat and boots with Dr. L. who has frequently been ribbed about his prolonged daily ritual of washing himself.

25. *July 25, 1959, Saturday, 12:05 P.M.* Ardis was at the kitchen table looking at a catalogue and thinking about what present she might get me for my birthday. At this exact point in her thinking, Lisa said, "24th of November, (Lisa's birthday)." There had been no immediate or recent conversation about birthdays, and my birthday was still several months away.

26. *July 29, 1959, Wednesday, 3:30 P.M.* While driving in the car with Lisa, Ardis was thinking again about Floyd's party and her reluctance to make a decision about going or not. At Ardis' ruminative moment Lisa, simultaneously again, repeated her earlier statement, "It's raining on Uncle Floyd's house." Lisa echoed her father's obstructive sentiments as far as Ardis might have been concerned. By so doing Lisa might also have expressed her desire for her parents not to leave her in the care of a baby sitter.

27. *July 29, 1959, Wednesday, 8:30 P.M.* Lisa had awakened and asked for assistance so that she could go to the bathroom. Ardis went into Lisa's room to help. At that point and between tasks I relaxed for a moment on Lisa's tiny yellow chair, rather than on a more suitable chair for an adult. The chair was completely out of view from Lisa and in the other room. While with Lisa, Ardis quickly thought, "I wonder what he's sitting on." At the time of this thought, Lisa said from the bathroom. "I want the yellow chair, I want the yellow chair." Perhaps Lisa felt threatened by her father's sitting on her favorite (and for her father, fragile) chair.

28. *August 4, 1959, Tuesday, 7:30 P.M.* Dr. Brown was phoning for a consultation and I was using the bedroom telephone. It was quite frustrating because the appointment book was not immediately available. Dr. Brown did not know of my predicament and these thoughts seethed solely within myself. At this juncture Lisa got out of bed, opened up both doors between our rooms, rushed to me and handed me her booklet entitled "Count The Baby Animals." Perhaps she acted out in motor fashion and attempted to ameliorate my frustration by perceiving the crude contents of my predicament and trying to remedy it in her own way, and at her own level. She chose a book by title and content more appropriate for my needs in recording data, like the day and time of an appointment, than had she chosen a book of more interest to herself like her other books on nursery rhymes, the gingerbread man, and so forth.

29. *August 7, 1959, Friday, 9:15 A.M.* Ardis, while cleaning the kitchen, was thinking of a dark blue Lincoln automobile. At this point Lisa said, "Mommy's car is black!" In point of fact, Ardis' car is blue. Ardis was pondering about automobiles since she thought the time might be propitious to turn in our old Ford and buy a new one. However, she repressed much of

this thinking. Perhaps Lisa, like her mother, was of the opinion that an automobile's color was of paramount importance. Possibly Lisa chose somber black as a symbol of her mother's dim prospect of getting a new car.

30. *August 9, 1959, Sunday, 9:15 A.M.* Ardis, while dressing Lisa, started to think of Irene Swenson, who is often at the house as a baby sitter. At that exact point, Lisa said, "(Mrs.) Swenson (Irene's mother) is coming tomorrow." Lisa is very attached to Mrs. Swenson and has many pleasant times with her.

31. *August 9, 1959, Sunday, 11:15 A.M.* Ardis was thinking of our friend, Les, and wondering if he would be over to visit in the afternoon. While wondering about this, she showed Eric a picture "that looks like Daddy." She frequently shows Eric pictures or gives him toys while she feeds him. While Ardis was showing Eric the picture, Lisa came from another part of the kitchen to Eric's high chair and said, "Maybe it looks like Uncle Les." Lisa has positive feelings for Les. There had been no recent previous mention of Les.

32. *August 11, 1959, Tuesday, 10:30 P.M.* Just before retiring I commented to Ardis, "Isn't Lisa dry through the night now?" Ardis answered, "No, every night I must change the diapers." I commiserated with Ardis whose household chores were endless and hoped that Lisa could soon be bladder trained for nighttime because this would make Ardis' tasks much lighter. The night of this sympathetic thought was the first time that Lisa was ever completely dry.

33. *August 14, 1959, Friday, 12:35 P.M.* While doing her household chores, Ardis looked out a highly situated window, beyond Lisa's view, and noticed a yellow car driving by. Ardis associated it with my father's yellow car. At this point Lisa said, "Mommy is not going to get a new car, just (the old one) painted." Apparently, a new car had much meaning for Ardis since it was a symbol of an improvement in conditions. Furthermore, she secretly awaited the day that she would have a car of her own and there would be no further conflict of two people needing the same car simultaneously. Possibly Lisa perceived Ardis' concealed despair about not having had a new car, as well as her happiness when able to borrow my father's yellow car. Lisa, by stating that the old car would be painted, might have perceived Ardis' reflection on the color with all its associational significance.

34. *August 23, 1959, Sunday, 10:30 A.M.* Ardis was thinking to herself, "Too bad Irene is at the seashore." Irene is a baby sitter and is most skilled in caring for Lisa. At the time this thought passed through Ardis' mind, Lisa was drawing on the blackboard. Ardis walked up to her and Lisa said, "Irene." As an associational catalyst it should be stated that Irene, as well as several other people, had spent time in the past drawing pictures at the blackboard; however, Lisa had not, either to Ardis' or my recollection, said

"Irene" at any previous time when she was drawing on the blackboard. Thus, the simultaneity of Ardis' unspoken thought and Lisa's verbalization, "Irene," would still have to be accounted for. The anticipated associations of the child might coincide quite closely with his parents'. Perhaps the telepathic event is frequently intermingled with this more readily recognizable associational response of a child who is identifying with his parents.

35. *August 23, 1959, Sunday, 4:30 P.M.* I was reading *Nothing So Strange,* an autobiography by the medium Arthur Ford (New York, 1958). When I am reading some journal or book, Lisa seldom comments. She had also failed to comment when I took her to the Medical or Public Library on previous occasions. Nevertheless, at this point she came up to me and said, "Miss Tubby's book." It was immediately after I had been reading about Miss Tubby in this book. Although Lisa had once, long ago, met Miss Tubby and seen her personal library, she was not aware of the nature of Miss Tubby's lifelong psychic researches, not more particularly of her friendship with Arthur Ford, or of my studies on telepathy.

36. *August 29, 1959, Saturday, 10:20 A.M.* While holding Eric on her lap Ardis thought she would turn his window air conditioner off because his room was getting too cold. While she was trying to make up her mind about doing this, Lisa entered the room and said, "Lisa is going to turn off the air conditioner; it's cool in Eric's room." Although it was cool in Eric's room, it was no cooler than usual, and Lisa had not said this before. Perhaps this event also illustrates the imperceptible merging of the usual means of communication and suggestion, with possible telepathic modalities.

37. *August 31, 1959, Monday, 5:45 P.M.* While standing in the kitchen near Lisa, Ardis was thinking of her expanding waistline. It was dinner hour and I was sitting at the table listening to the radio. At that point, Ardis had been pondering about how she could eat and gratify her appetite and still curtail excesses. Lisa asked me, "Daddy, do you want a cookie?" This might be interpreted as, "Daddy will you give me a cookie?" or telepathically extended via an identification with Ardis' unspoken wish for a cookie: "Will you please give me a cookie?—but you shouldn't—I'll gain too much weight." Lisa then crystallized the entire situation by saying: "Mommy can't have any (cookie); she is too fat!" Lisa echoed Ardis' ambivalence about eating and possibly censured her mother's oral desires with a revealing early oedipal quip.

38. *August 31, 1959, Monday, 7:00 P.M.* I had just finished speaking to my friend J. R. on the telephone, and Lisa was with me. Although Lisa had not spoken into the dictating machine in many weeks, the thought passed through my mind that it might be fun to have her try it at this particular time. However, this thought was negated by the equally valid feeling that, in the past, when I turned the dictating machine on and adjusted the record for

Lisa, she refused to speak. Therefore, I concluded it was best to remain silent. As soon as this matter was secretly settled, to my apparent satisfaction, Lisa blurted out "Lisa wants to talk on that thing (touching the dictating machine)."

39. *September 1, 1959, Tuesday, 4:20 P.M.* Ardis was with Lisa visiting a lady friend who was president of one of the women's clubs. While there, Ardis wondered whether this particular woman might be pregnant, since it appeared that she had gained some weight since Ardis last saw her. However, she was, by most standards, still slender, and Lisa who had seen many overweight women without commenting in the past, had never before met this particular one. While Ardis was silently dwelling on this subject that might also be a projection of her own conflicts in this area, Lisa was attempting to button a raincoat over her waistline. Although the raincoat did fit Lisa quite properly she said in a disgusted tone, "Too fat; too fat!" Lisa uttered this in reference to herself, but she also verbalized Ardis' overdetermined concern. If the woman was pregnant, she would have to resign as president, and Ardis as a member of the club nominating committee would be in a predicament, since a replacement was hard to obtain. Lisa might also have tapped a forbidden thought Ardis unconsciously harbored towards this other woman (the envy of pregnancy) as well as Ardis' concern about her own body image and my teasing her about doing "therapeutic exercises."

40. *September 4, 1959, Friday, 1:07 P.M.* Having finished with lunch, Ardis was thinking, "I wonder whether we should have corn muffins (tonight)." At that juncture, Lisa asked her mother, "Do you know where the 'Muffin Man' lives?" Lisa and Ardis, in the past, have sung the nursery rhyme "Muffin Man." At this time Lisa's appetite was gratified, and she was in a playful, friendly mood.

41. *September 10, 1959, Thursday, 10:00 A.M.* Ardis was wearing her opaque blue and white cotton bathrobe. She put her hand into her pocket and was wondering what she had in her pocket, when Lisa said, "I want that bandage." Ardis removed from her pocket what felt like a piece of scrap paper and then found out that it was a band-aid. Ardis' bathrobe is hung in her closed closet far beyond the reach of Lisa, and because of the hot weather she has worn it very infrequently, if at all. However, several weeks ago Ardis applied a band-aid to a particularly disfiguring furuncle on her face. She was very self-conscious about this disfigurement and has had poor results with the different treatments prescribed for her. Six weeks previously, when Ardis wore the band-aid on her face, Lisa (in her identification) insisted on wearing a band-aid also. Although the element of Lisa remembering that the band-aid was in the bathrobe pocket cannot be ruled out, it should be mentioned that Lisa, by mentioning the band-aid, was again touching upon a sensitive subject in her mother's life. At this stage, Lisa is very rebellious and

negativistic in her interpersonal relationships. Also Ardis is 5 feet 9 inches tall and Lisa is 3 feet 3 inches. Even if Lisa had access to Ardis' bathrobe, which she did not, it would be hard for her to reach high enough to put her hand into the pocket. Finally, Lisa does not in the normal course of domestic events have any cause to go into Ardis' closet.

42. *September 26, Saturday, 9:00 A.M.* While walking by the kitchen "intercom," it crossed my mind that an aromatic, hot cup of fresh coffee would be just right for the moment. However, this thought was squelched by the knowledge that the coffee that remained in the Chemex coffee maker would be quite tasteless, if not abominable, if heated up again. Moreover, it would take more time than was available to brew a fresh supply of coffee. However, this fleeting complex of thoughts was interrupted by my eye catching a jug of cider. It was particularly appealing, since the cider was cool and unusually appetizing with the moisture precipitating on the outside of the jug. However, I half suppressed this desire and vacillated with the previous thought of coffee. I then walked around the corner of the room and saw Lisa at the kitchen table. Prior to this, she should neither see me, the coffee, nor the cider from her particular position. Nevertheless, she gushed out almost simultaneously with my thought, "The cider smells very good." Lisa, like myself, was wide awake, enthusiastic, and in a state of well-being.

43. *September 27, 1959, Sunday, 3:20 P.M.* Ardis came downstairs with Lisa and Eric. Lisa sat on my lap, and I asked her what was going to happen that afternoon. She blurted out, without any apparent conviction or thought of what she was saying that "*Mrs.* Tubby is coming over." Although *Miss* Tubby was not coming over and has only been here on two previous occasions, Les, whom I met through Miss Tubby and who is one of her best friends, was coming over. These two people are associated intimately together in my mind. It is of interest that Lisa, who has never seen them together, nor apparently heard them discussed at the same time, also associated them together and possibly hinted at this merging by saying "Mrs." instead of "Miss."

44. *September 28, 1959, Monday, 4:30 P.M.* Lisa was having her supper and looking down at her plate. My mind associated to my secretary, Chabela, who was typing up the telepathic experiences with Lisa, and then I reflected on Lisa's pretty purple dress. It seemed particularly compatible with her red hair. The third association was directed toward the bowl of purple mums, and I thought, "Pretty, like those flowers . . . I wonder if Lisa will get this thought." Lisa, at that exact moment looked up and said, "I coughed on the basin (of flowers)." This was not so. Perhaps she said this as a symbolic expression of the intense sibling rivalry she then felt for her brother Eric, who was being fed by his mother. In order to accurately record this incident I rushed to my desk and put down the pertinent quotations. Although it was

still light outside, the paper I wrote on was not too well illuminated and caused equivocation as to whether to turn the lights on or continue writing under the existing conditions. As this flashed through my mind, Lisa entered the room and said, for the first time, "It is too dark in here!" Perhaps she perceived my irritation and attempted to remedy it.

45. *September 30, 1959, Wednesday, 11:45 A.M.* While sitting at the table, Ardis thought, "It's an awful inconvenience not having the dishwasher (which has been broken now for several days)." At that exact point Lisa got up from the table, went over to the dishwasher, pointed to it and said: "The Public Service man is going to fix the washer." Lisa was in positive rapport. Perhaps she clearly perceived her mother's predicament and wish.

46. *October 8, 1959, Thursday, 4:50 P.M.* While reading a magazine article about the new Premier of China, I noted that he had had four wives: One committed suicide, two were divorced, and the fourth was a pretty, young co-ed. As I looked at the fourth wife's picture, the thought occurred: "Ha, how ludicrous! Rascals! And they have mechanical minds!" (that a Communist who has women doing the heavy work of men should be interested in such a non-Marxist apostasy as beauty and fashion!). Lisa who was eating in another part of the room and could not see what I was reading, said, "That's funny Daddy, very funny." I asked her "What is funny?" And she said, "the radio (radiator)" and pointed to it. However, she did not explain in what way, nor how the radio (radiator) tied in. In this event she was unable to see me, and I had not laughed nor made any noise. Was her shouting of "radio" a tracer word indicating the telepathic event? Not quite comprehending the meaning of radio Lisa pointed to the phonetically similar radiator. The occurrence of tracer words that are associated with telepathic events frequently occur in therapy between the physician and the patient. Such commonly used tracer words implying a strong communication are: radio, electricity, superstition, television, telephone. Perhaps these words tag that part of the telepathic event which is in the preconscious and which with experience can be consciously recognized.

47. *October 10, 1959, Saturday, 7:15 P.M.* Lisa said, "I'm going to have coffee with Chabela." This was uttered at the exact time Ardis thought of having coffee. Lisa had never had coffee or any other beverage with Chabela, and this was strange, because Ardis thought of this on a day that Chabela did not work and it was also nighttime. Chabela's name might have been transmitted because I had thought about how Chabela was feeling in relation to her mother-in-law who was then acutely ill. Lisa might have condensed her mother's desire for coffee with her father's concern for Chabela.

48. *October 11, 1959, Sunday, 8:20 A.M.* Lisa was playing on the floor, and I asked her, "Do you know what? I have a surprise." Lisa answered, "I know, the pumpkin!" Lisa correctly guessed, to her father's dismay, that she

would receive a pumpkin. There was no previous mention of the pumpkin, and great measures had been taken to conceal this from her so she would be surprised.

49. *October 17, 1959, Saturday, 4:30 P.M.* Ardis was getting dressed for a wedding. It was a clear, bright, Fall day. She was wondering if it would be dark enough for a candlelight service. Lisa was sitting on the bed in the dressing room that is surrounded with eight windows, and as the thought flashed through Ardis' mind, Lisa said, "It is a little bit dark in that corner, I am going to put the light on." Lisa was in a friendly mood and quite excited about the wedding, because she had just been looking at pictures of her parents' wedding.

50. *October 18, Sunday, 1:05 P.M.* I was talking with Ardis about how some of our own card experiments had successfully duplicated the telepathic feats performed by Jacques Romano. While discussing this, the thought passed through my mind that "If our friend Les comes, Floyd (who was coming) would have to take a hint and leave so that we could get down to business with Les." At that exact moment Lisa said, "Uncle Floyd is not home, he is on an aeroplane going to Kentucky." Lisa correctly ascertained the fact that I was thinking of Floyd, and she condensed this with the "plane going to Kentucky" thought which correctly conformed to Les. Les has taken many plane trips to Kentucky. However, Lisa also rendered the useful and imaginative service of sending Floyd far away.

51. *October 18, 1959, Sunday, 5:15 P.M.* While walking downstairs from the third floor with Lisa, and holding on to her hand, I was afraid of hurting her arm because yesterday I played a game of "Tick-Tock" wherein I grasped her hands and gently swung her like a pendulum and hurt her. Although there was no strain to her arm as I held her hand, and she had not complained of pain, at the exact moment these thoughts flashed through my mind, she said, "Now let's look in Eric's closet (for the table we were searching for) and don't tick-tock Lisa any more!" She thus detected the painful experience for both herself and her father. Lisa was clear, bright and in a cheerful mood.

52. *October 18, 1959, Sunday, 8:05 P.M.* Lisa was drawing at the blackboard and Ardis wondered if Lisa was now of an age suitable for Nursery School. Lisa looked up at her at that exact instant and said, "Look what Lisa draws at school." Lisa had not previously associated school and the blackboard together.

53. *October 28, 1959, Wednesday, 12:00 P.M.* Lisa asked for a cookie and her mother told her that she could have one and that they would do something special in the afternoon if she was a good girl. Lisa then said, "I help make snowman." It was at the exact moment that Ardis thought of making a plastic snowman with Lisa. Three weeks previously Ardis received some

plastic foam decorations for making Christmas ornaments for the Women's Club. Lisa had not seen them since then, and it had never been mentioned to her in the past. This is perhaps another example of Lisa's correctly "guessing" her surprise.

54. *October 31, 1959, Saturday, 4:00 P.M.* While reading a magazine article my mind tripped on the last words of J. P. Morgan, who died in 1913, "I must go up the hill." I wondered what this enigmatic statement meant to a man who had so influenced the growth of our country. While I was pondering his last words, Lisa, who was playing at my side with pretzels on the lid of a can, said, "Go up the hill; go up the hill." When asked why she said this, Lisa remained quiet and looked straight ahead. Of course, Lisa is unable to read or write, and she had not uttered these exact words in the past. In her game and words Lisa faithfully acted out her father's perplexed absorption in a magazine article.

55. *November 1, 1959, Sunday, 3:45 P.M.* Coming upstairs from the basement, Ardis thought that she would telephone grandmother and thank her for taking care of Lisa. She was quite startled when she opened the cellar door and found Lisa pretending to talk to Grandma on the telephone in the hallway. Ardis did not tell Lisa or anyone of her intentions, yet Lisa correctly acted out the time, means and person of her mother's intended communication.

56. *November 1, 1959, Sunday, 7:20 P.M.* Ardis was looking at my appointment book for the coming month and her eye fell on November 24. She thought of writing "Lisa's birthday" at the appropriate line and Lisa said, "Draw a birthday cake!" Lisa was in a friendly mood. Although she might have associated the appointment book with her embryonic concept of time, and that in turn with her birthday, it should be pointed out that on many previous occasions when either her mother or father examined the appointment book and did not specifically think of Lisa's birthday, Lisa never commented. This might be another illustration of how telepathic communication is an extension or integral part of the usual means of thinking and perception. It would appear that telepathic reactions can work as harmoniously with the other sense organs and reflexes as they (viz. eyes and ears) work together.

57. *November 7, 1959, Saturday, 9:00 A.M.* Last night I had a dream of someone suddenly dying. I woke from the dream but was not frightened or upset in any way. The dream had the peculiar quality of not really belonging to me. It had such a different affect reaction for me that I gently woke Ardis and said with assurance that Lisa would awaken in a matter of seconds. Although Lisa's and our rooms were widely separated and the three doors were closed, this event occurred. Next morning when I asked Lisa what she had dreamed the night before, I thought to myself, "Isn't it wonderful that Lisa

has always been so verbal. And Eric, who has shown greater dexterity in mechanical skill than Lisa, is not by comparison as proficient in speech." Although Lisa could not remember what she dreamed, she picked up her father's peripheral thought and said, "Lisa can talk; I can speak!" Like previous, similar dream experiences (9, 12) it is impossible to state that there was no increased psychomotor activity which might have been subliminally perceived and reacted to. In the morning Lisa gave an answer that reflected her father's thought as well as expressing her own sibling rivalry.

58. *November 13, 1959, Friday, 6:00 P.M.* Lisa was playing with a cardboard paper towel cylinder, and while Ardis had her back to Lisa and was playing with Eric, she mused "Who could I invite to Lisa's birthday party?" Simultaneously with this thought Lisa placed the cylinder on top of her father's head and said to him, "Look at the birthday hat." As in previous examples (25, 56), Lisa was attuned to this significant affect-thought complex so that when her mother thought of Lisa in this respect it was quickly detected and emotionally exploited.

59. *December 12, 1959, Saturday, 8:30 A.M.* While in the kitchen Ardis is thinking of having her hair done "as it looks so awful." Lisa, who was playing on the floor with a Santa Claus, looked up and said, "I'm coming home from the hairdresser!" Lisa was in a friendly mood.

60. *December 22, 1959, Tuesday, 8:10 P.M.* Ardis asked me about wrapping our neighbor-children's Christmas presents. I offered the gratuitous comment that we had had no telepathic experience recently with Lisa. At that point Lisa started discussing a truck "with little cars in a garage" and then she immediately started talking about putting her cereal "in an oven, a stove." She said the pretended oven was broken and that Mr. Nelson, the handyman, would fix it. This was quite surprising to Lisa's parents because the present that was bought for the neighbor-boy, Paul, was a toy transport truck with little cars on it. Lisa's Christmas present was to be a toy stove. All these toys were put in separate cardboard boxes and then in a larger box taller than Lisa. All the boxes were locked in a closet of the examining room. Lisa had not seen the box or boxes nor had any inkling of our most closely guarded secret: what her own and the other Christmas presents would be. Yet, she had done such a good job of correctly guessing what the neighbor boy and she herself were getting that we quickly rushed to the room to make sure that in some way she had not gotten in or found out. However, everything was securely wrapped in the big box as originally put there.

61. *December 24, 1959, Thursday, 3:00 P.M.* Ardis said, "Lisa and I were resting. Lisa was holding a Santa Claus figure and having it pretend to ask her what she wanted for Christmas. She was more or less chattering to herself. I was trying to sleep and thinking about how Lisa and Eric have grown, and I mused, 'I have no baby any more.' My mind kept drifting to what peo-

ple had said about having your children when you are young. At this point Lisa blurted out 'Do you want Santa to bring you a baby sister?' This startled me as she had never mentioned a baby sister before in my presence."

62. *December 27, 1959, Sunday, 8:00 P.M.* Ardis and Lisa were sitting under the Christmas tree. Lisa in her play was holding a Santa Claus doll up to Ardis and asked "What do you want for Christmas?" Ardis was caught by surprise, but the first thing that came to her mind was the word "Car," but, before she could speak, Lisa loudly interjected, "You want a car for Christmas?" Ardis had not given a second thought to a car since obtaining a new one last September. However, a second car in the family would be of great value, since it would free Ardis from dependence on my office schedule. Lisa was in a friendly mood.

63. *January 5, 1960, Tuesday, 6:45 P.M.* Just as I was going to phone my telepathist friend, Jacques Romano, in New York, I silently associated to a joke that our mutual friend Mr. Newton told me. It was my intention to tell Mr. Romano that I had met Mr. Newton. However, it was essential that I see Mr. Newton in private because of some research I was doing on Mr. Romano, and I wondered if the latter would understand the reason for this and not be offended at my not inviting him. I thought Mr. Romano would be amused and matters smoothed over by a joke Mr. Newton had told me. While I was trying to recall the joke which concerned "Pittsburgh" (all that I could then remember), Lisa came up to me and shouted the word "Pittsburgh." The joke was about a shabby man in his 50's with an unkept beard. The bum went to the Baptist church but before he could enter, the minister asked, "Where was Jesus Christ born?" The man answered, "Philadelphia," and the minister threw him out. The bum then went to the Presbyterian church, and the minister asked the same question, and, when the bum answered "Pittsburgh," he was again thrown out. Finally he went to an Episcopal church, but the minister didn't ask any questions—he invited the bum in. So the bum asked the minister where Jesus Christ was born, and the minister said, "Why, Bethlehem," and the bum said, "I knew it was somewhere in Pennsylvania!" Lisa might have picked up her father's ambivalence toward Mr. Romano as epitomized in the joke he was trying to recall.

64. *January 5, 1960, Tuesday, 7:10 P.M.* While Ardis was washing the dishes she pondered about what she should have the cleaning lady do tomorrow. The first thought that entered her mind was to have the Venetian blinds and windows cleaned. Simultaneously with this, Lisa came up to Ardis and asked for a cloth to wash the windows. She was given the cloth and climbed on a chair and began washing the windows, saying aloud to Ardis, "Don't worry Mommy: I'll wash the window."

65. *January 12, 1960, Tuesday, 7:30 P.M.* While Lisa was getting ready for bed, Ardis was finishing a letter to her sister describing the opera she had

attended the previous night. She was thinking of all the fancy hairdos of the older women who were trying to look 25, but were obviously in their 50's. At this point, Lisa came up and wanted to comb Ardis' hair and play beauty shop. She ran and got a blanket to use as an apron and then pretended to shampoo her mother's hair. Lisa who was in a positive mood might have supported her mother's self-esteem as well as directed attention to a sensitive area of her mother's (and possibly every woman's) body image. How frequently is telepathy (empathy?) used in making identifications?

66. *January 13, 1960, Wednesday, 4:00 P.M.* While washing the dishes, Ardis was looking outside at the trees and wondering how long they would last with all the ice on them. Lisa came up and said, "The trees are crying for the children to come out." Ardis was saying to herself, shortly before her described thought. "The children need so much to get outside and get rid of some of their energy!" Lisa's statement was a metaphorical condensation of Ardis' thoughts and feelings.

67. *January 15, 1960, Friday, 12:00 Noon.* I was sitting with Lisa while Eric was howling because he was forbidden to play with the vacuum cleaner. Silently I thought to myself, "Thank God, Lisa isn't crying too!" At that point Lisa said, "Lisa doesn't cry!" How often might the expected associative reactions be telepathically catalysed? In this instance was the initiating force the sibling rivalry?

68. *January 17, 1960, Sunday, 12:40 P.M.* I was baby sitting while Ardis went to Church. When she returned I felt like telling her how good the children were, but refrained in order not to suggest to Lisa and Eric any implied alternative to good behavior. However, Lisa said almost simultaneously with the thought, "Papa was very good to Lisa and Eric!"

69. *January 19, 1960, Tuesday, 7:00 P.M.* While giving Lisa a ride in the wagon, I wondered if I should have my secretary phone Miss Tubby and ask her how to spell "Gurdjieff." Miss Tubby has a magnificent library on telepathy and clairvoyance and frequently from her vast experience knows the answers to many of my questions. Simultaneously with my silent thought, Lisa said, "All out with the crystall ball!" She was holding a rubber ball in her hands. Neither Ardis nor I had taught her the expression "crystal ball" nor had we ever heard it from Lisa in the past. However, Lisa said, "You taught me, Daddy!" She was in a friendly frame of mind. It would appear that the crystal ball might have symbolized Miss Tubby to me, and Lisa might have used this expression as a telepathic tracer.

70. *January 25, 1960, Monday, 6:30 P.M.* While having dinner with Lisa I wondered whether I should give her some milk. Hard upon my silent query, Lisa shouted, "Lisa wants sarsaparilla!"

71. *January 26, 1960, Tuesday, 1:30 P.M.* Ardis thought about phoning a neighbor lady to see whether she was home. It was her intention to take Lisa

and Eric over for the afternoon. However, she wondered when Eric would wake up. Simultaneously with this thought, Lisa said, "Shhh, Eric is sleeping." Lisa was very happy and friendly.

72. *February 7, 1960, Sunday, 2:30 P.M.* As Ardis was putting the lettuce away in the refrigerator, she thought to herself, "I'll have to take my fingernail polish off; it is all chipped." At that point Lisa came close to me and said, "Daddy, what color are your nails?"

73. *February 14, 1960, Sunday, 8:45 A.M.* We were having breakfast in the dining room, and Ardis and I were discussing Lisa's diet. We wondered if she was getting enough milk and, furthermore, we discussed keeping hard candy away from the children. We did not mention the word "candy" but spelled it out once. Ardis turned her head to the china closet to see if the bowl of white mint candies had been put back. At that point Lisa said, "I like white; I like white snow." This example might illustrate understandable associative memory processes and the combined suggestive effect of Ardis turning her head toward the blue bowl. However, did these processes work synergistically with telepathy?

74. *February 14, 1960, Sunday, 9:30 A.M.* For the fun of it I did a Russian Cossack dance to the accompaniment of "La Traviata" on the radio. However, it was a little difficult, and I wondered to myself "Am I getting too fat?" Lisa, who was in another corner of the room and had her back turned to me, was drawing on the blackboard. She then said loudly in reference to her drawing, "Tummy too big; tummy too big!" Lisa had apparently perceived a sensitive complex in her father's body image.

75. *February 20, 1960, Saturday, 3:00 P.M.* Ardis was dressing Lisa for her neighbor, Johnny's, party. While Ardis was tying Lisa's shoes, she thought to herself, "What a chore it is to get Lisa's snowsuit on. I wonder if she could go next door without her leggings?" At that point Lisa said, "I don't want to be cold!"

76. *March 10, 1960, Thursday, 10:50 A.M.* I was reading a letter from a physician friend of mine, asking me to write a letter of recommendation for a job. I was quite piqued because he addressed the letter, "Dear Schwarz" instead of using a more cordial greeting. This was not in keeping with the usual expressions of our friendship and the fact that he was asking me a favor. I was displeased but said nothing. Lisa ran up to me, showed me a paper she had in her hand, and said, "Bert! Bert!" in a very angry tone. Lisa seldom calls her father by his first name.

77. *March 11, 1960, Friday, 9:45 A.M.* Ardis was in the car with Lisa and looking for a parking place near the dentist's office. She drove past a good spot, thinking to herself, "It's too icy and once parked I would never be able to get the car out." At that point Lisa said, "Is your car stuck?" This illustra-

tion might also show the imperceptible merging of associative-telepathic processes.

78. *March 11, 1960, Friday, 10:45 A.M.* While walking down the stairs from the dentist's office with Lisa, Ardis noticed Lisa's shoes and thought to herself, "I should really have her shoes checked by some other salesman. I feel they are too big and I don't trust the judgment of the salesman we had." At that point, Lisa said, "I want a new pair of shoes."

79. *March 13, 1960, Sunday, 3:00 P.M.* Eric was riding the hobby horse and Lisa was holding on to the reins. When Ardis walked into the room, she thought to herself, "What a cute picture this would make." Lisa then blurted, "Take a picture of the children!"

80. *March 14, 1960, Monday, 6:30 P.M.* Ardis was clearing the dinner dishes off the table and Lisa was playing with her doll. Then Ardis silently thought about dessert. Just as she pictured to herself the oranges in the refrigerator, Lisa said, "I want some orange juice!" She usually refuses oranges when they are offered to her and only infrequently is she given orange juice at night.

81. *March 14, 1960, Monday, 6:45 P.M.* While Ardis was having her coffee, she was watching Lisa pretend to read. Ardis' mind had drifted to the reverie: "What fun it will be when Lisa can go to Nursery School." As this thought occurred to her mother, Lisa pretended to read about "a boy going to school."

82. *March 19, 1960, Saturday, 3:00 P.M.* While driving Lisa and Eric around town, we crossed Gates Avenue. At this point I thought to myself, "What is the last name of the neurosurgeon who lives a few blocks from here"? The name Woods came to me, but I confused it with another Woods family in Upper Montclair. While I was pondering this, Lisa shouted "Woods, woods!" However, she meant this in the context of "little Red Riding Hood and the wolf in the woods." Once or twice, almost a year ago, Lisa went to visit the neurosurgeon's family. However, she is accustomed to visiting the Woods family in the other part of town more frequently. Could this event have illustrated the intermingling of associative memory and telepathic processes? Lisa applied the word her father was groping for, but she displaced it to a context more immediately appropriate for herself.

83. *March 20, 1960, Sunday, 1:00 P.M.* Lisa was playing on the floor with her toys scattered around her. Ardis and I were having coffee. Ardis' mind drifted to a Woman's Club party where the different participants wore hats that were supposed to be suggestive of various song titles. She did not attend the party but recalled that the person who won the prize wore a child's tea set that she made into a hat. As Ardis was thinking about this, Lisa went to the other room where the toy box was and brought over the tray to her tea

set. The tray had a picture of a teapot on it. The child exclaimed, "Get a party ready; get a party ready!"

84. *March 23, 1960, Wednesday, 9:15 A.M.* Ardis was sitting at her desk trying to contact a lady on the telephone. When she was not able to get her she thought: "What have I done with my sun glasses? I'll need them before I go out as the sun is so bright." A few minutes later Lisa, who was sitting on the floor, started to complain about the sun in her eyes being too bright. The sun was not in her eyes and she was watching television. The dark, lined drapes were drawn at the windows. Lisa has not complained of the television being too bright in the past. The corresponding simultaneity of her thoughts to her mother's is to be noted.

85. *March 25, 1960, Friday, 7:30 A.M.* I was thinking of going to the Nursey to buy some pots for the morning-glory seedlings. However, there was the counter-impulse of whether it would be better to go tomorrow since the car had to go to the garage for repairs. I associated to the complex of the last time I went to the Nursery with Lisa and Eric, and how I bought Lisa a watering can. Simultaneously with these unspoken thoughts, Lisa grabbed her toy watering can and said, "Daddy, can I water the plants?" Lisa was in a friendly mood. She has never offered to water the plants before at this hour of the day.

86. *March 31, 1960, Thursday, 5:15 P.M.* Lisa and Eric were drawing on the blackboard. For no apparent reason, I suddenly felt a strong desire to eat a peanut. Concomitantly with this, Lisa starting chanting, "Lisa is going to draw a peanut!" It had been months since we had eaten peanuts at this time of day. And we had done so very seldom. If we had anything it would be pretzels or potato chips. Lisa was in a very friendly mood.

87. *April 12, 1960, Tuesday, 4:45 P.M.* I was standing in the reception room and chanced to think how beautiful the artificial red tulips were with the sun shining on them. I wondered to myself, "Are they really artificial?" At that point Lisa came running downstairs from another part of the house and, while still in a place from which she could not see the tulips, she said, "I want a red tulip to spin around." I was taken quite aback by this and asked, "What do you mean, you want a red tulip, Lisa?" "It's round (holding her arms and hands in a circle); it's round. I want a red tulip!" She became impatient when I asked her again what she meant and then I gave her a multiple choice question, "Is a tulip food, animal, flower or toy?" She didn't respond so I said, "All right, show me." She took me by the hand and led me upstairs to her room, opened the closet and then pointed to a red hula hoop. She distinctly said, this time, though, "I want my red hulip." (Condensation: hula plus hoop?) Later, when talking to my wife and secretary, I learned that at the time I was looking at the tulips Lisa puzzled them by saying, "I want a red tulip." Ardis later said, "This was strange and we looked at each other. I

said, 'What a silly request, for she hardly knows what a tulip is.' She started to cry so I sent her to you (physician) to have her ask again." Both Ardis and Chabela, my secretary, distinctly heard Lisa saying the word—"tulip." At the time of this event Lisa was in a very friendly mood. This might be an example of a warm feeling that Lisa's father had while in a relaxed, passive state, which she picked up without being aware of its origin and then transposed in her thoughts and feelings to something that would give her pleasure. The apparent simultaneity of her father's and her own verbalized thoughts would have to be explained on other than the usual sensory perception channels because of the distances involved and the architecture of our house.

88. *May 1, 1960, Sunday, 6:15 P.M.* While I sat on the green easy chair in the sitting room, Ardis suddenly got the silly thought of sitting on my lap. However, she repressed this and went over and sat on another chair. Whereupon, Lisa suddenly rushed over to me and said, "I'm going to sit on your lap, papa." I had just remarked to Ardis, "Isn't it strange, it's been such a long time since we've had any telepathic experiences with Lisa." Ardis laughed and explained her silent feelings. This is an interesting example, since Ardis never sits on my lap, and Lisa only does so occasionally. Furthermore, the event might have been unconsciously recognized for what it was by my remark. It is not often that I make such a remark and in this case it coincided with the situation between Ardis and Lisa. Did Ardis send to Lisa or vice versa?

89. *May 8, 1960, Sunday, 2:45 P.M.* Ardis and Lisa were upstairs in another part of the house, visiting with their friend Janet. I was reading Charles Richet's *Thirty Years of Psychical Research,* page 537. [The Macmillan Company, New York, 1923.] I came to this passage: "A child appeared who moved in the room just like a living child and was kissed by those present, and then returned to the medium and was gradually absorbed by him and disappeared, melting into his body." When I finished that sentence Lisa charged downstairs with her rag doll and said, "Dolly wants a kiss, she likes you so much and wants a kiss and hug!" This was strange because under ordinary circumstances, Lisa would remain upstairs with her mother and friend, and she is usually not so demonstrative. My first reaction was, "What a coincidence! Hadn't I just been reading about this?" I went back two pages and checked. Finally I came upon the exact area quoted, which I had just read when Lisa interrupted. Possibly Lisa acted out a crystallization in my thinking. Namely, it was at that point in my reading that it suddenly dawned on me that Richet had been describing many telepathic experiences that involved very young children. Lisa was in a friendly mood at the time.

90. *May 21, 1960, Saturday, 3:30 P.M.* Ardis, Lisa and Eric were visiting Ardis' parents in Minneapolis. Ardis was riding in the car with her mother, father, Lisa, Eric and their cousin on the way to the airport to pick up their

tickets, and Ardis thought to herself, "I haven't had a chance to see our neighbors the Baxters, and I've been home for ten days. I just have to see them." In a few seconds Lisa started jumping on the back seat, saying, "I want to see the neighborhood; I want to see the neighborhood." Ardis was amazed as she had never heard Lisa us the word "neighborhood" before.

91. *May 21, 1960, Saturday, 3:45 P.M.* Ardis was riding in the back seat of the car with Lisa, Eric and her cousin. Ardis' father was driving. Ardis was very concerned about how slow her father's reflexes were at the stop signs. "It always took him so long to start up," she said. "I was worried about his driving as he does so much of it every day, all day long. I was wondering how he kept from having accidents." Then out of the clear, blue sky, Lisa said, "I want to see the car crash."

Before an episode can be regarded as telepathic certain objections must be satisfied. Although the hypothesis of conscious deception can be excluded without further consideration in a study of this nature, the possibilities of paramnesia, hyperesthesia of vision, hearing, other sensory modalities, and chance must be accounted for. Paramnesia is an unlikely explanation for most of the described episodes, because they were recorded immediately after the incidents took place and before the surrounding factors and pertinent details were forgotten. However, it is regrettable that in the earlier stages of the investigation a lesser amount of surrounding data were recorded than for the later possible telepathic episodes. Although in many instances hyperesthesia of vision and hearing cannot be discounted, in these same instances the actual descriptions of the events do not exclude "uncontaminated" or partial telepathic processes. If telepathy is similar to other modes of perception and works in harmony with them, then study of these questionable borderline cases might have some significance for the understanding of such communication. The possibility that a particular situation could have been transmitted by a very subtle visual or auditory clue (unconscious suggestion) does not prove that this was the way the event was perceived. For instance in episode 79 Lisa's comment, "Take a picture of the children," could have been evoked by the sight of her mother's pleasurable facial expression when she saw Lisa and Eric playing with the hobby horse. And it might have been owing to associations and reactions similar to those of her mother that Lisa made a statement which perfectly matched her mother's verbatim unspoken thought at that very instant. That the child adapts herself to the world as her mother does, does not prove that these similar reaction patterns in the earlier stages might be dependent on a telepathic mode of communication. A striking identity of thoughts occurring almost simultaneously to agent and percipient is strong presumptive evidence of telepathy. Table 3-1 tabulates episodes that might conform the mid spectral areas, the borderline between

TABLE 3–1.   Telepathic-Hyperesthesia Spectrum.

Father	Mother
57	7
	64
	66
	73
	78
	84

an uncontaminated telepathic event at one end of the band and the usual means of sensory perception at the other.

The exact appraisal of chance coincidence depends on mathematical formulation. It would be difficult to imagine how such an accounting could be completely controlled with as many variables as occurred in these episodes without having to omit much data which on qualitative inspection appears striking. Nevertheless, it would be desirable to have some mathematical analysis so that chance coincidence could be appraised and the clinical data quantitatively analyzed.

Many of the possible telepathic episodes appear to conform to similar associative-memory processes in the parent and (identifying) child in response to a particular situation. The objection to the telepathic hypothesis in this case is similar to that of the hyperesthesia explanation. Namely the child, in his identification with the parent, will react similarly to the stimulus. The stimulus can be the situation that confronts the parent (agent) and child, and it can be perceived and reacted to on a completely unconscious basis. However, if, as might be the case, telepathic processes work in harmony with the other senses on a broad spectrum, then all borderline telepathic material should not be excluded. The examples in Table 3-2 illustrate this problem. It is impossible to determine whether they were pure telepathy, ordinary sensory perception and association or a combination of both.

Compilation of all the possible telepathic episodes revealed that they occurred 41 times between father and daughter and 50 times between mother and daughter (Table 3-3). There was no considerable difference between parents in the type of material that was transmitted. From a perusal of most of the described episodes it would seem that the parents were the agents and Lisa the percipient. However, it should be stated that this is not proof that the child did not think of the situation first but delayed speaking or acting until the parent responded to what he presumed to be his own thoughts or feelings. For example, in episodes 11, 59 and 65 the mother silently thought of hair and this was subsequently reacted to by her daughter. However, this is not proof that Lisa did not think of hair first, verbally responding only

TABLE 3–2. Telepathic-Similar Associative Memory.

Father	Mother	Grandmother
2	13	17
3	36	
21	45	
38	52	
44	62	
48	71	
51	75	
82	77	
	79	
	80	
	81	
	91	

after her mother's similar unspoken thought. Retrospective analysis of a series of telepathic drawing experiments demonstrated in many instances the fallacy of agency.

The often wax and wane pattern of the possible telepathic episodes might suggest another clue to their agency and origin (Figure 3-1). It seemed that the peak frequencies of telepathic episodes occurred at times when the father was finishing some psychical investigations. The March 1959 peak, when Lisa was 28 months old, coincided with the completion of a study on "Telepathic Experiments and Psychiatry";[174] the July-September 1959 period correlated with the completion of his investigations on the "Ordeals by Serpents, Fire and Strychnine."[172] Finally, the last peak coincided with the completion of a biographical investigation of a 96-year-old telepathist, "Jacques Romano Ninety-Six, His Unusual Life and Exploits."[181] These three psychic studies involved the outpouring of much energy, thought and affect. They chronologically coincided with the crystallization of much previous thinking on telepathy. These studies were major events in the family situation at the particular times of the increased telepathic parent-child episodes. The mother's increased responses at these times might have been a reflection of her husband's concern over these interesting and much discussed matters. The occurrences of these peak frequency episodes are also compatible with the observation that the telepathic event frequently corresponds to a preconscious thought-affect on the verge of emerging from repression and entering consciousness.[83,38] It might be supposed that in this way the telepathic episodes are to some extent influenced by conscious attitudes. Further support for this opinion is provided by the observation that there were more frequent telepathic experiences between this physician and his patients after sessions with the master telepathist, Mr. Romano, and this observation has also been independently reported by Ullman.[224]

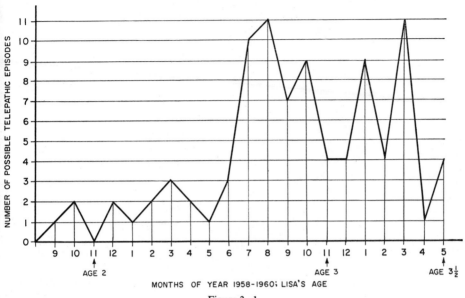

Figure 3–1.

TABLE 3–3.   All Possible Telepathic Episodes.

Father	Mother	Grandmother
1	4	17
2	5	
3	7	
6	8	
9	11	
10	13	
12	14	
15	23	
16	24	
18	25	
19	27	
20	29	
21	30	
22	31	
28	33	
32	34	
35	36	
38	37	
42	39	
43	40	
44	41	

TABLE 3–3.   All Possible Telepathic Episodes. (Cont.)

Father	Mother	Grandmother
46	45	
47	47	
48	49	
50	52	
51	53	
54	55	
57	56	
63	58	
67	59	
68	60	
69	61	
70	62	
74	64	
78	65	
82	66	
85	71	
86	72	
87	73	
88	75	
89	77	
	79	
	80	
	81	
	83	
	84	
	88	
	90	
	91	

The tagging of a telepathic episode by the use of various tracer words is another supporting factor for the genuineness of the phenomena. In these episodes such tracer words as "telephone," "radio," "talk," and even the father's use of the word "telepathy" are suggestive of the faint recognition by either agent or percipient of the occurrence of a telepathic event (see Table 3-4). This is entirely similar to Eisenbud's observation,[46] that "telepathic dreams (at least in analysis) are likely to incorporate in their manifest contents something that may be taken as an allusion to the very fact that they are telepathic."

In contrast to many later, more complex, responses several of the earlier episodes concerned food (see Table 3-5). Possibly this can be related to Lisa's very early oral desires. Apparently she was emotionally sensitized to her parents' thoughts on this subject since she correctly alluded to various foods at almost the exact instant her parents thought of them. This could be an important functional use of telepathy for the growing child of limited vocabulary.

TABLE 3–4.   Telepathic Tracer Words.

Father	Mother
1	55
46	79
57	81
88	

Another interesting observation is that occasionally Lisa gave similar responses to the agent's thought at widely varying time intervals. Some examples are: Lisa's use of the word "raincoat" for the grandmother's thought and, months later, she gave a similiar response to her mother's thought (17 and 24); Lisa's phrase "it's raining on Uncle Floyd's" (19 and 26) as a reaction to her mother's ambivalence about a dinner engagement; her comments on "birthday" when her mother thought of this at three separate intervals (25, 56, and 58); her condensed mentioning of a specific mother-daughter baby-sitting team when her mother thought of them (30 and 34); and finally the occasion of Lisa's "telepathic reading" of Miss Tubby's name from a book her father was looking at, and then at a later time Lisa's calling "Miss Tubby" in apparent response to her father's unspoken associations (34 and 43). These examples are similar to the finding that the percipient might be sensitized to certain stimuli and respond in an almost predictable telepathic manner.[174, 229]

The overall increase in frequency of telepathic episodes seems to correlate with Lisa's growing awareness of her environment and her differentiation in interpersonal relationships, as well as her parents' developing awareness and interest in such phenomena. This correlates with Lisa's growing interest in such abstract-cognitive functions as being able to "read" various story books. As Lisa learns to achieve more gratification for her dependency needs from psychic spheres rather than from the earlier more organic modes (food), her attention span in interpersonal relationships increases concomitantly with the frequency of telepathic episodes. These increased telepathic events also reflect the increased complexity of her expanding vocabulary and the development of various mental mechanisms.

TABLE 3–5.   Possible Telepathic Responses with Food.

Father	Mother
1	5
2	8
42	23
70	37
86	40
	73
	80

Although the total reported telepathic events are too few in number to break up into arbitrary classifications and then plot chronologically, it appears that the data closely correspond to Lisa's increased interpersonal awareness and identifications. Thus, many of the earlier responses concern food, and then, only later, people, body parts and various objects of particular social significance to the agents (parents) and Lisa (Table 3-6). In her developing identifications with her mother and father she learns to perceive correctly their innermost thoughts, feelings and conflicts. This process is in many ways similar to the poorly understood emotional contagion or communion (empathy; *13*) that exists between an infant and those who take care of him. When in rapport, Lisa has made statements that are complementary or sometimes embarrassingly revealing of her parents' wishes and feelings. For instance in episodes 37 and 39 Lisa quickly perceived her mother's weakly repressed sensitivity over her waistline, and in episode 41 she called out the word "band-aid" that might have signified her mother's memory of a disfiguring pimple. In example 76 Lisa startled her father by earnestly calling him by his Christian name, Bert, at the exact moment when he was silently annoyed over a letter he had received from a close friend who addressed him by his surname instead of more familiarly. In episodes 29, 33, and 62, Lisa perceives her mother's wishes for a new car. In episodes 11 and 15 she remarks upon her parents' (psychosexual) concern over hair-wave or moustache. In other examples Lisa demonstrates sibling rivalry with her younger brother (Table 3-9) and gives evidence of her developing oedipal stage (Table 3-10). It should be noted that three of these possible oedipal episodes are related to dreams (9, 12 and 57). She can perceive her parents' secrets and, when in a very friendly mood, she can almost pick their thoughts out of the air. For instance, she is very keen in perceiving information about her birthday (episodes 56 and 57), and such surprises as a snowman (53), pumpkin (48), or Christmas presents for her neighbor friends (60). In example 61 she either perceived or transmitted the wish for a baby sister. She can correctly use words or phrases that she does not comprehend, like "radiation" (20), "go up the hill" (54), "Pittsburgh" (63), and "red tulip" (86). These episodes of surprise, unusual words and phrases are listed in Table 3-7. In contrast to many of the other episodes, they are almost unique in that they offer few explanations other than the telepathic hypothesis. They are also interesting because they seem to have no particular symbolic meaning to Lisa. They are like foreign bodies since it was not possible to determine their origin. However such episodes might have much emotional significance since they dramatically threw her father off guard and forced him to take notice of the young child growing to womanhood like her mother.

TABLE 3–6.   Possible Telepathic Episodes and People, Body Image.

Father	Mother
6	4
15	11
16	14
18	19
20	24
22	26
28	27
32	29
35	30
43	31
46	32
50	33
57	34
74	39
76	41
85	45
	49
	59
	65
	83
	90

TABLE 3–7.   Possible Telepathic Episodes of Surprise.

Father	Mother
18	53
20	60
46	
54	
63	
86	

TABLE 3–8.   Possible Telepathic Episodes and Sibling Rivalry.

Father	Mother
44	60
57	
67	
68	

The use of various mental mechanisms such as condensation, displacement and projection were noted later when Lisa's vocabulary was becoming more complex and she was becoming more proficient in language. For instance, she perceived her father's unspoken associations of "Miss Tubby" with "Les" (43), and at a later time "Floyd" and "Les" were condensed in connection with their whereabouts and an aeroplane trip (50). She asked her father about his fingernails in response to her mother's unspoken queries about her own fingernails (72). And one time Lisa wanted a "red tulip" (86), but she did not really comprehend her statement which was apparently inspired by her father's thought. For in her confusion she substituted the neologism ("hula hoop") "hulip" for "red tulip." Finally, in episode 89 Lisa acted out through her doll (projection) the desire for the kind of affection that the father had just been reading about.

TABLE 3–9.   Possible Telepathic Episodes and Oedipal Conflict.

Father	Mother
9	37
12	61
57	88
89	91

From the perusal of all the data certain general impressions emerge. The various categories of possible telepathic episodes are arbitrary and show much overlapping. However, it would seem that in most instances the events took place when both child and parents were in a state of rapport. Little developed when there was no rapport or common meeting ground. The episodes often startled the parents and made them take notice of their daughter. The child, as far as could be determined, had no conscious awareness of the telepathic significance of the events. From the content of many of the episodes as well as the parents' surprised reactions, it can be conjectured that the infantile concepts of narcissism, omnipotence, omniscience and "mind reading" might have kernels of truth in telepathy. The possible significance of telepathic communication was noted by Freud[83] who commented: "One is led to conjecture that this may be the original archaic method by which individuals understood one another and which has been pushed into the background in the course of phylogenetic development by the better method of communication by means of signs apprehended by the sense organs."

Almost all the episodes occurred while the agent (or percipient) was preoccupied in a passive trance-like state. It was the agent's fleeting complex, existing in his preconscious thinking, that was apparently transmitted and perceived by the child, who, because of her own sensitivity to such data, responded. There was no evidence of any conscious control for any of the events. The episodes most often occurred at the intersection of the parents' and child's emotional needs. Analysis of the data reveals that when unmasked through an understanding of psychopathology, the episode is not irrational and devoid of meaning but serves a purpose in the interpersonal relationship between a growing child and her parents. Among other reasons, the emotional necessity of repressing such material of significance to both partners in the telepathic event gives the probably erroneous impression that it is a rare or vestigial oddity. Pederson-Krag stated that such communication might have been kept unconscious because, if the content of the communication were on a conscious level, there could have been many social complications from an awareness of erotic, antisocial, aggressive material.[144] Also if telepathic communications were the usual channel there might have been little need for the elaborate development of language and speech.

TABLE 3–10. Possible Telepathy and Mental Mechanisms.

Father	Mother
43	72
50	
86	
89	

It is just this point, however, that raises an intriguing question about the significance of telepathic episodes in various pathological conditions. It might be supposed that in certain pathological dissociations (schizophrenia, hysteria) disguised hostile and erotic impulses could be more poignantly perceived, and thus contribute to further splitting. A vicious cycle could be set up: viz., the dissociated patient could become more split by perception of unhealthy (i.e. hostile) material and thus become more vulnerable for further splitting in the specific areas to which he had been sensitized in his pathological, interpersonal and libidinal relationships. As a clinical observation, the author has had many more telepathic experiences in therapy with patients in dissociative states than with those in other conditions.

The episodes also demonstrate that the absent-minded or trance-like states of every day life appear to favor the occurrence of telepathy. At such times, the subject is preoccupied with material in his preconscious mind. This subjective state might be functionally similar to experimental states of sensory deprivation where the subject is isolated from the use of vision, hearing, touch and so forth. Thus it appears that the telepathic mode of communication could be an important emotional aid in maintaining mental equilibrium and adapting to severe stress. It would be interesting to investigate from this particular point of view the hallucinations and delusions occurring in such states of stress.

4
Possible Geriatric Telepathy

ABSTRACT: Although largely unrecognized, geriatric telepathy may
be a more common and widespread form of communication than has
been supposed. In later life, when impairment of hearing and sight,
social isolation and loneliness, increased dependency, brain syndromes
or other illnesses are so prevalent, patients may be unusually sensitive
to telepathy. Several examples are presented of possible paranormal exchanges in older persons, and also data from the life of Joseph Dunninger and from psychiatric practice. Telepathy occurring at times of
intense unconscious emotional significance may serve to bridge gaps in
interpersonal relationships and thereby diminish anxiety and improve
psychophysiological homeostasis. The interplay between telepathy and
related psi phenomena that interacts with the vicissitudes of aging is an
interesting field for further exploration.

Study of possible paranormal experiences in the elderly raises many provocative questions for the physician. He might wonder how such events happen
and what they are like. Are they rare or frequent, and what might be the
theoretical and practical consequences? In his well-documented monograph,
Karlis Osis,[141] the parapsychologist, analyzed numerous intriguing deathbed
visions involving older people; these data were obtained mostly from ques-
tionnaires sent to physicians and nurses. Nandor Fodor,[72] the pioneer parapsychologist and psychoanalyst, sensitively and critically scrutinized the
biographies of some well-studied famous mediums of integrity who had experienced many unexplainable episodes, presumably of the "psi phenomenon."* However, these and related reports are not always clear on the
persistence and extent of paranormal function during the aging of these mediums. Certainly Mrs. Piper,[77] perhaps the most intensively investigated me-

---

*A term coined to embrace extrasensory phenomena (thought transference and clairvoyance)
and psychokinesis.

dium in modern history, had numerous psychic abilities earlier in her life. Although she lived to age 91, little is said about her later years; for instance, it is not known whether there was either an actual or a spurious decline in her psychic abilities. Her original investigators—William James, Richard Hodgson, James H. Hyslop, and others—had long since died, and perhaps with their deaths there was a decline in the innovative approaches and interest in the problems that Mrs. Piper presented.

Another famous medium, Mrs. Gladys O. Leonard,[74] allegedly retained her abilities later in life. Eusapia Paladino,[76] a remarkable physical medium, demonstrated her telekinetic feats almost to the end of her life. Hereward Carrington, who studied Paladino for many years, once told Dunninger [24] that although she was prone to fraud, in almost every séance that he had had with her, 10–15% of the phenomena were genuine and unexplainable. The biographies of other famous mediums, such as D. D. Home [73] and Stainton Moses,[75] also contain a wealth of psi material that seemingly persisted to the ends of their lives. Throughout her long life, Mrs. Eileen Garrett,[118] who was studied by physicians as well as other specialists, had superior and extensively documented psi abilities.

In contrast to the classical psychic researches on mediums, much of which is connected with the study of the survival hypothesis, more recent approaches fully utilize psychodynamic and medical principles. Two gifted "sensitives" who can still demonstrate their practical skills as they age are Professor Tenhaeff's[214-216] famous paragnost Gerard Croiset who uses his abilities in the solution of crimes and archeological mysteries, and Henry Gross [176] the successful Maine dowser. No discussion of telepathy occuring in old age or at any other time of life can be considered complete without referring to the monumental contributions of four eminent psychiatrists: Jule Eisenbud,[53] Jan Ehrenwald,[37] Joost A. M. Meerloo,[126] and Montague Ullman.[225]

Studies of the youthful-appearing non-agenarian Jacques Romano,[181] indicated that his extraordinary psychic abilities persisted almost to the day of his death—and for all one knows, even after it. During my last visit with Romano the day before he died, he seemingly telepathically picked out of my mind all the particular sore points and polarized areas at that time (matters that I had never discussed with him)—and he was unaware of what he was doing. After I pronounced Romano dead in his bedroom (the next day), and I returned to his living room, I was shocked to see that his pocket watch, which had been on the desk and not running, had started.[178] Naturally, none of the other people in the room had touched the watch and there was no acceptable explanation for this event. Later there were also some possible psychic phenomena involving highly specific polarized complexes for the deceased Romano, some unusual patients, and myself.[177,179] For example, some possible telekinetic events included the crashing of an oil painting by Romano during my psychotherapeutic session with an unusual patient, and other similar telekinetic or conditioned spontaneous events.

There might be a parallel between the relatively simple early parent-child telepathy[184] and the more complex paranormal events in later life. As a child trusts and believes his parents, so older persons, mellowed with age, often have a similar attitude. Perhaps, though wiser and more reflective than the child, they are like the young helpless child in their need for communication with those on whom they depend. The older person's security is often threatened by an impaired ability to earn a living. This is often compounded by various disabilities including visual impairment and deafness; and the aged also suffer the effects of loneliness and social isolation.

Older-age patients who have various brain syndromes with concomitant memory deficits must communicate if they are to survive. While in such a minus state,[37] they also may be immersed in their world of remote memories and reveries, a world analogous to the day-dreaming and fantasy world of the child. For both the young and the old, such altered states of consciousness as the spontaneous trance-like states might be propitious for paranormal episodes. In addition to reacting to all the usual (often subtle) subliminal and suggestive methods of communication—including the usual introjection mechanisms—the aged, like children, keenly react to sensitive paranormal stimuli in a simpler, more direct way. This contrasts with the usual younger adult reactions which are characterized by elaborate psychopathological filters and disguises. The following examples from research and practice illustrate possible paranormal functions in older people.

POSSIBLE PARANORMAL FUNCTIONS IN THE ELDERLY

Dunninger's Demonstrations

In recent years I have studied Joseph Dunninger,[25] who has had a distinguished career as a world-famous magician and telepathist for more than 60 years. I have observed him perform various telepathic feats, such as when I drove him to his next-to-last public performance in a high school in Waterbury, Connecticut, on November 29, 1969. During that evening's demonstration he telepathically elicited myriad specific pieces of information from an audience that he, his family, my son, and myself had never met before. While on the stage he named serial numbers from social security cards, bills, coins, telephone numbers and addresses.

There were no confederates, and no one had written anything down. This performance was monitored by a tape recorder. No one has ever duplicated his feats. For example, in some instances through the years Dunninger passed out slips of paper to members of the audience and asked them to write down a specific question, for which they knew the answer. Then, if they chose, they could write down the answer which he gave them from the platform. If they didn't write the answer, he still usually gave the correct, precise information. At no time did the slip of paper ever leave their possession. On numerous other occasions, nothing was written. Thus in these ways the members of the audience through most of Dunninger's performances had an air-tight record of what happened. Unfortunately some of his purported telepathic demonstrations were so automatically and artfully mixed with showmanship that Dunninger himself often did not know when his demonstrations were completely genuine and when they were colored with extraneous material.

Some of the most amazing aspects of Dunninger's life have been his many spontaneous psi experiences with his own family, other people, and vairous members of my family. Also, during the period of my observations there were some unusual situations that I witnessed in his home, e.g., apparent phantom footsteps, crashes, possible thoughtography and telekinesis, and, spontaneous telepathy between us.

During his public career and in his private life, Dunninger ocassionally has made successful predictions. For example, as I corroborated from contemporary newspaper clippings in his scrapbooks, he correctly foretold Babe Ruth's record-breaking 60-home-runs season. He also predicted very closely —better than the pundits of the press services—the election victory of New York City's Mayor Jimmy Walker.

On Saturday afternoon, February 20, 1971, at an autograph auction at the Sheraton-Penn Pike Hotel, Fort Washington, Pennsylvania, Dunninger was unexpectedly called to the stage by his son-in-law (the auctioneer), Bruce Gimmelson, an antique dealer, and asked to predict the total receipts. Dunninger, age 79, who was unprepared for this (he had not been feeling well because of partial invalidism due to Parkinson's disease that was being treated with amantadine), perked up and agreed to try. According to Dunninger, his wife, two daughters and the son-in-law, he wrote on a piece of paper $41,740.00, and put it in an envelope, which was sealed and signed by four people: Bob Batchelder, Mabel Zahn, Manuel Kean, and Sol Feinstone. At the conclusion of the auction the 260 items were tallied up on the adding machine. The total was $41,740.00! In an article appearing in the *Ambler Gazette,* Ambler, Pennsylvania, Thursday, February 25, 1971, and headlined "Autograph Auction Draws History Hunting Collectors," Dorothy Drake wrote; "Dunninger lived up to the reputation of amazing, for he was only a dollar off in predicting the total amount of today's sale of $41,740.00."

Mr. and Mrs. Gimelson gave me the signed envelope and adding-machine tally slip. It was not possible for me to check personally with the four people who signed the envelope, but there was no reason to believe that the situation was any different from that reported, except that in her text Miss Drake was incorrect, and Dunninger's written prediction precisely matched the tally slip. (This event might not be unlike the well documented case of precognition cited by Nobel prize winner, Charles Richet,[152] in which a M. Gallet predicted the exact vote for the election of M. Casimir-Périer as President of the Republic of France.) My confirmation and study of the Dunninger auction prediction (February 20, 1971) took place February 24, 1971, during our weekly sessions. The accounts as given me by Dunninger, his wife, and younger daughter coincided completely with the facts that I ascertained independently from his older daughter, son-in-law, and the newspaper account (February 25, 1971). It should be stressed that Dunninger had no explanation for his feat but was rather nonchalant, as he is for most of his psi skills.

Hanging On

After consultation on an elderly male patient with chronic brain syndrome, right hemiparesis, congestive heart failure, and azotemia, I debated when writing my note what to say about his right upper extremity. At that precise point, the patient, who had not said much before, asked me about his right upper extremity. The patient died a few days later, and I wondered whether his concern was sent to me about the one area of his many disabilities regarding which he was most sensitive, or whether he had picked up my thoughts? Unless the event was coincidence, could the patient with his clouded sensorium have been reaching out telepathically for support and sustenance? He was hanging on and trying to survive.

The Injection

An 85-year-old disoriented woman had a defective recent-and-remote memory, spoke incoherently, and threatened to pull a knife on the nurses. Because of her senile delirium it was hard to have any meaningful communication with her. While sitting by her bedside and thinking about her situation, I recalled a similar case that had a telepathic tinge,[177] and wondered about possible telepathy in this instance. My next thought, while sympathetically concerned about my patient, was the likelihood of an untoward chlorpromazine hypotensive effect following an intramuscular (gluteal) injection. At that point the patient, for the first time overcoming her confusion and momentarily dropping her defensive tirades, said: "Somebody put it in here (pointing to gluteal area) and it hurts." Did I pick up subliminally or telepathically the patient's sore gluteal area, or did my queries about the possibility of another painful injection immediately evoke a telepathic response in the fearful, sensitized-to-pain patient? Pain can be a telesomatic response.[180]

Telepathic Busybodies

The patient was a 74-year-old woman who was hospitalized for years because of involutional melancholia. When I first saw her, she had been transferred to a nursing home. Because of a disability from an old hip fracture, she was restricted in her activities and needed a walker. A biospy had recently been performed for lymphoma of the left eye. She was upset over this procedure and the necessary follow-up x-ray treatments. However, she had no conscious awareness of the malignant nature of her illness.

In many previous psychotherapeutic sessions there had been much telepathy. One day the patient began her talk with: "My grandson's girlfriend (a nurse at a local hospital) will soon return to the hospital. I look forward to having her care for my husband, as he will have surgery on the fifteenth" (removal of uric acid tophi from both elbows). During the long pause, my thoughts drifted to my visit the day before in another town, with my childhood friend B. K., who lived in an allegedly haunted, remodeled old Dutch farmhouse. In our conversation, B. K. mentioned the recent marriage of a white Canadian nurse from one of the hospitals in my town, to a Negro. He said that he had heard about this from Scouting activities and wondered how common interracial marriage was in Montclair, which has a sizable black population. While I was thinking of this, the patient said: "Ann (daughter) tooted the horn Saturday when she drove by your house. She saw you raking leaves. She was on the way home from the wedding of the Canadian nurse and the Negro."

After a long pause I thought that perhaps we might be establishing telepathic rapport, and that I would attempt to prove it by telepathically sending the picture in my mind's eye of a white bride in a nurse's uniform and the groom who looked like the black entertainer, Sammy Davis, Jr., who is blind in one eye. At that the patient said: "It is hard to know what to put on these days: it is cold, then warm, the x-ray place was busy—goodness!" The patient might have been attempting to approximate my thought of the half-blind entertainer with x-ray treatments of her eye and the fear of being blinded. I again attempted a clear focus in my mind's eye by seeing a black groom and white bride on top of a conventional wedding cake. The patient said: "Those flowers are from St. Peter's Church. My daughter-in-law brought them yesterday." Since we seemed to be tuning in, I thought I would send the patient (or did I receive?) a mental picture of her son who, though older than I, had graduated from the same college. The patient said: "The maid (in the nursing home) personally brings Fred (son) a cup of coffee when he drives in and she sees him." It now seemed certain that we were tuning in. In my mind's eye I next saw a saxophonist and drew a picture of it and wrote musical notes, though the patient could not see what I was doing. She countered with: "Should Dr. Cyrus (ophthalmologist) come in?" This was unsuccessful telepathically, but I still felt certain we could communicate in this way so I thought, I'll do it again, darn it! I saw the saxophone and this time "heard" the music. The patient chimed in with: "Was the music going when you came in? Was it to cheer up the patients?" (She was referring to Muzak, frequently noted in the halls, but not being played the day of this interview.) My next thought was the *Newark Evening News,* which I clearly visualized. I was certain this had something to do with the patient's trend of thought. She then said: "They have medicine to stop chicken pox itching; Mrs V. told me they gave it to her son for this." Nevertheless, I believed I was correct and the next time I would succeed with my thought about the *Newark Evening News.* The patient continued: "Mary W. read in the *paper* that a 35-year-old girl had chicken pox and died from it. I'll try to think of *news* to tell you." I swished my tongue around my mouth (an enclosed area) and tried to "project" the taste of salt. Then the patient said: "I told Dr. Johnsen (radiologist) that I don't see how they can do it (radiation treatment) without injuring the eyesight." Perhaps the patient displaced my projected sense of taste to her threatened vision; however, I decided to try again, but this time I swished my tongue inside my mouth and vividly sensed "sweetness" because of the associatively noted sugar on the patient's tray. She continued: "A friend has claustrophobia, you could never take her in that room" (x-ray room where patient had her treatment). I was stuck in an elevator one time on the third floor, and a couple that was with me got panicky. It was my friend, and since then she wouldn't ride one. She gets panicky in her son's Volkswagen; she drives a Lincoln. I don't like heights." My thoughts were, 'Whose ideas are whose?' The tongue swishing around the mouth (anatomically, a confined space) could be compared to the patient's associations with claustrophobia, i.e., being trapped in an elevator as the tongue is fixed in the mouth. My mind then drifted back to B. K.'s 200-year-old Dutch house haunted by Negro slaves. I could mentally hear their ghostly walking around and the cool breeze-like effects that were described to me by B. K. and his family. The patient said: "Mrs. P. has a new roommate, from Montclair, who is not well and in bad health. The aides (Negroes) take them out walking too quickly; they can't go fast; they get chills and die(!)." In this exchange the patient or physician criss-crossed associatively to Negroes, cool chilling effects, ghosts, and death. These intuitive of possible telepathic cross-associations might have indicated the patient's struggle to survive and her desperation in seeking my full attention. For my part, this patient sought my professional help at a time when I was looking for a challenge—something different from the usual type of material. Although I seldom saw these elderly chronically paranoid patients for any length of time, the family (husband, son, daughter, and grandson) were so decent to deal with that I wanted to help them as well as the patient. She got along well for many months, during which time there were numerous subliminal communications that seemed to burst into telepathic episodes, even on rare occasions, the telepathic "pulling" of Christian names out of thin air. Following the death of her husband, she again sank into the depths of a depression from which no combination of drugs or psychotherapy could rouse her. If there was telepathy at this time, there was little or no awareness for it. She had lost the will to live and she died.

I wonder how many other elderly patients with chronic brain syndromes, senility and paranoid ideation might basically have a problem of undue brain sensitivity to heteropsychic telepathic stimuli. It is not a question of subliminal vs. telepathic stimuli, but of how the two processes work together —like our eyes and ears, with all their interrelated central-nervous-system connections.

Nos Morituri Te Salutamus

Many years ago I saw a depressed, confused, elderly widowed restaurateur-cook, who had originally responded to electroshock treatment. However, several months afterward there was a recurrence of symptoms, and her family transferred her to a nursing home. While there, except for minimal hypertension and transient episodes of confusion and poor memory, her health was fair. Late one night, three years after admission to the nursing home, Harold, her son-in-law, excitedly phoned me from the family restaurant. He reported: "I was asleep in the easy chair and was jolted awake early in the morning by hearing my mother-in-law knocking at the back door and shouting, 'Hey Ethel (her daughter), hey, Ethel!' I looked at the clock; it was 3:30 A.M. I got up, and examined both doors (to the restaurant) and put on all the lights. I wondered, 'What's wrong here? Did mother get out of the nursing home?' I woke up Ethel from a nightmare." Ethel, who lived in a separate wing of the building farthest removed from where her husband Harold was, said: "In my dream I was yelling 'My God! My God!' I was in the kitchen, looking at the back door and had a dreadful feeling that it was an atomic attack. I couldn't move, and was paralyzed. So were Harold (husband) and our two helpers."

When I interviewed Ethel on the telephone she said, "When I awoke, Harold told me about the knocking and mother's calling my name. He asked if I had heard it. He insisted on my accompanying him to the back door. We turned on all the lights and searched the place but found nothing. We couldn't account for this. Harold was never that way before, and I couldn't get over it. At his insistence I called the nursing home first thing in the morning to find out if mother was all right." This was also the first time during her mother's confinement that Ethel had telephoned at such an hour to inquire about her mother's health, which had not changed since her admission. Ethel continued: "The nurse who answered the phone was very surprised and said, 'You surprise me, for I was wondering whether or not I should call you. Your mother was very sick last night, about 2:00 A.M. How did you know about it? Your mother fainted and couldn't be aroused for several minutes.' "

Again, at Harold's insistence (even before Ethel's call to the nursing home), Ethel made special arrangements to visit her mother the next day, Saturday, usually the busiest day of the week for the family restaurant and a day Ethel never went on a visit to the nursing home. When she did visit her mother that Saturday morning, the then fully oriented mother who apparently had no awareness of the previous night's events, asked Ethel if Harold and the granddaughter were coming later. Then, at 3:20 P.M., almost twelve hours after the unusual nocturnal visitation, the nursing home telephoned Harold to report that his mother-in-law had just died.

This premonition was verified later by direct interviews of Harold, Ethel, and P. G., the chef, who knew about what had happened. When Harold was asked if he ever had any similar previous experiences, he recalled how, 30 years previously, a bird kept trying to get through the window and refused to go away; the following day a member of his family died. This was indeliby impressed upon Harold's mind because 3 years afterward he had a similar experience and he was stumped for an explanation. This baffling type of situation has been explored elsewhere.[111,189]

Ethel's father died when she was a young child and her mother, who was of foreign origin, had struggled in raising Ethel and her two older brothers. The younger brother left home as a teen-ager and was seldom heard from for many years. The older brother a chronic alcoholic, never worked but was supported by the mother, Ethel, and her husband. The mother, Ethel, and her alcoholic brother never had striking previous psi experiences. Harold (Ethel's husband), was of old American stock and had been orphaned as a small baby. For him life might have meant survival. He might have harbored much resentment toward his mother-in-law for his intolerable situation, as both he and Ethel worked hard to make a success of the mother-controlled restaurant, only to see the fruits of their labors squandered and imbibed by the ne'er-do-well older brother.

For diverse but complementary psychodynamic reasons, it might be speculated how both Harold and Ethel were sensitized to the mother's approaching death, as much as the mother was herself. Possibly the mother, through this dramatic form of presumed paranormal communication, prepared her daughter and son-in-law for what was to follow within 12 hours. In this way she sought (and received?) some forgiveness for the past and for her previous destructive permissiveness toward the parasitic son (and brother).

Because of their early life, catastrophic losses of parents, and their seemingly interminable years of hard work and bondage to an unjust situation in the family restaurant (which was owned and controlled by the long-lived mother), Harold, Ethel and the mother, through their collective traumatic monition of the mother's crisis (her fainting spell), may have found relief, surcease and permanent release from an otherwise nearly unbearable plight.

This transaction is similar to the telepathic drawing experiments[174] in which several people were involved and volleys of drawings were sent and received. It was impossible to reconstruct who were the senders and receivers in this triangle involving a possible telepathic dream, telepathy, telekinesis or telepathic auditory hallucination, or possibly, even a telesomatically-induced death.

The Revival Meeting

The following incident occurred during the treatment of a 38-year-old registered nurse, a physician's wife. Originally she was brought to my office in a state of hypomania, by her father. During her manic depressive illness she had three hospitalizations with courses of electric-shock treatment. However, under a regimen of lithium and psychotherapy she showed gradual improvement, and at the time of this incident she had been syntonic for many months.

The facts of this report were fully confirmed by the nurse's physician-husband, whom I have known for many years. It pertains to her father, age 63, who had carcinoma metastatic to the brain and throughout his body from a primary lesion of the lung. The diagnoses were confirmed by the findings on pneumonectomy, neurological examination, brain scan, and roentgenography. The father was hospitalized after he had alternated between stupor and coma for many weeks. While in the hospital, the family visited him daily. Although his sensorium was clouded, they scrupulously avoided saying anything in his presence lest he be disturbed. Despite the importunities of other family members, the father's wife, because of presumed severe past emotional difficulties, refused to permit her husband's transfer to a nursing home: "I don't want him, or anyone else, to think that I railroaded him into a nursing home to die, as I did his mother."

The nurse-daughter was very attached to her father and in many of her sessions she frequently recalled how: "My father delivered me. The doctor came for my (twin) brother who was born *after* me." One day the daughter came to her session and was glowing: "Father came to, and sat up. He took over, and got himself admitted to the nursing home. He knew nothing of one insurance policy running out and of the litigation over his bills with his major medical insurance company. The hospital cost $145 a day, 75% of which was covered by the insurance, but the major medical maintained that his present illness (that led to pneumonectomy) was the same one he had at first and the clause said that if you heal in the two interim years you win (and the insurance is valid for a "second illness"). But between my father's original operation and current hospitalization, his doctor had sent the insurance company a bill for $20 for a checkup, which they claimed was for treatment of the original illness and that is why we had the litigation and such backbreaking expenses.

"At the very beginning of his illness he said that he was going to get up into a chair and go into the sunlight. For weeks, the most he could do was just occasionally blink his eyes in recognition. He had stopped eating. Yet he came to and got out of the hospital one hour before the insurance was used up—the 120 days which are allowed. He didn't know of this when he entered the hospital, and we had just found out about the used-up insurance one day before father came to. He had been alternating between stupor and coma for 14 weeks. He had two hyperthermia attacks and a fever of 105°. He stared for days on end, and he also had hemiplegia. We were very upset because the major medical refused to pay and the other insurance for the hospital was used up."

"Yet on Saturday father sat up in bed and called my husband by his nickname, asked about his stocks, the twins, the other children, and their birthdays. Mother, who had gone to the hospital for fourteen weeks and had gradually seen father sink into a coma, was convinced that it was a miracle: 'God made him sit up and come to.'

"Father got into a chair and asked me to wheel him outside. He looked at the trucks speeding on the highway for a half hour. At the time I put him in the chair he told me: 'This is your birthday.' My husband had told him in the morning. Dad ate two full dinners though he had been on a liquid diet for six weeks. Mother was going to (legally) seal all his stocks and bonds, house and boat. She was dumb-struck that Dad knew exactly what stocks he had and their prices at the time he became ill and was hospitalized. He remembered what he said when he went into his office. My brother checked his statements and found out that Dad was right.

"Sunday he said his side was paralyzed but that he was going to swing his arm in the air. 'You know why?' he said, 'Because I fought it. I might go down, but I'm going down swinging. Now I can move my finger.' Dad said that now he had accomplished what he wanted. Then he slipped back into coma, and in a short while he was dead.

"On Monday my mother said: 'Oh, I feel so relieved. My conscience doesn't bother me that he is in a nursing home.' Something must have happened to his brain. We were all so careful, because my father's ears were his eyes, and for that reason we never talked even outside the hospital door. For all this time mother blocked our desire to put father in a nursing home, but now he could go because of his unusual revival which was perfectly timed, for now he was completely covered by insurance."

This example might illustrate how subliminal and possibly telepathic and other factors might operate in a terminally ill, stuporous-comatose patient and account for a spectacular revival that brought great peace not only to the patient but to his guilt-ridden, emotionally disturbed wife, and other members of his financially harassed family. The near-precise timing and clinical response were unusual. The patient's arousal and behavior answered the most urgent needs of his family. He psychophysiologically (and physically?) rose to the occasion. It is beyond the purpose of this report to speculate on various possible pathophysiological mechanisms, involving the interplay of emotion, subliminal and psi awareness, and extension, progression and regression of such factors as the tumor, edema and hemorrhage.

This patient's dramatic arousal is similar to that in the report[157] of an 11-year-old boy who was in a state of adrenocortical collapse and intelligibly echoed from the depths of coma the thoughts of his physician: "I live; therefore I am," with a profound statement for one so young: "Nothing is more important than life."

5
Possible Telesomatic Reactions

The psychosomatic significance of various illnesses is well established. This paper explores the possible telepathic mediation of psychosomatic or "telesomatic" reactions.

Under controlled laboratory conditions, using sensitive mathematical methods, telepathic communications have been demonstrated by J. B. Rhine[151] in America, S. G. Soal[206] in England, and others. Although many of the early investigators of telepathy were physicians, until the advent of psychoanalysis, psychiatry had relatively little to contribute to parapsychology. Since Freud there have been scattered psychodynamic studies.[21] Notwithstanding considerable conscious[50] and unconscious[126] resistance to this potentially revolutionary body of data, it is still a paradox that comparatively little investigation by psychiatrists has been undertaken. It has been suggested[158] that parapsychology would have more to offer psychiatry than *vice versa*.

In one of his earlier papers, Eisenbud[44] mentioned the likelihood "for a telepathic stimulus to occasion an asthmatic attack or any other set of physiological events." Although he asserted that he had "seen several examples of psychosomatic developments on a telepathic basis," he offered no examples. In a different detailed psychodynamic study[176], it was shown how a patient's incapacitating psychosomatic illnesses might have been induced (or at least strongly influenced) by a "sick" relationship with a telepathic mother. Examples in this same study and elsewhere[181] further show the tie-in of psychophysiologic factors and telepathy.

Despite Dean's laboratory experiments[20,19] and Cadaret's intriguing review,[11] little has appeared concerning the practical, clinical aspects: possible telesomatic reactions. To date these essentially parapsychologic studies emphasize (a) the use of physiologic measures to define conditions under which ESP occurs, and (b) physiologic measures used as means of registering ESP responses. I reported[184] a series of 504 presumed parent-child telepathic episodes showing many possible telesomatic and motor-acting-out responses.

In these, it looked as if the parent's or the child's thoughts caused somatic motor (or autonomic) reactions in sender or receiver. The usual criteria for telepathy are uniqueness, simultaneity, actual or symbolic equivalence of thought and feeling, and telepathic tracer effects. Often it can be shown how the presumed telepathic episode will often recur in an almost predictable manner when the psychodynamic-situational constellations are similar. Psychiatric study technics are involved in unconscious mechanisms, manifold nuances of interpersonal relations, and various trancelike states of altered consciousness. Both psychiatric and laboratory physiologic investigations suggest that telepathy offers an attractive hypothesis for the understanding of psychosomatic diseases. The following cases present some possible telesomatic reactions.

Case One

"Last night, for the first time in years, I had a severe toothache. I told my wife about it at 7 A.M. and shortly afterward made an appointment with my dentist. At 10 A.M. my mother phoned to say she was having an extraction that day. Her last extraction was years ago. No one in my family knew about mother's trouble. When I saw my dentist later that day there was neither discernible disease nor reason for my complaint. I have had no recurrence since then. Could I have picked up and somatized my mother's repressed anxiety over her trip to the dentist?"

Case Two

The 38-year-old father of two children was awarded custody of them following his divorce nine years ago. Although the wife had left him on occasion in the past, she always returned and never threatened to take the children. During his psychiatric interview he said, "Even today, I don't understand it. At the time of our divorce things were at the worst. I was scheduled to work on Saturdays. One Saturday I left the house at 6:30 A.M. and got a third of the way to work when I suddenly became very ill. I had abdominal pain, and the cramps were so severe I couldn't drive. I rolled out of the car but when I turned around to go home the pain stopped. Because of this I decided to start for work again, but once again (for the second time) the pain returned. I then decided to go home. By the time I got to the house I had no pain, headache, or perspiration. It wasn't until the next evening that I discovered my wife's packed suitcases. I had no awareness of this at the time. She would not leave if I were around. I later learned that she had intended to take the children. I think it was because of this fact that I had the attack. She was most annoyed that I came home and was underfoot."

In this example the patient's security was threatened. He might have tele-pathically picked up this threat by his somatic reaction. Through being forced to return home he saved his children. The pains left twice, but only upon his decision to return home.

Case Three

A women in her middle thirties with an old disability from poliomyelitis had been treated both in Holland and in the United States by the renowned Dutch healer,[146] Croiset the Clairvoyant.[214-216] Croiset asserted that he could influence muscular contractions: eversion, inversion, and dorsiflexion of the right foot. In a light trancelike state, he indicated the patient's appropriate muscular reaction by the direction of his outstretched hands. The patient's eyes were not on his hands. In fact, Croiset was in another room and it was impossible for the patient to see whether (and in what direction) he was "stimulating" her. Unfortunately it was also impossible for the observer to check precisely when and how Croiset was stimulating.

This American woman (who was in close rapport with Croiset) was seized with acute "fast heart rate, abdominal cramps, diarrhea" and malaise in Tar-rytown, New York. She connected her autonomic reaction "to Croiset" but did not fully understand it until four days later. At that time, following an interview with the physician, she learned that at the approximate time of her reaction Croiset had unexpectedly landed (from a paragnostic Australian crime-sleuthing trip) at John F. Kennedy Airport in a state of collapse, with severe abdominal pain and malaise. Although he was expected to arrive in America several days later than his actual arrival, this was not definite and was never confirmed.

The woman's somatic reaction was not related to any similar illness for any member of her family or friends. It can be conjectured that the woman's abdominal reaction and half-awareness of Croiset, which coincided with his acute distress and unexpected proximity, might have been telepathically me-diated—a way of telling her that the man upon whom she had pinned such high hopes for help was close by and in danger. And in turn, Croiset, alone in America and acutely ill, in his desperation, might have thought of his kind friend and patient with the old disability.

Case Four

A 10-year-old boy had a convulsion 5 years ago and nothing since. Because of this (plus an associated moderate, generalized dysrhythmia on the electro-encephalogram) he had had yearly tracings and had been on anticonvulsant drugs in the interim. On the morning of his annual electroencephalogram, he had his second seizure. Contrary to their usual practice, the parents did not tell their son that they had planned to bring him from Atlantic City to Montclair for the electroencephalogram. It was wondered, therefore, if these kind parents could, by their uneasiness, have triggered their son's seizure through subliminal, unconscious means, or possibly telepathic psychophysiologic stimuli. There was nothing unusual in the patient's immediate history to account for this seizure.

Case Five

A 13½-year-old girl with temporal lobe epilepsy was meticulously studied for 8½ years and reported by my collegue, Dr. B. A. Ruggieri.[157] My contact with the patient was limited to performing serial electroencephalograms. These all showed marked generalized dsyrhythmia and right temporal focal sharp-wave changes. Once a typical seizure occurred during the recording. Clinically the patient had hundreds of major and minor seizures and had been difficult to manage with drugs and psychotherapy. The latter was given for depressive reactions. During one of the sessions, telepathic and telesomatic exchanges occurred between the patient and Dr. Ruggieri. For example, Dr. Ruggieri experienced a "severe but momentary abdominal cramp. The thought went through my mind, 'I hope she does not get a spell,' since her convulsive disorder frequently manifested itself as abdominal epilepsy. I had experienced the cramp as my own but mentally associated to my patient's problems. Immediately thereafter this girl began to stare straight ahead and make swallowing movements. When it was over, she described her feelings: 'It felt as though my stomach was about to blow up.' Later when the daughter described this incident to the mother, the latter asked. 'Did you tell the Doctor you had this spell?' and the girl reportedly answered, 'I didn't have to, he sensed it'. "

Dr. Ruggieri continued, "One day, while I was talking alone with this girl's mother, I was surprised when she spontaneously told me that on several occasions through the years while away from her daughter she had sensed that her daughter was having a convulsion and, on checking the matter as carefully as she could, she had found that her daughter had indeed experienced a convulsive episode at that same time. From my interviews with the daughter it was apparent that she had some emotional problems with her mother. Repeatedly in the past the mother refused to see a psychiatrist for the benefit of her daughter if not herself. However, the mother's history and my own experiences with the patient made me wonder about the possibility of either the mother telepathically detecting her daughter's seizures, or telesomatically causing them."

Case Six

A young Army wife was unexpectedly hospitalized for threatened abortion. Her mother (who was 56 years of age and hundreds of miles away) developed uterine bleeding at the same time. The older woman's last menstrual period had occurred eight years previously. She thought this was unusual because six months before this episode she had had bleeding when her second daughter, who lived more than one hundred miles away (and had no immediate contact with her) went into labor. The third episode of unexpected uterine bleeding occurred while the older woman was in New Jersey. At that time, her first daughter was in California. She had given birth to her baby seven weeks before the expected date. The older woman was not immediately aware of the relationships between her three bleeding experiences and her two daughters. She told her physician at the time because they seemed to be such strange coincidences. Twenty months after the last episode of bleeding, the older woman had a massive hemorrhage. Uterine carcinoma was diagnosed and she had a successful hysterectomy. Her episodes of pathologic uterine bleeding coincided with major obstetrical changes in the lives of her two daughters and might have unconsciously directed the older woman's attention to her illness.

The two grandchildren who were associated with the odd bleeding had congenital anomalies, and the earlier (the first born) grandchild also had anomalies. Possibly the grandmother had not developed her carcinoma at this time. Of the five grandchildren born during this period, the only one free of anomalies was also the only one *not* associated with the grandmother's bleeding. The last born was after the grandmother's hysterectomy (and of course, her incapacity to respond with bleeding)—if there was any relationship at all. Detailed genetic investigation of both daughters and their families failed to uncover any reason for these four tragedies.

This woman's husband, a very successful businessman, came from a "telepathic" family and at times had himself been aware of his involvements in various telepathic episodes.

Case Seven

During his psychotherapy, a 36-year-old businessman had many physician-patient "telepathic" episodes. He had a sadomasochistic relationship with his alcoholic, hostile, competitive, domineering father, who was also his boss. After years of abuse, and threats of being fired or quitting, the patient surprised everyone by leaving his father's employ and seeking work elsewhere. He took great precautions so that his father would not know where he sought work and block him. Some prospective employers were doubtful about hiring him because of their knowledge of the father's precarious health, family loyalties, and so forth. Finally he obtained a new job at a marked increase in salary. Only his wife and the prospective new employer knew his secret. The new job involved much soul searching since it was with a competitor of his father's in a different state, hundreds of miles away, and would mean major changes in his life—the final manifest separation from the unhealthy destructive dependency on his father. He later learned that at the approximate time of his agonizing decision, and while awaiting the call from the new employer, his father had a second coronary thrombosis. The first such attack was nine years before. This event, so fortuitously timed, shifted all the complex relationships and at the "zero hour" the patient had a change of heart and returned to his family company. However, this time he was put in full charge, as his father was now forced, on his physician's advice, to retire. It can be wondered if the tyrannical father had an (unconscious) telepathic awareness of his son's major decision and responded somatically when no other response might have sufficed.

Case Eight

While receiving psychotherapy for a depressive reaction, a 33-year-old physicist had many "telepathic" episodes with his physician. He also had some presumably telepathic dreams. A late afternoon dream vividly portrayed almost all the specific, detailed (censored) circumstances of his physician's anxiety over an unanticipated trip to a New York airport to see the acutely ill Croiset. The other dream apparently detected in surprising detail his physician's daughter's surprise birthday gift of an old-fashioned fourposter bed and canopy. A third episode was the physician's waking from a sound sleep in the early hours of the morning by the physicist patient's telling him telepathically, "I'm alright now—had abcessed tooth-extracted." Earlier that day the patient telephoned the physician because of a toothache. His own dentist had previously examined him and told him there was nothing wrong with the tooth: the same advice he had received from a Midwestern dentist four months ago when he had a similar toothache. The physician advised his patient to see another dentist, and no further thought was given this until the veridical nocturnal episode.

In his sessions the physicist was aware of some of the face-to-face patient-physician telepathy and contrary to the usual custom, these communications were explored in treatment. Because of his interest in telepathy, one day the physicist participated as a subject, in one of Dean's well-controlled laboratory tests for telepathy.[18] The presumed episodes were monitored with the plethysmograph. On two separate occasions the physicist got attractive responses: pronounced transient tachycardia and change in vasoconstrictive states when a specific sender looked at a card saying (or symbolizing) "mother." It was hoped that with additional experiments a statistically significant result might be obtained. The patient had some deep-rooted problems with his mother. The telepathic response did not happen with other names.

During one of the experiments the successful sender was disturbed over some unanticipated extraneous sounds on his earphones. The patient, who was in a different part of the building and had neither earphones nor other connections with the sender, responded to this unpleasant intrusion in the same telepathic-physiologic way: "the biggest reaction . . . ever seen. It leads us to try better." With a different "cold, sourpuss sender" there was no evidence for telepathy.

In therapy the patient became aware of the superficial similarities between the successful sender and his mother. Both had a gushy, smiling effusiveness. Following the second successful telepathic-physiologic tests the physicist became depressed. He did not know why until therapy, when he recognized that he repressed his rage toward the successful sender who risked his life, on the trip back from the laboratory. The sender, in the physicist's opinion, was a reckless automobile driver. This dissociation of the sender's reckless driving was similar to the physicist's pattern of repressing all anger toward his mother's analogous behaviour.

This interesting laboratory and clinical datum justifies the speculation that with the passage of time various psychosomatic states could develop or be precipitated where there is an unhealthy parent-child telepathic rapport. That might apply, for example, to possible paroxysmal tachycardia, hypertension, hyperthyroidism, acute peptic ulcer, ulcerative colitis, and so forth. As indicated in the example of the physicist, all commonly recognized communications and those that occur on an unconscious, nonverbal basis could, *via* telepathic mediation, be vastly complicated by somatic shortcircuiting.

From these examples, it would appear that telesomatic reactions are part of a continuum of interhuman relatedness—physiologic expressions of telepathically sent thoughts, behavior, and affect. The process can be partial for any one of these areas or (as in these examples) complex. The telesomatic reaction occurs on an unconscious level and is almost totally out of the participants' awareness. Unless the data were carefully collected and scrutinized with a telepathic hypothesis in mind, the event could be entirely missed. Identification of telesomatic reactions is facilitated by the tracer effects which appropriately tag the events. Since the telesomatic reaction happened out of awareness clinically and also in one cited well-controlled laboratory test, it can be supposed that it might occur much more often than is commonly thought. Hence, it is worthy of serious consideration from both the practicing clinician and the researcher.

SUMMARY AND CONCLUSION

The hypothesis for telepathic mediation of psychosomatic (telesomatic) reactions is illustrated by eight case reports. This interesting area of investigation is thought to have much potential and theoretical value for the understanding of the cause and treatment of psychosomatic illnesses, pain reactions, and so forth.

CLINICAL STUDIES ON TELESOMATIC REACTIONS

In a previous study[180] the concept of telepathically induced psychosomatic reactions was reviewed and eight possible examples were presented. Since little clinical data have been reported on this subject in the interim, this report presents additional examples which might be of interest to the general physician.

In recent years there has been a revival of interest in psychic healing, the use of hypnotism, and acupuncture in the treatment of various ailments.[63,220] Although there are many popular accounts of well-known healers and mediums who have devoted their efforts to the alleviation of a variety of diseases, there has been a dearth of controlled observations by physicians. Eisenbud,[49] in his review of the British psychiatrist West's *Eleven Lourdes Miracles*, concluded that "because of the untrustworthy nature of the evidence, one can never know for certain whether they [unusual healings] actually did or did not [occur]."

In carefully controlled statisically analyzed studies, the physiologist Grad *et al.*[93] discerned psychic healing effect on induced wounds in rats, and in related experiments Grad[94] found a significant effect on the growth of barley seeds. In a different vane, Bagchi,[1] a neurophysiologist, has given much fascinating material on possible paranormal physiological effects observed in India.

Although there have been popular accounts of alleged unusual effects by psychic surgeons like the controversial Dr. Tony (e.g., Harold Sherman's *Wonder Healers of the Phillippines,* Los Angeles, De Vorss & Co., 1967) of the Phillippines, there have been no critical studies published by physicians, to my knowledge. My interviews of some physicians who had witnessed such unorthodox treatments yielded conflicting opinions. Recently I studied two people who had lived in Dr. Tony's home and had been "helped" by him. After reviewing their photographic color slides and other data, it seemed that these were clinical examples, although handicapped by difficulties, which merited first-hand investigation. For example, one woman, who was intelligent, honest, and free of relevant psychopathology, had pictures of the painless "psychic" removal of her obstructing, chronic nasal polyps.

Another celebrated psychic healer was the late Arigo, in Brazil, who has been studied by Puharich.[148] Hopefully Puharich will soon publish his detailed observations in medical journals.

Perhaps the reasons that physicians approach alleged psychic healings with such great caution are: (1) the dangers of fraud, superstition, quackery, and psychopathology; (2) the poor quality of the reports, with lack of suitable controls; and (3) their own experiences in practice, where they can observe occasional instances of "spontaneous" or transference cures for many diseases and psychosomatic reactions which are as wondrous as the "cures" of the popular accounts. Thus, the criteria for the alleged "Healer's cures" must conform to a high standard before they can be recognized as worthy of study. For example, the psychodynamic aspects of pain make it an ideal symptom for psychic alleviation by laymen and physicians. The subjective response of pain has a diverse etiology which can be relieved by placebos, suggestion, psychotherapy, drugs, surgery, and various combinations of subliminal and possible telepathic influences.

Although suffering from the drawbacks of all anecdotal material, Henry Gross,[176] and Jacques Romano,[181] apparently had the ability to often relieve pain that was refractive to orthodox measures. They also performed healings throughout their careers. Mrs. Krystal,[176] an insulin-dependent diabetic, had illness-related, presumed telepathic, episodes between her physicians and herself. Many of the events in a physician-patient's[176] life and his physical deterioration were presumable telepathically detected (or telesomatically induced?) by his "sensitive" mother.

In the scrapbooks covering his 60-year career, Joseph Dunninger,[24] had many testimonials from physicians acknowledging his successful hypnotic treatments in a hospital and clinic affiliated with Columbia University College of Physicians and Surgeons. Perhaps one overlooked reason that some hypnotists like paragnosts Jacques Romano and Joseph Dunninger were sometimes spectacularly successful whereas others were not, was the existence of the unconscious telepathic (telesomatic) effect. Furthermore, Dunninger also recalled many telepathic experiences with his mother, who had syncope (or temporal lobe epilepsy?) for many years. Wherever he was traveling, he invariably picked up her seizures. In some cases his awareness of them may have been responsible for his obtaining first aid and saving his mother's life. Study of examples of parent-child telepathy[184] might yield many clues for understanding telesomatic reactions.

In *The Curious World of Twins*[88] there are some extraordinary examples of unusual coincidences or possible telepathy and telesomatic reactions. Moreover, it is not unusual to read in the papers, or rarely note in practice, how a devoted husband and wife, although separated by distance, die within hours of each other—as if they had possible psi awareness of what was happening to their mates.

A simpler, practical approach to the intriguing problem of psychic healing might be through the back door, where the complex variables that exist in healing can be curtailed: that is, through the study of presumably telepathically precipitated illnesses. Eisenbud[44] and Jung[79] clearly foresaw this fascinating possibility. The following examples illustrate this.

1. NURTURE

After a woman gave birth to her first child she was dry. Because of this and other reasons the baby was cared for by her sister, who lived miles away. However, when the infant started incessant crying and screaming, the mother, at her home, developed sufficient milk. Although coincidence and other factors might be considered, I wonder if this could be an example where the baby's hungry screams may have precipitated his mother's necessary telesomatic response. For her part, the mother might also have been influenced by an unconscious sibling rivalry, namely, resentment over her failure to produce milk and over the fact that her infant had to be mothered by her sister.

2. FOOD PSYCHIC-DYNAMICS

A new waitress at the restaurant was given a verbal order for stuffed peppers but of the many items on the menu she brought me "the incorrect," but telepathically correct and unconsciously wished for, Salisbury steak. When I asked her about the error, she offered excuses not unlike posthypnotic rationalizations.

This example from the psychic-dynamics of everyday life might be extended to pathological mechanisms where a mother's deep-seated confusion about food in reference to feeding her infant can be telepathically carried over into later life where the child might develop eating problesm, obesity, or other conditions. For example, possibly some cases of obesity are refractive to treatment and understanding because the telepathic hypothesis is overlooked. That is, the early parent-child confusion and a destructive, subtle, permissive attitude for food might be caused by the mother's telepathic-subliminal sending of her secret, unconscious wishes to her child which are contrary to her conscious thoughts and statements. "I don't want you nibbling all the time" (while her mouth waters for the delicious chocolate cake in the icebox). By analogy, the late Adlelaide Johnson[155] in her conferences

presented data showing how some instances of obsessive-compulsive vascil-
lation and indecisiveness might be ascribed to the mother's confusion in
handling her child during the habit-training period. The child develops guilt,
not for the act, but toward his parent because he does not do what the parent wants him to do (unconsciously and telepathically).

3. PREGNANCY

During a quiet interlude of a psychotherapeutic session with a young woman
who had an hysterical character neurosis, I was startled when she blurted
out, "I predict a boy for you." When asked why she said this, she insisted, "I
am positive you said your wife is pregnant!" I was dumbfounded since I had
said nothing at all, and I was not aware of any such event, and her comment
was completely out of context (and unwanted). While I was wondering if
this could be telepathy, the patient continued, "Maybe I'm getting to be a
medium—I associated to the last time *I* was pregnant—I knew I didn't hear
your voice coming out of the walls. I am quite crushed. How ridiculous. I
feel I'll go back to my concealed tomb. You don't want me—telepathy interests me. When my son hurt his hand and when my mother died I (telepathically) knew it."

At the conclusion of the session I jokingly mentioned this obtrusive foreign-body thought to my wife, and was shocked to learn that indeed she was
pregnant. The patient discovered my wife's secret and perhaps showed her
oedipal ambivalence towards myself and others in her life as well as jealousy, and resentment toward my wife and myself.

4. DIABETES MELLITUS

While at home Mr. K. was very upset because he felt that something horrible
had happened to his 20-year-old diabetic son who was hospitalized in a
semiprivate room. Against his better judgment, the father felt compelled to
phone the hospital at 8:15 A.M. His premonition was correct even though
the patient in the adjacent bed answered the phone and said, "Joey is all-
right." However, the father insisted that this was not the case and that the
nurses should immediately waken Joey. It was then discovered that Joey was
in insulin coma which, as was subsequently learned, must have developed at
3:00 A.M., when, in error, he was given an overdose of insulin. This situation had not happened to Joey before in the hospital. But the father, on several previous occasions had had experiences where he might have
telepathically apprehended his son's impeding hypoglycemic reactions. For
example, once Joey's father and mother were in line at a New York theater,
many miles from home, when the father suddenly informed his wife that

they must leave immediately and telephone their daughter to get help for Joey, who was in trouble. This was shown to be the case. The father also recalled possible telepathic and telesomatic episodes with his identical twin brother during World War II.

5. PAIN AND THE ESCAPE

A middle-aged woman came to her psychotherapeutic session and said: "I saw stones and twigs while walking down the street and said to myself, 'Nellie, be careful.' I was trying to figure out why I was worrying about walking; I looked down on the path and wondered why my leg bothered me. I said to myself, 'What could happen if I hurt my leg and couldn't walk? This (fear) is silly.' When I got home my [teenage] son phoned to say that he had badly injured his leg on the glass coffee table (and had to have it sutured)."

This patient recalled other possible telepathic examples with her schizophrenic son. Once, during her treatment in New Jersey, I learned how shocked she was over the morning newspaper's headline of a "Russian roulette" murder. She was acutely fearful that her son, who was then hospitalized in Florida, would "commit a horrible crime like his best friend had just done (who murdered his brother)—there but for the grace of God goes Billy." Billy might have picked up his mother's horror that he would lose control of himself and do something "wrong" like his friend, for, at the time of the mother's panic over him, he escaped from the mental hospital where he had been doing well for an extended period of time. In a phone call to me, the hospital confirmed this unexpected and ticklish situation, for they took great pride in the care they gave their patients and it was a long time since anyone had escaped from the closed-locked division. Could this mother have telepathically sent her sudden fear that something horrible would happen to her son and in this way have given him the impetus for losing control of himself and escaping?

6. MARITAL HEART FLUSTER

When a 58-year-old physician, Dr. I came for his psychotherapeutic session, he said that six days previously he became acutely ill with an attack of auricular fibrillation (heart arrythmia). He had to take the drug quinidine every hour. He developed side effects of dizziness and diarrhea and his cardiologist friend advised him to quit drinking and smoking and ordered him to bed for two days. While fearful of dying, and home in bed, Dr. I received a telephone call from his estranged wife, whom he hadn't spoken to since her birthday, three months earlier and before that he hadn't any contact with her for several months. He was curious about why she had called him at this distressful time, and in particular, why in her conversation with him she beat around the bush. For example, she asked Dr. I how to prepare truffles, and she also asked Dr. I how his friend the cardiologist was. Since the cardiologist whom she seldom mentioned in their marriage before, never got along with Dr. I's wife, he felt this question was odd and it sent chills up and down his spine. The cardiologist, who was divorced himself and hated Dr. I's wife, had advised him never to marry her. To the best of Dr. I's knowledge, it was impossible for his estranged wife who lived at a distance from him, to know about his acute heart arrythmia, and these factors were born out in other ways. For example, later that same day the wife telephoned again and the tape-recording answering machine took her message. Dr. I, rather than have his sleep disturbed, and being curious about his wife's rare call—two in one day— returned her call and became quite suspicious because she was out of character by being cozy and friendly toward him. He knew that his wife couldn't know about his poor health since that was a secret shared between his friend the cardiologist, to whom he referred patients, and himself. It was imperative for his own practice as well as any possible divorce action that no one should know of his sudden distress.

When asked about possible precipitating factors for his heart arrythmia— the first in five years, and only the third in his life—he initially ascribed it to the drinking and smoking, which upon detailed questioning was no different than his usual pattern. Then it was apparent to him that there was a shift in his relationship toward his wife. Rather than being submissive and depressed as he was before his attack, he became angry. He could no longer forgive himself for marrying her and ignoring the advice of his cardiologist and his own best judgment. He recalled all the things he had done for his wife and her children by her previous marriage, and the little to nothing that she and her family had done for him. For example, he remembered that the last time she had seen her, 5 months earlier, when he drove to her summer home on Labor Day, rather than greeting him and affecting a reconciliation, she threw him out of the house at midnight and he had to drive a long distance, on crowded holiday highways, exposed to drunken drivers, etc.

It can be conjectured that his wife might have telepathically tuned in on her husband's heart crisis since she, still being married to him, was the beneficiary of his estate, and by re-establishing contact at this time she was exploiting his precarious situation for her own good. However, it can also be wondered if the wife might have telepathically apprehended her husband's shift from resignation and depression to anger, and his decision to go through with a divorce—all radical changes in his stance which affected her interests—and precipitated her counter reaction: a wish to get even and a need to restore the status quo of his dependency upon her.

Could his wife's possible telepathic awareness of her husband's plight have stirred up her own thinly veiled ambivalent, destructive wishes—coming in for the kill—and stirring up more stress than he could handle and bringing about the telesomatic solution: his incapacitation with the cardiac seizure?

In addition to the superficially outlined psychopathology, one might wonder about the possible psi talents for Dr. I which might have sensitized him for this cardiac seizure. Once, in a previous session, the physician-patient remarked that in his home in Europe, as a boy, he acted as a medium for seances attended by his parents and relatives. He also had some telepathic episodes during his psychotherapy, and shortly after the heart arrythmia he reported an alarming experience. He received a phone call from a former girlfriend, a married woman from whom he hadn't heard in a long time. It was arranged that they would have a clandestine meeting in a parking lot, and that he would then take her out for a drink. She agreed and said that she was in a public phone booth on a highway, only five minutes away. Dr. I had to be careful because he was fearful his estranged wife would find out about his girlfriend and the divorce action would be jeopardized. And he was also concerned about his married girlfriend's welfare. Hardly did he hang up than the phone rang again, and an unrecognized man's voice said: "You talked to my wife. Listen to me, I know you'll see her in a few minutes." The man repeated the message and then started screaming. In his psychotherapeutic session Dr. I interjected: "My heart stopped. He was saying the truth but without any definition. I never met him and didn't know who he was. I dropped the phone back on it's cradle. It rang again. I put the tape recording machine on and it recorded his strange voice again—neither masculine nor feminine. I jumped in the car and drove to where I was to meet my girlfriend. When I told her about the call, and asked if it could be her husband, she said it was impossible. To prove that it was not her husband, we drove to my home, from where she called her husband and I listened in on an extension." Subsequent contacts with the girlfriend also confirmed that the mysterious caller was not her husband. Dr. I was completely flustered.

Perhaps his experience is similar to the not unheard of situation where a "wrong" phone call is received by somebody of the same name as the person being thought of, or sought at the time, and yet not the person in question—possible nominal telepathy. In Dr. I's case the match was such an extraordinary coincidence that it makes on wonder about the possibility of telepathic nexus—Dr. I (and his girlfriend?) had so much anxiety over his forbidden actions that he, a natural paragnost, broadcast his indiscretions and nearly brought about his ruin. Dr. I, apparently by displacement, was the recipient of a "wrong number" call from an infuriated husband at the moment of his planned illicit tête-à-tête with his girlfriend. Further examples of this possible telepathic, and at times possible telekinetic, telephone effect and related paranormal audio tape experiments are further explored elsewhere.[157,200]

II: PSYCHIATRIC EXAMPLES OF PSYCHIC-DYNAMICS

6
Built-in Controls and Postulates for the Telepathic Event

Fundamental to the understanding of telepathy as it occurs in the psycho-therapeutic doctor-patient relationship are the criteria for the telepathic event.[37,39,44,126] Despite careful documentation of the supposed telepathic event, with its similarity and near-simultaneity of thought content, its uniqueness and the identifying tracer concepts, certain objections are frequently raised. These include inadequate observation, coincidence, similar doctor-patient thought-affect responses to subliminal stimuli, and lack of discernment for the subtle, unconsciously determined associational processes. These necessary criticisms may have caused some of the psychiatric literature on telepathic events in psychotherapy to seem extremely prolix.[21] Indeed, presumed telepathic events are often obscured in pages of apologia to prove whether there actually was a telepathic event, instead of being fully and dynamically explored.

Thus, the problem of what factors might provide a suitable milieu for telepathic rapport, and might augment or retard the telepathic process, is left in limbo, and the study of telepathy via clinical methods can easily become discouraging and stagnant. The reader of such articles on telepathy could understandably become perplexed and confused with often boring, quasi-obsessional details.

For the past 10 years (1955–1965), the writer (B.E.S.) has made firsthand psychiatric investigations of several gifted paragnosts. In the course of these studies he learned a technique of unmasking psychic (mostly telepathic) events as they occurred in psychotherapy and daily living. From apparently only occasional telepathic occurrences in the years 1945–1955, which were not particularly heeded or were brushed aside as coincidences, the writer from 1955–1965 had learned to recognize and on occasion presumably "send" telepathic thoughts.

During the 1955–1965 span, when 2013 patients were seen in psychiatric consultation and many subsequently received short-term or prolonged psychotherapy, 1443 telepathic events have been recorded. In everyday life involving the writer's two children, ages 9 and 7, his wife, and himself, 542 telepathic events have been noted. Also during this period some of the writer's physician colleagues have "learned," through discussions of telepathy, a similar ability to recognize telepathic events. These physicians have contributed experiences from their own families and their patients.

Most of the presumed telepathic data for the writer and his friends meet the criteria as described in the literature. However, the sheer mass of presumed telepathic data and the apparent ability to develop modest telepathic talents in oneself and others who hitherto had seemingly not possessed such ability still do not fully answer the criticism concerning the validity of a presumed telepathic event.

In select instances, one possible way of answering such criticism might be the research method of collaborative psychiatric investigation.[104,201] In this multilateral technique the patient and several members of his family are studied concurrently by separate highly skilled physicians over varying periods of time. During the course of psychotherapy the therapists meet frequently to compare all the data about their patients. In this way many previously inexplicable psychopathological reactions can be fully explained, and, furthermore, predictions of future behavior can often be made with uncanny accuracy. Although such a refined method of obtaining all the details of interpersonal and intrapersonal communications for an entire family is more desirable, for this particular application it is not only impractical but would still probably not provide sufficient information to "prove" or "disprove" a presumed telepathic event.

I

A built-in clinical control in the study of a telepathic episode is the finding that the experient* will telepathically respond in a predicatable manner to certain stimuli at varying times. For instance, a 3-year-old girl gave identical responses to her mother's and father's silent thoughts at different times.[173] And in a series of psychodynamic drawing experiments in telepathy[174] it was noted that "in many of the instances described, when very similar targets were used at widely varying times, the responses given were also similar to the earlier percepts." In the drawing study further built-in controls were af-

*Heywood, R.: ESP: A Personal Memoir, in a footnote p. 35 quoting Professor Dodds who suggested the word rather than "percipient." (E. P. Dutton & Co. Inc., New York 1964).

forded by the highly specific response to the spontaneous use of a red crayon rather than a pencil or a pen.

Further evidence for built-in controls is afforded by the recurrent type of "errors" made in some clinical telepathic experiments. For instance, in thinking of a card test the experient will often confuse the visually similar numbers 6 and 9 (upside down 6), 3 and 8, and the phonetically similar ace and eight. This is such a common "error" that upon ocassion a young girl has learned to correct herself by giving the second choice: e.g., the 9 instead of the first-called 6. As another example of built-in controls, Jacques Romano[181] would often astound his audience by not only correctly calling the card the experient thought of but the alternative card he first had in mind. Also, if the experient was instructed to think of a particular deceased person, Romano would amaze his audience by telling the experient many facts not only about the person that he had in mind but also about the first person he thought of. These so-called "errors" can be quite meaningful and give clues to the telepathic process, which has similarities to memory mechanisms.

The modus operandi of these so-called telepathic "errors" is also quite familiar to Joseph Dunninger,[24] and still further support is provided by many of Professor Tenhaeff's shrewd observations.[214,215] He has brilliantly shown how some so-called "errors" produced by the paragnost in his attempted solution of various crimes are really parapsychological successes. Professor Tenhaeff also notes that some of his paragnosts "specialize" in certain types of crimes, for which they have a built-in psychopathological sensitivity. For crimes out of their range of sensitivity they have no particular telepathic prowess.

Thus, support for built-in telepathic controls is provided by the oft-noted fact that the professional mentalist can to some degree develop his telepathic abilities in a way completely harmonious with his purpose, the paragnost who works on various crimes has his particular flair, the outstanding laboratory experient can achieve striking statistical success in calling cards, and in a manner appropriate to his occupation a psychiatrist can develop particular telepathic abilities.

The following case from psychotherapy illustrates some aspects of built-in telepathic controls.

A young businessman, a bachelor, sought psychiatric help because of anxiety and extreme shyness with women. Part of the patient's detached character defenses could be ascribed to his relationship with a very hostile, competitive father. Throughout the patient's formative years his father was preoccupied with business and was seldom at home. The father, a self-made man who always worked long hours, unfavorably compared his son to himself. The patient's mother, who was partly blind, was neglected and ridiculed by the father. She had an ungratifying marital relationship and confided all her intimacies and problems to her son. He had to cater to his mother and repress all his rage toward her (and his father). Possibly as a consequence of these relationships with his parents, the patient, an only child, was quite socially withdrawn, distrustful of other people, and particularly frightened of the opposite sex. This attitude was apparent in the patient's transference to his physician in many of the earlier, twice-weekly psychotherapeutic sessions, during which only five telepathic events occurred prior to the 45th session.*

The night before the 45th psychotherapeutic session the writer (B. E. S.) was dining and had a cocktail with a colleague, N. B. The writer was quite happy to visit with his friend N. B. because of a trying day noteworthy for two traumatic events. First, a paper of his on telepathy was rejected again. Rather than accept "defeat" the writer felt more than ever in an "I'll show the world" mood. Second, the writer had told his friend N. B. about the odious necessity of setting very strict limits on Britt Marie, the Swedish mother's helper for his children. Although Britt Marie was engaged to a boy in Sweden, she wanted to have fun with American playboys. The writer, who felt morally responsible for Britt Marie, tried to make light of the situation that could be dangerous for her (and the writer) by jokingly telling N. B., "I'd like to send Britt Marie a dozen roses from Sweden and say they are from her boyfriend to remind her of her vows."

Also in the course of the evening the writer told N. B. of a previous experience with traveling clairvoyance that involved a patient N. B. had referred to him. This former patient and the current bachelor patient were very similar in their temperament and psychopathology. While describing the earlier traveling clairvoyance experience to his colleague, the writer sat back and once again tried to see in his mind's eye what people would flash before him.

Later that evening, when the writer returned from the restaurant to his home and signed in with his answering service, he was stunned to learn that at the approximate time of his joking reference to Britt Marie, her fiancé had telephoned her from Sweden, for no apparent reason. It was felt that it could have been a long-distance telepathic episode because of the specific psychodynamics which beautifully served the needs of Britt, her fiancé, the writer and his family (triangle).

The following morning began with a surprise, for the bachelor patient opened his 45th session with: "I was talking to a date last night and strange things happened. You [B. E. S.] appeared as an apparition at 9:30 [approximately time of narration to N. B.]. I fantasied, does he want me as a son? The apparitions mean I'm reaching a point of progress when these things

---

*In the writer's experience with most patients if some telepathic events do not occur in the early sessions of treatment, he doubts the strength of the transference and the patient's unconscious motivation for help.

must come out—I've never had apparitions in the past—the apparition was over the girl's shoulder [patient dining in New York City]. She is a divorcée and intellectually stimulating. I have a feeling of comfort in communicating with her. The apparition came and went two or three times. I had only one cocktail and some wine but I was not high, and I never had apparitions before with it [alcohol]!"

It seemed plausible that the occurrence of the apparition was quite suitable for both the patient's and the physician's needs. It related to the physician's two splitting traumas. For after the rejection of his paper on telepathy he was motivated to show the unbelieving world and after an unpleasant scene with Britt Marie he was party to a complex, triangular telepathic event between Sweden and America. Furthermore, the apparitional quality of the experience was specifically and spontaneously related to a previous success of traveling clairvoyance involving a patient similar to the bachelor.

The patient's needs were well served by the spectacular projection (visual hallucination) of the apparition of his physician. The telepathic triangle of baby-sitter, fiancé, and doctor corresponded to the triangle of patient, girl friend, and doctor. The apparition of the physician at a critical moment in the patient's life could have symbolically substituted a good father, the physician, for the past introjected, hostile one and aided the patient in his attempt to master his anxiety. The patient in his needs complemented his physician's scanning for a suitable subject to accomplish his emotionally overdetermined purposes of traveling clairvoyance. Both experiences occurred late at night and might have been physiologically synergized by the moderate use of alcohol.

In subsequent psychotherapeutic hours, the 45th session and the apparition loomed as a crisis point in the patient's treatment, for it heralded a more intense transference. The patient, who had hitherto been most cautious in discussing events of great poignancy in his life, became more open.

The next major psychic episode occurred the night before the 65th session when the writer, during sleep, had spontaneous traveling clairvoyance. He could recall only the subjective sensation of leaving the body and traveling. This was the first time this had happened to the writer since this patient began his treatment. This experience seemingly correlated with the writer's 6-year-old daughter's waking up at 2 A.M. screaming. There was no apparent reason for this unusual coincidence. However, because the writer was unaware of what events in his life might have precipitated the experience, it was conjectured that he reacted to an oedipal nightmare of his daughter and that she initiated the train of events.

When the patient came for the 65th session, he said: "The night before last (the time of the writer's traveling clairvoyance) I awoke with a real start. Somebody was in the room—I was really frightened and jumped out of bed.

It took me more than an hour to get back to bed. There was another person by the bed, a man, a robber intruding over me, about to smash me. I had to fight or run until I realized where I was."

It seemed that this episode had features similar to the cluster of telepathic experiences surrounding the 45th session. However, in contrast to the anxiety-allaying aspects of the 45th session, the affects for patient and doctor as brought out in the 65th session were of unpleasantness and fear.

The patient's material during the 65th session and the immediately preceding hours contained examples of his mother's seductive comments on "sex rings." He was becoming very upset over his dawning awareness of his own repressed anger at his mother. His growing ability to express anger made him recoil in fear lest he be punished in retaliation for such thoughts. However, it was felt that this, the fear of expressing anger, was only a background factor. The specific precipitating incident of the patient's projection of the terrifying unknown phantom prowler [or in such a complex transaction, possibly the physician's apprehension of the patient's distress and a reaction with his daughter or other permutations] was that the patient was acutely primed for the unusual and uncanny. In his company's golf tournament earlier in the day, prior to the experience of the phantom prowler, the patient obtained a hole-in-one for the first time in his life. All at once the shy, retiring bachelor, who seldom played golf and who was relatively unknown in his company, received much acclaim for his "luck." Rather than bask in such glory, he shunned all the attention lest he be envied his success (hated by hostile, competitive father) as in his earlier life situation. The patient projected his fears, as in the previous example of the apparition where another triangle (oedipus situation) existed, but this time his experience was also telescoped with the experiences of the physician and his daughter, who with the patient composed the triangle. All three parties to the event were suddenly awakened from their sleep, an optimal time of physiological readiness for such experiences.

The third similar presumed telepathic episode with built-in clinical controls* occurred on the night before the 163rd session. That evening the writer's colleague N. B. paid a surprise visit for the first time in more than a year and a half. The writer was amused because he had just been discussing N. B. with a mutual friend, and he concluded that N. S. telepathically summoned (A). N. B.'s possible telepathic involvement became more apparent when he stated the purpose of his visit. After asking for the use of the writer's copying machine for some routine invoices, N. B. came to the point of his visit by mentioning a patient of his who, at that time during the sum-

---

*For the reader's convenience, each relevant psychically charged tracer event in the following constellation will be lettered in the text.

mer season, had won 20 daily-double horse races (B).* N. B., who knew of
the writer's interests in psychic research and specifically of the traveling
clairvoyance experience with his former patient and the more recent apparitional experience with the bachelor patient, was bubbling over with details
about this "lucky" woman and some of her strange characteristics.

Another catalyzing motivation for N. B.'s visit that evening was his noting
recent newspaper headlines about the writer's father, who had bought one
lottery ticket on the New Hampshire Sweepstakes many months previously
and had won a top prize (C). N. B. and the writer joked about such freak
luck and dilated on the chance probabilities of winning a lottery or correctly
predicting horse races. This was difficult because both N. B. and the writer
(like his father) did not bet on horse races, let alone attend them, and they
were totally unfamiliar with the vocabulary of the race track.

While still in a mirthful mood, N. B. and the writer reserved the strongest
guffaws for the name of the horse that won the race for the writer's father:
Roman Brother. For N. B. knew of the "pact" between the extraordinary
jolly paragnost Jacques *Romano* (D) and the writer. If anyone could come
back from death it would be Jacques Romano, a man who had performed
many spectacular telepathic feats throughout the years and who even joked
about breaking the bank at Monte Carlo. Also on one occasion N. B. was
such a highly successful subject for one of Jacques Romano's "spirit read-
ings" that some members of the audience actually screamed at the shock of
an apparent transfiguration of N. B.'s deceased father (E).

A third presumed psychic tracer event that evening was also compounded
with the horse-racing situations. It pertained to a colleague of N. B.'s and
the writer. Once this colleague, before the writer knew anything personal
about him, was the subject for a most remarkable "spirit reading" by
Jacques Romano. When the writer drove Romano from New York to Montclair earlier in the day, he was told several of the details of the reading that
was to take place later that night. After such a demonstration this colleague
described an unusual, apparent precognitive dream (F) in which he foresaw
all the winners of a whole day's horse races. He followed up his dream by
going to the track, placing his bets and pyramiding his winnings exactly as
he had dreamed it. This man, in all other ways a skeptical surgeon, also told
the writer about many lifelong telepathic experiences with patients, but the
uncanny experience of the precognitive dream became the focal point of
friendship between this colleague and the writer. In the surgeon's final illness he once intimated to the writer that he would attempt to contact him
(after death) if he could. For several poignant reasons he would have had

---

*The writer subsequently confirmed this information from interviews with this person and
others. Furthermore, while under his observation she continued her successes and won 44 daily-
doubles for the season. She is under study.

strong motivation to do this. Although the writer never told this colleague, he wondered about an unusual subjective experience of traveling clairvoyange (G) that involved his friend shortly before his death.

The writer thought no more of the experiences with the surgeon friend until a few months after his death when the aforementioned turn of events dramatically directed his attention to horse racing again. Although the unusual circumstances surrounding the horse race were intellectually dismissed as coincidences, the writer was emotionally intrigued with the farfetched symbolism of the horse race and the possible communication from Jacques Romano or his surgeon friend. It was thought plausible that if coming back were possible, there might be many obstacles and difficulties so that even what seemed on the surface ridiculous coincidences and the like should be scrutinized.

While discussing these strange events and coincidences with his friend N. B., the writer was also quite perplexed about an unexpected recent upswing in his telepathic researches. For the very day before his father's horse won the sweepstakes, the writer met with Dr. Ralph S. Banay who, unaware of the extent of the past rejections of the writer's telepathic studies, discussed with him the possibility of devoting an issue of *Corrective Psychiatry* and *The Journal of Social Therapy* to the subject of medicine and psychic research. Quite surprised and enormously elated with this completely unanticipated opportunity to contribute an article on telepathy to a psychiatric journal (H), the writer did not wish to jeopardize such an assignment by telling Dr. Banay what was pending the next day with the horse race. He reasoned that if he did, Dr. Banay would certainly have ample reason to throw up his hands and conclude that psychic research, which is so often a frustrating hodgepodge of unusual events and coincidences, of the real and the unreal, could not be worthy of publication in his psychiatric journal.*

Thus on the eve of the 163d session with the bachelor patient the writer

---

*No matter how well the process is "learned," not infrequently the most relevant telepathic thoughts are dissociated from until retrospectively recognized. Such a pertinent thought on the rim of consciousness but completely dissociated from until the preparation of this manuscript concerned a close friend of Dr. Banay's and the writer's: the Rev. Timothy V. A. Kennedy, M.D., a priest-psychiatrist, who died while attending the Ecumenical Congress during the year. Through his abiding interest and practical suggestions, Dr. Kennedy encouraged these psychic researches. He discussed and read many of the protocols; and although his death was unexpected, from many previous conversations and mutual experiences with patients it seemed that he, if survival was possible, would attempt to communicate. On one of his last postal cards, Dr. Kennedy wrote about his recent visit where he was "seeing Padre Pio the stigmatist" (Winowska, M.: Das wahre Gesicht des Pater Pio, pp. 149, Paul Pattloch Verlag/Aschaffenburg, 1961). Dr. Kennedy and the writer often discussed various alleged psychic abilities of Pater Pio (I) and once considered traveling to Italy to study him. The odd point of this is a previous, rather striking telepathic communication, purportedly from the late Dr. Kennedy, and this event related to the symbolism of Roman Brother, the winning horse. To the writer, a Protestant, Roman Brother was the perfect symbol for Dr. Kennedy (J).

was excited over several new developments in psychic matters. Once again the specific motif of traveling clairvoyange was apparent and overdetermined.

In his 161st psychotherapeutic session the patient reported that since his last session his grandmother had died. In his 162nd session the patient described the funeral, which took place on the weekend. He saw his parents for the first time in several weeks and became incensed over his mother's martyrdom. She "had to pay all the expenses for her mother's funeral rather than share them with her poor baby brother. Grandmother always gave him money until he was 40." Along with his anger at his mother for her masochistic permissiveness toward her shiftless brother, and his more acute awareness of the undermining effects of his mother's similar role with his hostile, aggressive father, the patient became anxious and fearful of a retaliatory expression of anger. His behavior toward his mother had shifted, and it seemed as though a new kind of relationship was forming.

In his 163d psychotherapeutic session, the morning after the aforementioned galaxy of psychically charged events in his physician's life and the first session after the shift in his relationship with his mother, he reported: "As I climbed into bed I had an apparition of someone starting to fight—a large black figure—fear of looking—I'd be shot."

For the third time, the concatenation of spontaneous, psychically exciting events in the writer's life was unexpectedly related to specific events, fears, and needs in the patient's life. These highly charged experiences for both patient and physician, which might have been traumatically crystallized in the episode of the phantom prowler, were quite similar to the specific events surrounding the apparition reported in the 45th session.

Possibly the death motif interwoven in the physician's psychic tracers as well as in the patient's real life accounted for the terrifying aspects of his experience. As in the previous episodes, this event occurred late at night when thresholds are lowered and a moderate amount of alcohol might have unleashed some of the ecstatic fantasizing aspects.

Another cluster of possible telepathic events in connection with the apparition and kindred experiences occurred one night several months later. While the writer was struggling for the best way to organize for publication the notes of these telepathic transactions, he commented to his wife, "I wonder how this (notes on apparitional experience) will be picked up? There are no secrets in the unconscious." In the very next session the bachelor-patient reported his dream "of the night before last [the time of the writer's comment]—holding a session but with observers—not clear it was your tape recorder—other people with tablets beginning to take notes. I said, Oh no—the whole deal is off. If it's going to be this way—I refuse." When asked about the meaning of this dream, his only comment was "A difficulty in communicating—I think my own case is unusual and distinct—in a peculiar, detached way I think this." Again as in previous sessions, the patient had no conscious knowledge of the extent and significance of the many psychic transactions.

The final incident in this series of built-in controls occurred the day before the 195th session. Earlier that day the writer was discouraged to learn that his psychobiographies of paragnosts had been rejected. His convictions of the worth of his studies were bolstered, however, by a startling confirmation of a telepathic death dream that occurred five days previously. He had seen "proof" in the local newspaper obituary page and had received further corroboration from a long-distance phone call. The third psychic tracer occurred late that evening before the session with the bachelor-patient when the writer's colleague N. B. phoned to report two psychically significant experiences. One of his reports was a follow-up on the woman who could apparently foretell the outcome of horse races and the other was a telepathic experience between an emphysematous patient and his wife and N. B. When the writer told N. B. of his labors over this manuscript, he jokingly asked what fictitious initials he'd want. Because of the spontaneous recurrence of an unusual concatenation of near-specific psychodynamic prerequisites for an apparition-like experience, the writer confidently wondered aloud about what would happen the following morning with his bachelor patient.

Early the next day, in the 195th session, a striking telepathic parapraxis was noted and the writer was confidently awaiting confirmation of what had happened the night before. The patient immediately complied: "That early session with Louise, dinner with her . . . a vision over her shoulder . . . I was startled. I never saw a vision. It was like a religious miracle . . . a saint appearing in a halo of light. This was quite unique."

When asked, "What do you remember about it?" he said, "The apparition was opaque, full, living color . . . it stayed for a little while . . . not a flash. I was startled and awestruck. I knew who it was . . . it never occurred before or after."

When asked why he brought this up at this particular session for the first time since the apparition had originally occurred 21 months ago, he said, "I got concerned about the amount of time I've been involved here." The patient had mild influenza; was discouraged and angry with his physician possibly, among several reasons, because of his unconscious awareness of the scientific use of some of this highly charged material. Again in this event, as in the previous ones, the patient's needs complemented symbolically through telepathy the life situation of his physician. Possibly with the mild influenza the threshold of consciousness was lowered and highly significant events that occurred earlier in his treatment were telepathically recalled.

The constellation of spontaneous noncognitive events associated with his experience had their parallels in the previous apparitional reactions. The patient demonstrated with built-in clinical controls by responding in his usual, almost predictable fashion. However, from the first apparitional episode to the experiencs of the phantom prowlers and finally to this unusual flashback experience, there was a noticeable decrescendo effect. What had originally burst forth as a spectacular surprise and repeated itself in the wake of an avalanche of psychically related incidents had gradually subsided to an uncomplicated telepathic event almost pallid by contrast. In its effect on the unconscious mind the spontaneity might have been diminished through repetition. The motivation for some of these experiences, in their unique aspects, had lost much of the initial fervor.

Any one experience by itself might have shortcomings for the telepathic hypothesis, but the recurrence of similar events when the emotional constellation with the implicit needs and splitting, anxiety-provoking situations for both patient and physician were in harmony (built-in controls) made the case for telepathy compelling. At no other times did apparitions or the like occur with this patient, and in the writer's experience this is an almost unheard of type of event to occur in psychotherapy.

II

Another way of supporting the validity of a telepathic event that occurs in psychotherapy is provided by the analogy to Koch's postulates:*

1. "Constant association with the suspected organism with the disease" might be compared to a telepathic event that satisfies the criteria of similarity and near-simultaneity of thought and the occurrence of tracer words.

2. "The suspected organism must be isolated from the disease tissues and carefully studied in pure culture" can be likened to the occurrence, after the initial telepathic transaction, of a second or additional telepathic event during a psychotherapeutic session (or consecutive sessions). This volley, or cluster effect, might be regarded as tending to confirm the genuineness of the presumed first telepathic event.

3. "Organisms from the pure culture must be innoculated into healthy animals or plants for the production of the characteristic symptoms of the disease under investigation" can be related to the purposeful and successful telepathic transmission of a clearly held thought, affect, auditory or visual symbol during a psychotherapeutic session where postulates 1 and 2 have already been satisfied. This might demonstrate the state of telepathic rapport.

In this way the satisfaction of the telepathic postulates might tend to en-

---

*Wilson, C., and Haber, J. M.: An Introduction to Plant Life, pp. 222, Henry Holt & Co., New York, 1939.

dow particular telepathic events with a high degree of credibility. The following case, although derived from a psychiatric examination and not psychotherapy, might be illustrative of this.

Example

While having breakfast with his wife and for no apparent reason, the writer berated a colleague B. T., a very capable internist, for referring only chronic brain syndrome problems for psychiatric consultation. The last such patient this physician referred, several months ago, presented many annoying complications for the writer. After the writer's secretary reported for work later that morning, the internist B. T. called to refer a patient with a chronic brain syndrome. This incident seemed to be a common example of telepathic summoning where the writer was unconsciously aware of his colleague's thoughts (or vice versa) and they were telepathically detected and interpreted in the described critical way (or vice versa). This particular type of presumed telepathic event happened not infrequently with this particular colleague through the years.

The patient was seen later in the day in the living room of his home. He was an 81-year-old blind, wizened man of Dutch patroon stock, who sat in his chair picking at his clothes and pleasantly humming and whistling parts of old-fashioned tunes. He did not speak and apparently could not comprehend or answer any questions and commands from the physician. Similarly, the patient made no sensible response to his wife's attempts at mediation. The patient also appeared oblivious to his wife's comments about his progressive mental and physical decrepitude.

Because of the presumed telepathic summoning by the patient's physician earlier in the day, the writer reflected upon a situation of several months ago when there had been unusual telepathic exchange with an elderly patient who had a chronic brain syndrome. The physician also recalled how Jacques Romano was quite telepathically successful with a few brain-damaged patients.

On a whim, the writer decided to try a telepathic experiment with his elderly patient. Although such a notion seemed preposterous, the feeling was acted on. The writer's first thought was of the number 74, his own house number, a figure that could be clearly visualized and held in mind. Immediately after this thought the patient muttered his first audible words, "30 days —30 days."

Taken aback for a second by the patient's numerical response to the sending of a number, even though it was not the exact number, the writer quickly thought of "Beautiful light—cheer of Christmas." Hardly was this "sent" than the old man turned his eyes up toward the bright white ceiling (the room was dark) and smiled.

Rather intrigued by this unusual exchange but still not satisfied because of the approximateness of the responses, the third thought of the volley sprang before the mind's eye. It was Indian relics, a childhood hobby of the writer's. Before the writer could decide on a clear mental picture of either an arrowhead, a spearhead, or a tomahawk, the patient suddenly became agitated and tried to get out of his chair, muttering incoherently and reaching toward a dark, oaken box on the table. His wife restrained him and then lunged out of her chair, saying that the patient wanted to show the writer the box. She opened it and there was a tomahawk inside. When this (transaction) was appropriately acknowledged with a "How very unusual!" the patient and his wife retreated to their former statuses and postures.

In this example the first telepathic event was motivated by the dual tracer concepts of the telepathic summoning of the patient's physician (or vice versa) and the memory of the previous telepathic exchange with a different patient with a chronic brain syndrome problem. Although the second response of turning the eyes upward at the ceiling was nonverbal, it was appropriate to the writer's thoughts and followed immediately after the first possible telepathic event, thereby tending to confirm its validity. The third episode of the Indian relic, which was a motor-acted-out, near-direct hit from the physician to the patient (or from his wife and various permutations), made the likelihood of telepathy still more creditable. Thus in analogy to Koch's postulates, the suspected event was recognized (isolated) duplicated (cultured), and finally in a rather clear-cut fashion the process was strikingly confirmed by sending a telepathic inpression (injection).

Unlike examples from psychotherapy where the patient has a clear sensorium and is in command of his intellectual faculties, this patient was blind and had severe mental deterioration in association with his chronic brain syndrome. His physical impairments made the likelihood of subliminal stimulation and all the other frequently cited objections very remote as possible alternative explanations to telepathy. The chronic brain syndrome case is appealing in its simplicity, for it avoids many of the problems of telepathy as they occur in psychotherapy, where variegated surrounding data must be presented to support the possible telepathic-psychodynamic relationships. The occurrence of telepathy in a chronic brain syndrome patient provides a clinical example of Ehrenwald's hypothesis of how telepathy might be favored in states of the minus function such as sleep, trance, and so forth.[36]

COMMENT AND SUMMARY

One might wish that there had been more data about the psychodynamics underlying the various events. The writer also regrets that more could not be stated for, rather than weaken the validity of the telepathic hypothesis, it would have vastly increased its plausibility even if it jeopardized anonymity. Often it is the most negative, poignant, tender, and personally revealing events which contribute to the telepathic exchanges and which are withheld.

This conscious (or unconscious) withholding factor is related to the manifold reasons for resistance to psi in general.[50,126] It is not the disbelief of what is so true emotionally and telepathically revealed, but the fear of recognizing in an unmasked form the most genuine, deepest nuances of the interpersonal relationship, the implicit hostilities, and the evidences of sentiment, warmth, and affection. Most of the described episodes of presumed telepathy, psychic tracers, and their surrounding emotional complexes seem to be characterized by such deep-rooted, sincere motivation, and a confidence based on numerous successful previous experiences.

Although the telepathic aspects were never recognized by the patients and were never disclosed to them in order to keep the treatment on keel, some of the comments came as close as possible to a conscious recognition of what had happened. All the events between patients and physician had their complementary aspects and psychodynamically were always significant communications. The occurence of related unusual coincidences and other possible psychic experiences, and even at times a retrospectively identifiable similar dramatis personae, in actuality or symbolically, served as fuel for the ensuing events. It was a slice of time, as if time could be sliced like a sausage with the "random" spatial arrangement of the events and coincidences corresponding to the various seasoning ingredients in relation to each other and the particular plane of the cutting. What actually happened was illustrative of Jung's concept of synchronicity[110] where the coincidence of events in space and time has been hypothesized to have a meaning more than mere chance: "A peculiar interdependence of objective events among themselves as well as with the subjective (psychic) states of the observer or observers."

These experiences might have their practical, clinical value in various psychopathological and psychophysiological (telesomatic) reactions. One might wonder how the telepathic hypothesis would be applicable to an instance where a crazed assassin is telepathically triggered in his fiendish mission by some sick person who is knowingly or unconsciously in rapport with him. The theoretical and philosophical significance of such clinical telepathic events probe into the nature of man and his ancient history, his folklore legends of ghosts and luck, apparitions, and the supernatural, and his most searching view of himself and the cosmos.

The problem of criteria for the recognition of telepathic communications as noted in clinical psychiatry is briefly reviewed. A specific type of uniqueness, that of built-in controls, where a spontaneous telepathic event will recur in an almost predictable manner when the spontaneous constellation of psychodynamic forces for patient and physician are similar, is illustrated by a patient in psychotherapy who telepathically perceived an apparition or its equivalent at five disparate times. In a second example, concerning a patient with a chronic brain syndrome and advanced physical and mental decrepitude, a volley of apparent telepathic communications between patient and physician took place according to hypothetical telepathic postulates where a presumed telepathic event was noted, confirmed by a second or additional telepathic episode, and finally made more creditable by the successful, conscious sending of a telepathic thought.

7
Telepathy and Pseudotelekinesis in Psychotherapy
The Four Faces on the Tiles

"Thoughtography"—the photographing of thoughts on polaroid camera film —has been brilliantly documented and explored by Eisenbud.[51] Thoughtography presents some of the most challenging and mystifying of data. The implications of this study for all of science, and psychiatry in particular, are revolutionary.

Possibly related to thoughtography are the data of spirit photography, the image of Christ on the Holy Shroud of Turin,[232] and the alleged lightning engraving of human images on ordinary window glass.[35] Unfortunately much of this data is controversial, at best. The difficulties were well illustrated by Bernard S. Finn, Curator, Division of Electricity of the Smithsonian Institution, who kindly wrote in reference to the window pane image of an old lady which was reputed to be part of the museum collection, but which could not be located or identified: "Until we actually see such evidence I am afraid that it will be difficult to offer any explanation to account for these phenomena. It seems most unlikely that image registration could occur in glass that was not previously treated with photosensitive materials." However, he enclosed a reference[99] which gave several instances where lightning storms were associated with various odd pictographic impressions of humans.

This report is about some unusual telepathic episodes, in particular about a woman patient in psychotherapy who experienced a sudden unanticipated recognition of faces on four ceramic kitchen tiles. At the exact time of her

144

experience an experiment concerning telekinesis and thoughtography was under way in her physician's home with the cooperation of Joseph Dunninger.[24] The patient had no knowledge of her physician's research activities and what was planned for that evening.

Saturday night, March 5, 1965, seven physicians, two dentists, a chemist, and their wives came to a party at the writer's home in Montclair, New Jersey. The guest of honor was Joseph Dunninger. He arrived at 8:30 P.M., one hour later than expected. Although none of the guests had any idea of what was planned, I hoped that Dunninger might be encouraged to demonstrate some telekinetic phenomena or thoughtography. In my previous interviews with him, he had recalled how on some occasions he had shattered a thin wine glass by means unknown to himself. He also described some unusual spontaneous telekinetic experiences from his varied and fascinating life.

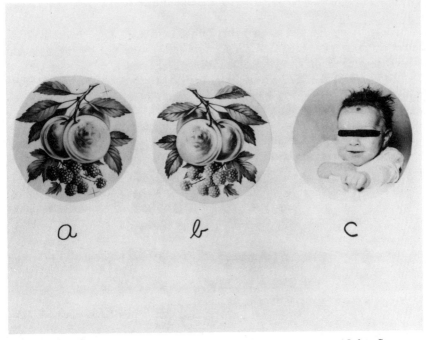

Original   Finished Tile   Infant Son

Dunninger had once shown the writer a scrapbook picture of a purported spirit hovering over a coffin containing the body of a recently deceased medium. Dunninger had been given this picture by Houdini, his close friend.[97] Although Houdini exposed countless psychic frauds, he never could explain this "spirit picture." Dunninger also recalled how once, years earlier, a newspaper editor concentrated on one of many photographs while a picture was taken of Dunninger's head. When the film was developed it showed a reasonable facsimile of the photograph the editor had been looking at.

When Dunninger arrived in Montclair, he reminisced about these episodes and many other extraordinary paranormal happenings from his long and illustrious career. Despite the availability of various wine, champagne, and beer glasses, a small marble statue of Hippocrates, and a polaroid camera, Dunninger was not in the mood for an experiment in telekinesis or thoughtography. He seemed tired from a busy week, but, being a great artist, he gallantly visited with the guests and performed some intriguing feats.

II

Five days later, on Thursday, March 10, 1965,* the physician's patient, a 30-year-old housewife, began her psychotherapeutic session in a rather excited way.

"Queer things happen to me. Remember two years ago when I had my house done over by the interior decorator—tiles were put by the sink and stove—they're all pink—and the middle one showed a picture of fruit, I walked out into the kitchen Saturday night (March 5) and a picture of a baby had come through! It had a birthmark on the head—on each and every one of the peach tiles! I asked my husband to look, to check whether I was

---

*On this same date which was the physician's son's seventh birthday, psychodynamically complex presumed telepathic-telekinetic events took place involving the son and Mrs. "Krystal" (Schwarz, B. E.: Psychic-Dynamics, pp. 161, Pageant Press, New York, 1965). While the wife was preparing the birthday party for later in the day, her husband begged for her opinion concerning promotional ideas about Mrs. Krystal that his publisher was pressing him for. Just as he was reading to his wife: "A beautiful, high official's wife explosively became aware of her psychic abilities early in marriage and learned how to exercise some control of these uncanny talents for the benefit of her husband and circle of friends—," there was a loud explosion that paralyzed them.

It was a quiet day, no one else was home, and all the doors and windows were shut. The top of a No Cal soda bottle had blown off. The wife and husband searched the kitchen for the cork and then heard another crash as a hypodermic needle fell to the floor. The needle had been owned originally by Mrs. Krystal. After her death it was given by her family to her physician. She was a diabetic who used such needles for insulin injections.

The bottle that exploded was No Cal ginger ale. As a diabetic, Mrs. Krystal used only artificially sweetened soft drinks. There were eight bottles of intact club soda next to the No Cal. As I was dictating this episode immediately afterward the door bell rang, and the physician shouted to his wife that this would be telepathic in some way because of all the excitement. It was a telegram from Mrs. Krystal's son and daughter-in-law, from their home in Florida, wishing Eric a happy birthday. They had never sent him a telegram before: in fact, this was the first telegram he had ever received. Later in the day, in addition to much high-quality telepathy with patients, the physician received a phone call from Dr. Louis Cartnick, who had not phoned for two years. Dr. Cartnick did not know it was Eric's birthday. He was Jacques Romano's partner; after Romano's death he had taken over the pharmaceutical business. Jacques Romano, who never had any children of his own, was very fond of Eric and was his godfather.

seeing things. It looked like Roderick [son] with a birthmark when he was born [had corrective plastic surgery at ten weeks of age]. My husband worried and said I should go in and look at Roderick—he was congested.

"It was in the evening, while I was doing dishes at 8:30. I was going to call you as my first thought. I never noticed it before. I thought I was imagining things, or that it was a warning that something would happen. I went in and even woke up my son that night. I'd never buy a tile like that. I want perfection. I looked all over for that tile . . . a decorative wall tile that would blend in.

"Why would it come out after all this time? I've had it two years this spring. The tile behind the cake box and not under the rays of the [recessed fluorescent] light is seldom washed, but it is the same. Peaches [the tile fruit motif upon which the faces appeared] are my favorite fruit. No one could paint over [the tile]. [The fruit motif] was baked in. I took bleach and everything [steel wool, detergent, soap].

"It's my son, or a dried up old man. My girl friend said it was a warning, that I wanted babies very badly. I still think of the baby I didn't have. It's [tile] still the same: I look at it every day, it's a shiny baked glaze."

From the patient's comments during subsequent sessions, it was evident that this event had taken place as she described. All members of the patient's immediate family, friends, neighbors, and employees had seen the tiles and come away puzzled and in awe. Prior to this specific time, no one had ever "seen" a face on the four decorative tiles. After this date there were four faces.

Because of the patient's extraordinary claim the tiles were inspected and photographed with a polaroid camera. Also, the writer inspected pictures of the various members of the patient's family who might have been psychodynamically related to the faces on the tiles. Because of the "spooky effect" of the tiles, the patient made arrangements for their removal from the wall.

Because of the unusual coincidence of the planned experiment for telekinesis and thoughtography and the patient's experience with the tiles, it was important to establish how and when the faces appeared on the tiles. After two and a half years of searching in the United States and England it was possible to track down the mystery. The artist who designed the fruit motif on the tiles was located and he wrote: "This image was created accidentally when I designed this pattern. In fact, since this pattern is a reproduction, and has gone through the process of plate making, retouching, and printing, I can hardly call this design my own any more, and [I] did not try to convey any inner thoughts of myself, my family, or anyone else." The illustration shows (a) the artist's original picture; (b) the finished tile with the projected face; (c) a picture of the patient's infant son with the birthmark.

In the patient's psychotherapeutic sessions she related her experiences to her thwarted desire for another baby, and to the "reconciliation" with her father who had been unkind to her in her formative years and who died when she was young.

From the patient's further comments and from study of her husband's and her own family photograph albums, the tile faces with the birthmarks seemed to be a projection and condensation of (1) her son as an infant with a birthmark in the approximate area, and (2) her father with whom she had identified her son; and (3) her husband's bald, deceased, intensely disliked and penurious employer-uncle. In her sessions the patient seldom mentioned her son's earlier disfiguring naevus pigmentosus. She was quite anxious about her own blemishes and had once received plastic surgery for cosmetic reasons.

The projection of the faces on the tiles was a telepathic illusion,* and, like most telepathic communications, it symbolized highly significant, anxiety-laden situations that served the interests of both physician and patient. Her experience might also be viewed as a transference reaction which symbolized her wishes and telepathic unconscious awareness of her physician's researches. For example, she might have thought, "Pay attention to me. Look what I can do. I can do better than the famed mentalist you are studying." Her unusual experience nearly answered a research hope for the physician. In a most surprising way it was a successful wish-fulfillment even if displaced from the target area of Dunninger and telekinesis.

Paranormally this patient was a rather unusual woman. In the course of her prolonged period of treatment she had much telepathy in face-to-face, physician-patient confrontation. For example, many sessions had one to three telepathic episodes, and in one session there were seven discrete episodes. The difficulty in reporting such data is in defining the cutoff point in presenting the complex exchanges of thought and feeling. Much of telepathy in psychotherapy is a continuum involving a complex associational matrix. There are problems in presenting accounts of clinical telepathy in a lucid style, free of quasi-obsessional piddling and in a succinct enough manner to convey the uniqueness and emotional impact.

Prior to the tile episode, the patient once apparently invaded her physician's unconscious (or vice versa) and accounted for a most unusual telepathic dream that pertained to the unexpected death of her husband's hated and meddlesome uncle.

---

*It should be emphasized that the artist did not draw a face in the original design for the decal. He assumed that following the processing of the tiles (during which the size of his original design had been markedly reduced to fit the tile) the combination of colors and forms were such that when the tiles were presented as a finished product for sale, it looked as though there was a face drawn on the peach. Despite all this, nobody ever noticed the four faces until the night, and specific time, of the experiment for thoughtography with Dunnigner.

On another occasion the patient had a premonition of death. "I awoke and said [to my husband] I knew someone was going to die—a terrific intuition, like I had when Roderick had hurt his hand." Later in the day her favorite aunt whom she hadn't seen or heard about in years died. The patient's mother had died when she was young and this aunt was a mother-surrogate until she completely rejected the patient for marrying someone she (aunt) disapproved of.

After this completely unanticipated event actually happened, the patient became very upset. On the night of the death, while thinking of the aunt and the possibility of her "return as a ghost" the patient, unable to fall asleep, got up and went down to the kitchen to have a cup of tea. "I turned the switch on and the bulb blew out with an explosion of sparks and fire and the glass lampshade [2 mm thick and 20 cm in length] cracked and shattered. This had never happened before [nor has it since]—it scared me because I was thinking of someone who had died!"

In psychotherapeutic sessions after the tile pictures, the patient continued to have much telepathy in her treatment and some rather out-of-the ordinary experiences. For instance, when she returned home one night, she was quite shaken because, as she described it to her husband at the time she saw her "neighbor lady standing in the front hallway with all the lights on behind her. This was at 10:30 in the evening." She told her husband about this because of the odd hour and the woman's lingering at the door. The next day she was shocked to learn that the neighbor she thought she saw had actually died a few hours previously.

Another unusual event happened one night, when the patient and her husband were in Hawaii. While having dinner in a fashionable restaurant, she was certain someone was present at the dinner table. She could not free herself of this conviction. "I felt somebody was looking over my shoulder. It was driving me crazy—every two minutes I was looking back—I was annoyed —but nobody was there!"

At the time of the woman's Hawaiian experience, her physician in New Jersey, while visiting with a colleague H, told him of a puzzling, weird, purportedly telepathic dream that he could not interpret. H, trying to be helpful, asked, "Miss Tubby* died, didn't she?" The writer said he had neither

---

*Miss Gertrude Ogden Tubby, secretary to Professor James H. Hyslop, founder of the American Society for Psychical Research, and formerly secretary to the American Society for Psychical Research. Four days after this inquiry, a friend, Mrs. Nancy Crawe, phoned to say that Miss Tubby (at the time of the weird dream that was nearly synthesized by H's question!) had taken an unexpected turn for the worst, was put into an oxygen tent, and had just died. At the time of Miss Tubby's death an unusual possible telekinetic event occurred. Of twenty postal cards on the bulletin board, a particular card—and the only card of telepathic significance, mysteriously fell off the bulletin board. Mention, and a written note was made of this because of the odd

seen nor heard about her in a long time. H knew of Miss Tubby but had never met her. Neither he nor the writer had discussed Miss Tubby in a long time. She had been hospitalized for a few years with a chronic brain syndrome and until near the end her condition had been unchanged.

Supporting this presumed New Jersey-Hawaii telepathic episode was the fact that at the precise time of his patient's restaurant experience the physician was thinking about her. Although he did not mention it to H, the physician was thinking about how, earlier in the day, he had taped a radio program, "The World of Susan Bond" on WMTR, Morristown, New Jersey.

He was reluctant to tell his colleague H, about the radio show on which he had discussed his patient's psychic mystery of the faces on the tiles.

It should be stressed that it was only after much hesitation that he mentioned on the taped radio interview the peculiar faces-on-the-tiles episode involving Dunninger and his anonymous patient. Although the physician had the patient's permission to pursue the matter scientifically, he had never before publicly mentioned this patient-related psychic episode. The patient had no knowledge of the radio program since at the time of the writer's invitation and the taping for the broadcast, she was in Hawaii. Allowing for the six-hour time gap between Hawaii and New Jersey, it seemed possible that the patient might have been telepathically sensitized to her physician. While she was asleep in Hawaii [4–5 A.M.], her physician at the radio station in New Jersey [10–11 A.M.] was wrestling with the ethics of the tile-face problem that directly involved her. He was fearful of being asked questions about her psychopathology and the possible bearing it had on the faces. It was essential to preserve her anonymity. Thus the patient's presumed telepathic hallucination of "someone being present at the dinner table," while she was in the Hawaiian restaurant, was temporally and specifically related to the physician's turmoil much of that day and his late evening discussion with his colleague of (1) the associated Tubby events, and (2) his suppression of the anxiety-laden news of the radio show about the patient. The New Jersey episode had multiple telepathic tracers: Dunninger, Miss Tubby, the odd faces on the tiles, and thoughts of the patient who was quite telepathic herself. As

---

circumstances. However, this event was unsynthesized until the news of Miss Tubby's death. One evening, a week later, H, after hearing of his nearly correct synthesis of his friend's dream, wanted to exploit his strange ability. This episode and various other incidents related to Miss Tubby were discussed. When H left, and the writer was alone in his house, he shouted out half boisterously, "Miss Tubby, if you are around in any shape or form, make yourself manifest!" He immediately turned the foyer lamp off by a pull-chain switch and went upstairs. He had hardly walked up a flight of stairs when the light went on spontaneously. Quite shocked to say the least, he examined the lamp switch and so forth, but could discover nothing to account for the peculiar event. The facts of Miss Tubby's final illness were verified by interviews of the hospital's nursing staff and physicians.

reported for other psychodynamically studied telepathic hallucinations and illusions,[177,183] the episode was overdetermined for telepathy.

COMMENT AND SUMMARY

Mere descriptive details of psychic events are of limited value. They seldom tell much about the people involved—their psychopathology, motivations, physiology, and so forth. By contrast, telepathic episodes during psychotherapy offer an unusual opportunity for understanding in statu nascendi how psychic events take place, what influences them, what purposes they might serve, the kind of people involved, their psychophysiology, associative processes, and so forth. Dynamic psychotherapy, which is based on a thorough knowledge of the unconscious mind, is indispensable for the research and treatment of emotional and psychosomatic illnesses. It is ideally suited for the study of telepathy.

Professor Tenhaeff[214-216] and others have successfully employed psychodynamic techniques for exploring telepathy. Tenhaeff's brilliant studies have illuminated the psychodynamics underlying the paragnost-consultant relationship. He has been the leading pioneer in demonstrating under good scientific conditions, the practical applications of paragnostic skills for solving crimes and archaeological mysteries, and for locating missing people and objects.

It is probable that the influence of parapsychology on psychiatry will be enormous. These few reported telepathic examples from the psychotherapy of one patient, which are not isolated instances, give some indication of the potential scope of this influence. It should be clear that psychic events are no less complicated than what happens in psychotherapy. Despite the formidable problems, any chipping away or correlation of psychopathologic and psychic data would appear to have practical value.

Meerloo[124] and others[21] have shown the multiplicity of purposes that telepathy serves: viz., increased mating urge, needed intensification of communication in family relationships and in cases of physiological decortication. As indicated in this report, telepathy might be an emergency or survival mechanism that prepares the person (or organism) for changes. By having events impinge on the outer fringes of awareness, he has time to adjust through unconscious mental and psychophysiological processes and thereby establish a more stable equilibrium. He is then able to ward off the possible traumatic effects of being surprised by sudden changes in his physical and inter-personal environments.

The telepathic episodes that seem to follow splitting experiences might reveal how the organism is prepared for these otherwise damaging sudden changes. This remarkable process, which is usually beyond conscious recognition, might frequently occur in people. By preparing for changes and warding off excesses of anxiety telepathy could make behavior proceed more smoothly. By unconscious resistance to an awareness for telepathy—the difficulty of unmasking the telepathy of everyday life—the person is somewhat protected from chaotic impulses that could lead to endless confusion, etc. Telepathy, like dreaming, has a highly significant practical function in interpersonal relationships.

8
Precognition and Psychic Nexus

PART 1

Telepathic episodes and physician-patient telepathic dreams are not rare during psychotherapy. Reports about these, telesomatic reactions, and other psychic matters are becoming more frequent in the psychiatric literature. However, there are few carefully documented presumptive precognitive dreams.[66,95] Many purported precognitive events are, on deeper study, most likely telepathic, if they are psychic at all. This was the case in the series of vivid dreams related to the death of a renowned parapsychologist.[179] This problem of telepathic versus precognitive is also illustrated in a related study of telepathic psychodynamic drawing experiments.[174] In the study, with a volley of drawings, complex telepathic crisscross effects were observed between sender and receiver. However, the data could also be interpreted as precognitive: what the percipient thought he had telepathically received was really a precognitive impression of the sender's next drawing.

I

Background

At the time of his death Les Egbert* was widely recognized as "Mr. Woolen Yarn Industry." In addition, he was not only a successful executive vice-president of the Columbia Minerva Corporation but also an author, playwright, and psychic researcher. The writer met him in 1958, when checking on some of the psychic data presented by Jacques Romano.[181] In addition to independently verifying many of Romano's unusual experiences, Les de-

---

*Hereafter referred to as Les.

scribed some of his own extraordinary psychic events. For example, in 1935 he lived in a haunted house where there were such happenings as: "lights going on and off, water overflowing a vase, manuscript floating off a table, doors opening and slamming, table tipping, shades flying up, raps, the dog running and howling as if panicked for no apparent reason, the family seeing the dog being 'let in' the house three times in one night when the door was locked from the inside and there was no ordinary explanation, the young son waking up screaming, and apparitions."

The bizarre events subsided with psychiatric investigation of the Egbert family by Titus Bull, M.D., who for many years was associated with the American Society for Psychical Research and was also Director of the James H. Hyslop Foundation. The Egberts were referred to Dr. Bull by Miss Gertrude Ogden Tubby, former secretary to Dr. Hyslop and for years Secretary of the American Society for Psychical Research. Dr. Bull, who advised the family without fee, concluded that Mrs. Egbert was a "sensitive" and should abandon seances and experiment in the occult. When Les's son was interviewed as an adult, he faintly remembered some of the unusual events of 1935 and confirmed his father's account. Many others among Les's longtime friends and business associates vouched for his truthfulness and recalled the unvarying and consistent details of his narrative. It should be emphasized that such accounts, unless truthful, could make a person vulnerable to ridicule. Les had nothing to gain by telling these matters to his friends.

In numerous meetings with the writer Les appeared to be quite telepathic himself, even though he was unaware of many of the exchanges. Possibly this was one reason why he was such a successful sales executive: making decisions, "second guessing" the minds of competitors, and being almost prescient about what products would appeal to the public for the coming season and which ones would fail. He once recounted a precognitive experience in which the astrologer told him that his son, who was then in the armoured force ready to embark for the European Theater of War, would never see the conflict. At the last moment a freak accident occurred and, as prophesied, the son missed combat.

During the course of their friendship the writer witnessed other psychic events with Les. For example, the jovial Les once "visited" the writer and his wife in the middle of the night by traveling clairvoyance. Les's memorandum written at the time, April 7, 1958, stated: "Tried to reach Bert at 3:00 A.M.—was to awaken him and make him realize who it was. At 4:15 I wakened and had dreamed I was at Bert's. The dream was so real I thought, 'I planned to go mentally and not physically'—I remember a large white screen—flat—thought I talked to both—very jolly—wrote Bert I tried to reach him."

The attempt was apparently reacted to (as recorded at the time): "At approximately 4:00 A.M. Ardis [the writer's wife] awakened and saw a figure standing by the pink chair in the bedroom. It had on a 'brown tweed coat' and there was an aura about it." Neither she nor the writer knew that Les owned a brown tweed sports jacket. "When visiting yesterday (April 10, 1958) Les identified the large wall map of the United States in the electroencephalographic laboratory, saying that this was the 'large white screen'." He had never been upstairs in the house before this.

Among Les's precognitive experiences several of his friends recalled how, "on a hunch," Les once violated his lifelong business habit of frequent commercial air travel and refused to take a certain flight from Cape Cod. He later learned that the plane had crashed and everyone was killed. Another example that Les told many friends about was his recurrent (later proved correct) proscopic dream of his ancestral home in Scotland, the Ross Priory.

From 1958, until his death in 1966, Les organized and was active in an oil prospecting company in eastern Kentucky. In addition to availing himself of the best advice of geologists, he also had the unique services of the successful Maine dowser, Henry Gross,[176] whom the writer was studying. Thus, because of their many common interests, Les and the writer established a firm friendship.

On December 26, 1966, Sunday, the day after Christmas, the writer attended a party at Les's home. This was his first visit there since Les's return from a trip to England and Scotland where he had discovered that his ancestral home, Ross Priory, was exactly as he had dreamed previously. He showed numerous pictures of it. At the time of the party Les had laryngitis.

Then the writer neither saw nor heard anything about his friend for 20 days. As was learned weeks later, soon after the party Les left his New Jersey home for Florida to recover. According to his wife, Les was happy and healthy in New York City on Thursday night, January 13, 1966. His business associate, Miss Nan Comstock, Editor-in-Chief of McCall's Needlework and Crafts magazine, had an appointment with Les in his office the next morning at nine o'clock. She was surprised to find how ill he looked and learned from Mrs. Rosamay Winston (Les's assistant) that although he had been working all week he complained of nausea and seemed sick.

Presumptive Precognitive Dream

The writer awoke at 6:00 A.M. on Friday, January 14, 1966, and told his wife (as recorded later that morning) about "an odd dream, that had a tag of prophecy to it. President De Gaulle committed suicide and a Negro senator became acting president of France—advance notice of what would happen in three to four days."

The obvious interpretation of the manifest content did not carry any feeling. However, the dream was so odd and tracer-laden for prophecy that the writer violated an axiom of psychotherapy by writing it at 8:05 A.M. during a session with [paragnostic] patient F.[177] Associatively, F. compelled the recording of the dream because in his psychotherapy he had numerous telepathic episodes, some spectacular recurrent apparitions, and psychodynamically overdetermined telekinetic events, as for example the Romano oil painting crashing to the floor, and office Venetian blinds violently shaking.

At 7:30 A.M., before seeing F. at 8:00 A.M., the writer looked at several greeting cards his wife had recently purchased with thought of our next-door neighbor who was then fearful of having a stroke. When she showed the writer one of the funny get well cards, his reaction was, "Ha, this would be fine to send Les; but no, it's ridiculous because he is all right, and psychiatrists don't fool about such matters!" No further thought was given to this conversation.

Later that Friday afternoon, while answering a letter from a lady who had heard me on an all-night radio show a few weeks previously, I kept thinking of Nan Comstock's nephew, Arthur, one of the guests at Les's recent party. My thought was that Arthur, who was well informed on the situation pertaining to the Panama Canal Zone, would be an interesting man to be interviewed by Long John Nebel (WNBC). I had hardly finished writing Long John's name to the woman when Long John Nebel telephoned from New York, inviting me to appear again on his all-night radio show, this time on the following Tuesday. His guests were to be Alan Jay Lerner, co-author of the Broadway musical about psychic matters, "On a Clear Day You Can See Forever," and Jess Stearn, newspaperman and author of psychic books. My reaction was that my association about Arthur for the Long John show was possibly an incorrectly synthesized telepathic apprehension of Long John's intentions concerning myself.

The following day, Saturday, at 10:00 A.M., while in the public library, I received a call from my office telling me to rush to the Montclair (N.J.) hospital special care unit to see my friend Les, who was in acute prostration. He had been brought to the hospital by ambulance from his New York apartment the day before at 4:30 P.M. The arrangements were made by his friend, Nan, who had first thought her nephew Arthur could drive Les to the hospital. This was at the approximate time of Long John's telephone call to the writer and the writer's thoughts of Arthur. As was later learned, and confirmed from the hospital records and interviews with the family, friends, and the attending surgeons and physicians, Les had developed acute abdominal pain at approximately 9:00 A.M. Friday (January 14, 1966) with associated vomiting and diarrhea. When I saw him at the hospital, he was in an oxygen tent. Perhaps because of his intense pain, prostration, and confusion, it was impossible to communicate with him verbally.

My instantaneous reaction on hearing the news from my office was the dream! It assumed an immediate and horrible significance. All at once the pieces fell into place. Les, the tall, thin, man of aristocratic Scotch background, who was the *president* of our company and responsible for our joint interest in the oil explorations, as well as other interesting research projects, was symbolized by "President De Gaulle." The "Negro Senator" and successor was associated to Les's son and heir apparent. In contrast to his father's fair hair, eyes, and skin, the son was of a swarthier complexion with dark eyes and hair. The Negro was linked to a past magazine article which stated that De Gaulle's successor would be a virtually unknown Negro senator from some caribbean island possession of France. Like the "Negro Senator," the son was obscure and untested to me at least, in reference to our oil drilling venture. Although a capable and versatile scientist and former university instructor, the son had no previous experience as an entrepreneur and president of an oil exploring company.

It was immediately evident to my wife, to me, and to Les's physician, who knew of my dream, that the prophecy of "committing suicide and death in three to four days" pertained to Les's acute illness (pancreatitis). His own body tissues were being painfully dissolved with pancreatic enzymes. Les had no previous pancreatic difficulty.

On January 16, 1966, Sunday, when there still was hope for improvement, the writer told his dream to two other physician friends of Les's who knew about many of his past psychic experiences. However, Les's general condition and the associated peritonitis worsened so that he died on Tuesday, January 18, 1966, at 11:15 A.M. The diagnosis of acute pancreatitis with peritonitis was confirmed on post-mortem examination.

At the precise time of Les's death in the hospital, a drug retail man in my office presented me with a black notebook and decorative apothecary jar, lettered in black, *Pro Dolore,* and filled with the analgesic, Darvon.

Later, at 1:30 P.M., my editor friend, Mrs. Joan Jesurun, telephoned while I was thinking of her. She had been critically reading my manuscript on Jacques Romano, and I had not heard from her in two weeks. Joan, who was afflicted with arthritis, was very upset because she had recently fallen and badly injured her knee. In her opinion, the most helpful analgesic was Darvon.

II

Associated Possible Psychic Events

For reasons described elsewhere,[179] it seemed desirable to search for all possible psychic phenomena involving the physician and his patients, as well as friends, before, during, and after Les's illness and death. His unexpected fatal illness had a splitting effect on me and, because of our friendship and business interests, it seemed well to attempt a clinical evaluation of possible telepathic effects. This method of applying psychodynamic insights to a series of telepathic events seemed worthwhile in a previous volley of spontaneous psychic experiences.[179] Superficially, this method is somewhat analogous to the often spectacular and sometimes tedious classical psychic researcher's cross-correspondence studies with mediums.[221] However, whereas the classical studies are replete with detailed cognitive material, imposing affidavits, and so forth, there is an almost total absence of attention to psychodynamic, psychophysiological, and historical details of various personally charged material.

In their psychotherapy, patients are used to talking about intimate personal matters, often relatively without censorship, Thus despite many complex variables such as subliminal, suggestive factors, and the like, it still seemed worthwhile to search for possible telepathic leakage in the spontaneous life situations that were actually happening before one's eyes.

It was hypothesized that Les, who had deep significance to the writer, might through some kind of unknown affinity, have psychically or telepathically "come through" the physician's patients in the various psychotherapeutic material, associations, and so on. Therefore, I undertook to read all patient records for telepathy from December 31, 1965, to January 18, 1966. Nothing unusual in connection with the death came to light. For the reader's convenience the major psychic complexes are numbered.

1. As was learned almost one week after Les's death (January 20), Les entertained some friends in his New York apartment on December 16, 1965. Nan Comstock, who has had many past validated psychic experiences, told fortunes and attempted "reading cards." Nan recalled how Les's wife got "the ace of spades next to the ten of spades." Nan was inwardly horror-struck and felt certain that the cards pertained to Les. However she attempted to cover this up by telling Mrs. Egbert that "a woman friend would die in three days to three weeks." The tension abated when, coincidentally or not, one of Mrs. Egbert's close woman friends died unexpectedly in three days. Although Nan's statement was made on January 18, 1966, Mrs. Egbert told the writer (independently at a different time from when Nan told him) that she was certain in Les's apartment on December 17, 1966, that she would never see her husband there again. She recalled saying the words out loud without realizing it.

2. On January 11, 1966, the writer's nine-year-old daughter, Lisa, made what was for her a most unusual statement. Since Lisa's and her brother Eric's parent-child telepathic episodes[184] have been recorded from babyhood, this comment was written at the time, although the interpretation of it

was unknown. Completely unrelated to any known events in her life, Lisa told her mother and me, on the night of January 11, 1966, "Something tragic will happen." The next afternoon Lisa returned from school very upset because a classmate fell out of a swing, was knocked unconscious, and was taken to the hospital by the police ambulance. The record of January 12, 1966, said: "I [writer] didn't give this any credence because Lisa [several days ago] overheard us (mother and father) discussing Jeanne Dixon, Washington prophetess. I had received the book [as a gift from Les Egbert], which Lisa had looked at. However, Lisa had never said anything so boldly before. She had not read or looked at it [the book] in the past few days. For the record, this coincidence is included to see where, if any place, it leads [!]."

PART II

On the morning of Les's death, four patients were seen and two of them had six telepathic episodes with the physician.

3. Later that evening, on the all-night Long John Show (January 18–19, 1966) the unfolding assortment of psychic events was further compounded. The broadcast was about Alan Jay Lerner's (and Burton Lane's) Broadway musical on psychic matters, hypnosis, and a psychiatrist, "On a Clear Day You Can See Forever." Based on a vivid dream, Les had once written a play, "The Boy Who Lived Twice," which was produced on Broadway in 1945. It was about psychic matters, a psychiatrist, and hypnosis; its motif centered about an original piano concerto. At the time of this play Les renewed his friendship with Jacques Romano, who advised the cast and particularly the actor who had the role of the psychiatrist for the hypnosis scenes.

This odd coincidence of Les's psychic play and Lerner's psychic musical, as well as the precognitive dream and Jacques Romano, was mentioned on the all-night show.

Several days later the writer received a letter postmarked Ireland on the day of the all-night show. It was from Romano's old friend, Swift Newton.* It was the first note from Newton to the writer since Romano's death in 1962. It was wondered if because of the very hectic (splitting) day, Newton was telepathically summoned across the Atlantic. It was very unlikely that he would have heard a local New York radio show at that hour of the day in Ireland. Certainly no mention was made of this.

4. Buoyed up with coffee, the writer, at 8:00 A.M. (January 19, 1966) listened to his patient F.[177] recite a presumptive telepathic dream that vividly portrayed his physician's ordeal on the radio show. In the session there were

*While writing this part of the manuscript, the author received a letter from Swift Newton, postmarked Rome. This was the first letter since the one mentioned above and stated ". . . your Christmas card . . . has been tucked away to answer 'some day' and this is the day."

also some direct-encounter telepathic episodes. The fact that there was no physician-patient telepathy with the other patients for the remainder of the day was attributed to the writer's lack of sleep and exhaustion.

On the morning of Les's death four patients were seen, two of whom had six telepathic episodes with the physician. For the eight patients that were seen from January 20 until the time of Les's funeral on Saturday (January 22) there was one telepathic dream, sixteen telepathic episodes, one possible telesomatic reaction, one possible precognitive experience, and one rather striking telepathic visual hallucination.

5. On January 21, 1966, Friday, at 8:00 A.M. patient F came into the office with a broad smile on his face. He could hardly restrain himself from laughing when he described how a "very odd thing had happened!" Since his last visit he had received a letter from the well-known, bearded Commander Bullhead (pseudonym), the president and living trademark of an internationally famous beverage concern.

In some way Bullhead had learned about the bearded F , a junior executive in a different industry. Although F had not applied for any employment elsewhere, Commander Bullhead had requested an interview with him for possible consideration as a vice-president in his company. F and Bullhead had never met. The strange and possibly humorous precognitive feature of this event was that more than two years ago when F returned from an ocean-sailing vacation with his new beard, the physician had quipped, "It's just a matter of time until Commander Bullhead will be contacting you!"

6. During the noon hour, on Friday, the day before Les's funeral (January 21, 1966), the physician, in his office, expressed strong reservations to his wife about the religious services planned for the next day. He joked that he could better visualize the coffin in his consultation room, with the somber rites conducted there, than anticipate an unfeeling, cut-and-dried type of service elsewhere. This very private (and sacrilegious) wisecrack was linked to a family joke of long ago. A patient (seen in consultation for alcoholism) upon first entering the physician's office had remarked, "Doctor, you have a very beautiful and spacious office!" The physician thanked her, but then was floored by her next statement, "My husband would love to see your office. It would be just perfect for him. He's a funeral director!" It was a story that Les Egbert had heard and chuckled over.

On January 25, 1966, Tuesday, a phobic woman patient, who had not been seen for two weeks, came to the office quite upset. She had recently returned to her job in a bank after an absence of many months. While out to lunch at noon, on Friday, January 21, 1966, she had a most disquieting experience; the only one of its kind in her life.

But first, it might be interjected that in her psychotherapeutic session, while she was describing another matter, the physician thought of poor Les dying. He revisualized the grim hospital reception room scene on Saturday, before the death. In his mind's eye he clearly saw himself talking to Les's son and noted how the son's winter *coat* was on the couch beside him and the writer was wearing his heavy leather *overcoat*. At that affect-laden, hovering vivid complex of death and coats, the phobic patient said, "Went out with Frank (president of the bank and friend of her husband). We put our *coats* on the chair. It was weird, almost as if a body was there. It was a man in a coffin. When you have a body next to you it's difficult—I'm nervous when I get into a restaurant anyway— and it was disconcerting having *that* next to me. It resembled a body in a coffin! As I sat there I could see this in the background. It was 12:30 in the afternoon. You'd better believe it. You had to keep looking back. I kept telling myself it was ridiculous. It was just two coats there. I can't account for these crazy things—I had one Rob Roy—the body was there before the cocktail—after it—it went away. I kept saying to myself. "I know they're coats. It's ridiculous!" But, out of the side of my eyes, the side of my head, or whatever . . . that silly vision kept coming in. In minutes it was over. I was very glad. It stayed five or ten minutes, but it seemed like hours."

The patient, who came from a city many miles away, was in a town more than 10 miles away from the physician's office when this episode occurred. She had no knowledge of any of the aforementioned events in her physician's life.

This patient, whose own life was haunted by many tragic deaths when she was young, was a very dependent person. In her psychopathology, she isolated herself from contacts with others. For these and many specific and detailed reasons, it was conjectured that, like Professor Tenhaeff's paragnosts,[214-216] she was poignantly sensitized for psychically apprehending such a tragic event in the life of her physician. She dramatically projected in her vivid telepathic hallucination her physician's grim joke. Her experience was in emotional resonance with her physician to whom she was bound in transferring her dependent feelings and longings. Her experience might also have been interpreted as a means of mastering the threatened separation of the future (death). Her projection could also be viewed as a repetition of her past tragedies. It condensed her underlying ambivalence of fear and dread of her repressed hostile wishes for what might happen. This was manifest in her anxiety over her new job and boss.

Extrapolation of the effects of such an in vivo, telepathic, visual hallucination to other areas might include such questions as (1) how common might telepathic hallucinations be when recognition is given to the role of psychodynamic distortions and so forth? (2) what possible relationship could such a clinically bizarre experience have for behavioral aberrations, exalted states of inspiration, creativity, religious ecstasy, and so forth?

For most of the patients, much of psychotherapy was essentially passive, and leading questions were never asked. It was impossible to probe every moment of the significant events in the patients' lives during the time under study. Although desirable from a research point of view, it would have been therapeutically contraindicated to explore this interesting area. However, unless some study of this kind were made, taking into account various defense mechanisms, and the like, one could not *a priori* invalidate the hypothesis that many additional interesting telepathic communications for current and past patients did not happen.

It would seem that telepathy might be noted more often (1) if the telepathic hypothesis were seriously considered as a possibility, and (2) if there were a complete accounting of significant events in the lives of specific patients to see what the data are and how and in what way the various episodes happened or dovetailed with the situations in the physician's everyday life. It should be evident that in this spotty sampling much apparently valid material was uncovered.

During seances spectacular telepathic material is sometimes spoken by the entranced medium. Unfortunately, these otherwise first-rate psychic (and psychodynamic) data are vitiated because there are defects, such as poor controls, inadequate records, untrained observers, and so forth. Nevertheless, there is enough truth and success in this ancient practice to warrant use of a psychodynamically analogous method: the study of frequent letters from a patient who was in strong transference to her physician. These are described below.

7. While a dependent, disturbed patient was in a split, dissociative (near trancelike state), it was hypothesized that some meaningful telepathic material might "come through" her letters. At the time of Les's final illness and death and over a period of several months, the physician had been seeing an ex-nun who was rather telepathic. She had several presumed psychic experiences with members of her family as well as many episodes with her physician. A college professor, she had sought medical help for depression which was related to prolonged social isolation. It was her habit to write her physician almost daily letters about her thoughts and feelings. Although the content of her letters seemed always well organized, the liberality of expression suggested a process not unlike the autochthonous outpourings of automatic writing. Her letters from January 12, 1966, until January 22, 1966, were carefully studied. On January 12, Wednesday, she wrote Christ's words spoken from the cross, "Eloi, Eloi, lama sabachthani?" Perhaps sacrilegiously for herself, she stated that Christ's agony lasted only a minute but her problems had lasted three years! She had never written in such a strong fashion before, and there did not seem to be sufficient change in her actual life situation to

account for her desperation. There were no notes for the 13th and 14th, but on the 16th she wrote about a (possibly telepathic) dream [with her physician] and on the 22nd of January, at the time of Les's funeral, she wrote:

> John Ciardi's little allegory in the *Saturday Review,* "Refugee Angel"–I don't understand all he's driving at but I know the feeling–"If I think hard enough, shut here in my own will, dark, I believe I could re-invent myself as a thing, a moat would be enough: I have survived ambition. I tell myself and then I know. I've been gulped down into the same pride I rose in once–that insistence on being real, always that insistence among other dreams of nothing."

With imagination the patient's quotation could be construed as an epitaph for Les. Although she had previously written about deaths that happened in her life, she never wrote so sensitively as in this possibly telepathic displacement from an event in her therapist's life–about which she had no knowledge.

This most inexact, "far out" research approach is included not so much for the data, but rather as an attempt to define a possibly useful technique for future studies. The idea is simple–if it is but considered–and there is no dearth of clinical material.

8. On January 27, 1966, the writer–who is not a dowser and has no major dissociative phenomena–checked the nylon dowsing rod that Henry Gross[176] had used in Kentucky on the Les Egbert expeditions. When he unlocked the door to the cabinet that contained various memorabilia, he was shocked to discover that one of the twigs of the strong forked nylon rod was broken. The last time he had seen the rod intact was in December, 1965. Detailed questioning of all the people in the house confirmed that no one had opened the cabinet and broken the rod. There was no sign that any of the other numerous fragile objects in the cabinet had been displaced or broken. It was perplexing because the dowsing rod was the symbol *par excellence* of the writer's friendship and exciting Kentucky adventures with Les Egbert, which through death had now come to an end.

Comment

Various psychic data and multiple telepathic tracers surrounding a possible precognitive dream are documented. The near-specific and at times spectacular relationships of events which occurred, mostly at the unconscious level, minimize coincidence as an explanation for most, or many, of the episodes. Any one event might be dismissed as coincidence, or as an example of the telepathy of everyday life. However, the concatenation and the quality of all possible varied psychic episodes seem to give some kind of meaningful picture of complex interhuman communications. There seems to have been a continuum, or psychic nexus, involving many people and types of phenomena.

The particular chronology for the various life events suggests that at the time of the possible precognitive dream, Les, although ill, was not in acute distress. As in an example already cited,[179] it would seem that there was much to suggest the physician's unconscious telepathic awareness of his friend's (and many other's?) anxieties. Possibly, by some kind of virtuoso unconscious diagnostic technique, a dream was conjured which came true in the way and time predicted.

However, the prophecy of death in three to four days is more difficult to explain as telepathic unless, in some way, there was a telepathic pooling or condensation of knowledge of several people, which was unconsciously and correctly synthesized in the dream. This type of "precognition" would really be a heightened or quasi-laminated form of telepathy. It would be entirely akin to the hypothetical telepathic processes occurring in the creations of genius.[178] The telepathic hypothesis for "precognition" would posit possession of a highly developed and unconscious skill—on the order of the mathematical feats performed by idiot savants.

Presentation of the precognitive dream without the allied psychic nexus would strip it of much of its strength and present an incomplete picture. The separate parts would not be pieced together into a more meaningful whole. It can be conjectured that if a wider-scoped, more psychodynamically oriented technique were applied to the study of seemingly isolated proscopic events, precognition might be more commonly recognized.

If any one was a candidate for psychic experience of this type, it was Les Egbert. By personal experience and sustained keen interest, he was deeply immersed in psychic events and had an open, nondogmatic outlook concerning such strange happenings. His preconscious mind (and his friends') was well prepared for what might have happened. For example, there was his repeated proscopic dream of his ancestral home and his lifesaving precognitive dream of the airplane crash. His psychic experiences formed focal points of communication—emotional resonance—with the writer's research interests. Their friendship was originally formed through their mutual interest in the paragnosts Jacques Romano and Henry Gross, both of whom had precognitive experiences.

The psychodynamic approach to the psychic nexus indicates the existence of a highly meaningful relationship as demonstrated in individual telepathic episodes. A useful purpose is served and there are practical clinical implications—for example, the causes and treatment of various behavioral states, psychosomatic reactions, and so forth. This approach emphasizes anew how the detailed setting of a psychic episode should not be considered apart from the experiences and unconscious life of the participants.

Just as serial dreams have much added significance and practical value in the treatment of a patient, so serial psychic events contribute to the overall understanding of the treatment procedure.

A study of the varied synchronistic episodes in the psychic nexus might some day yield answers to the questions: (1) if the events were foreseen could they have been prevented? (2) Could the awareness of such episodes have suggestively (iatrogenically?) or telepathically contributed to the illness (telesomatic reaction, suicide, homicide, etc.)?

In reference to this report of a spontaneous nexus, brief mention might be made of other techniques used in studying precognition. Many laboratory experiments are often so intellectually contrived that they may exert an inhibiting effect on precognition. When high scores for precognition are obtained in the laboratory, they are usually so rare and of such low order that the data are barely sufficient for detailed analysis and comparison.

A further difficulty in the laboratory research is that the necessary precautions and design of the experiment to guard against fraud are *sui generis* suggestive of distrust and suspicion: they unwittingly suggest fraud. Furthermore, any (unconscious) suspiciousness on the part of the parapsychologist in reference to the paragnost could exert a negative influence on this psychic process. Ironically, a form of negative telepathy might suppress the very thing being sought. Much has been written about the possibility of fraud in experiments, but all to little about the no less serious and subtle problem of an unconscious fraud complex.[51,90] One is no less easy to identify and manage than the other.

This unfortunate dilemma for psychic work might be obviated by training more investigators who have a profound understanding of the unconscious mind. Thus, more emotionally sophisticated experiments could be devised. Another possibility might be the selection of people for psychic research who, in addition to their other qualifications, have a past history of psychic experiences themselves. Furthermore, one could attempt through psychotherapy to further develop their aptitude and awareness for telepathic episodes. The baker uses yeast so that the cake will rise!

One of the promising methods of study of precognition is the combined clinical-experimental approach so brilliantly pioneered by Professor Tenhaeff in his grab (or chair) test. In one such experiment* conducted between Utrecht (the Netherlands) and New York, certain relevant methodological problems became immediately evident: namely, the renowned

---

*As translated by Mrs. Cornelia H. L. v A. Matteson. Data has not been analyzed.

paragnost, Gerard Croiset, in his original proscopic impressions (in Utrecht) for what was to happen weeks later (in New York City), might have been compromised by ethical considerations, such as the need for preserving privacy for the subject in the presence of an audience, and so forth. In addition, because of the necessary conscious censorship, the gifted paragnost might have (unconsciously) inhibited the full measure of other proscopic impressions. For example, as in many reported experiments Croiset, who is very sensitive to criminal matters, might naturally focus upon such data from the proscopic experiment. Needless to say, being a fine man of high ethics, he would be reluctant to state any off-color or quasi-criminal data about the projected consultant. This was borne out from direct observation of some of Croiset's telepathic-clairvoyant impresssions as well as from study of Jacques Romano. In many instances Romano withheld poignant data. The subjects did not so much fear that Romano was "wrong" as that he was right and that he knew more than he said publicly.

This difficulty pertains, therefore, to validation of the prophecy when questioning the consultant. The obstacles are similar to those existing with the original proscopy. If the consultant were quizzed in reference to residual specific features (the censored material the paragnost withheld), many of the events are so attenuated and vague as to be meaningless, and others are so potentially traumatic either directly or symbolically for the consultant that he has much conscious reluctance and unconscious resistance ("forgets") to recall the specific events.

The experimentally and superficially trivial events that might appear to the consultant and public as a total failure might actually have been the most successful part—if only the facts were known. Because of distortion, withholding of information, unconscious resistance, and the like, there are many difficulties in bringing them to light. Despite these difficulties, some of Professor Tenhaeff's published tests with Croiset have been spectacularly successful.

The nexus of spontaneous psychic events poses compelling problems for future clinical investigation. The unraveling of the psychic nexus would seem to offer much promise for a better understanding of man. Like the galaxies, it has unlimited dimensions. Psychic-dynamics provoke concepts that challenge and question our understanding of what man is, who he is, and his place in space and time.

9
Synchronicity and Telepathy

"Synchronicity takes the coincidence of events in space and time as meaning something more than mere chance, namely, a peculiar interdependence of objective events among themselves as well as with the subjective (psychic) states of the observer or observers."[109] Synchronicity, in addition to having, as someone has said, "a causal vertical connection between happenings and a horizontal connection between events," might also involve telepathy. An understanding of the possible connection between synchronicity and telepathy would appear to have practical value for the physician in psychotherapy. Many possible clinical examples and discussions of the ramifications of this connection have appeared elsewhere.[36,37,44,45,69,126,177-179,181,184,186,214-216]

The following four vignettes, which are not rare and which were chosen from many other possible examples, illustrate clusters of apparently related and meaningful episodes. It should be emphasized that the presumed telepathic aspects of the reported happenings occurred in a continuum. For the purposes of this report there had to be a cutoff point; consequently, many temporally related patient-physician telepathic episodes that preceded or followed the reported happenings were omitted.

1. THE CASE OF P.J.

P. J., a middle-aged housewife, sought help because of a severe depressive reaction. Her problems were related to the recent death of an adolescent daughter, her husband's excessive drinking and her son's antisocial behavior. In the course of psychotherapy there were countless sessions with single or multiple telepathic patient-physician episodes. In one session the patient tearfully recalled a college love affair of years ago. Later that same day of her treatment, she was shocked to learn that the one person in the world who knew of the secret affair of long ago had phoned from Florida to New Jersey to ask how she was. The patient hadn't heard from her friend in a long time.

Four years later, while thinking over patient-physician telepathic episodes with P. J., I recalled the Florida-to-New Jersey example and tried to remember the name of P.J.'s Florida friend, but failed. It was a kind of memory exercise game where recall of an emotionally overdetermined name was a valid check of my own alertness and therapeutic involvement. I purposely avoided going to the files to find the name. While driving to my summer vacation cottage and mulling over this "forgotten name," I picked up a young hitchhiker. It turned out that this man had the surname that I was seeking and, moreover, that he was a nephew of the person in Florida. I hadn't picked up a hitchhiker in years, nor have I since then. This person and that name had not crossed my path before, nor have they since.

In the course of protracted treatment, P. J. had a schizophrenic reaction and was hospitalized. After her discharge and more extensive office psychotherapy, she gradually seemed to have found herself. Her son, who had collaborative psychotherapy with his mother, had also made progress and ceased his delinquent acting out. P. J. completed her requirements for a teaching certificate and managed to finance the son's education in a private school far removed from the corrupting influence of her then-separated alcoholic husband.

One day, while visiting him in a New England summer camp, P. J. was stricken with a ruptured cerebral aneurysm. Her physician phoned me in reference to my data on P. J. Moved by this poor woman's tragedy, I immediately penned her a note, but subsequently learned that she had soon died of the disease. I heard nothing more about either her son or her husband.

One day three months later while driving about town, I chanced to pass P.J.'s former home. I mentioned to my wife how my former patient had lived in that house, how she had had such heartbreaking tragedy, how she had worked hard to get on her feet again and provide for her son, and how at the moment of success she had died. "Poor W (son), I wonder whatever happened to him? Did he slip back under his father's influence'? Was P.J.'s father (W 's grandfather) able to help him?"

Two days later, at 3:00 P.M., the doorbell rang while I was in my office. My secretary became upset when she found a state police detective inspector at the door, seeking information about P.J.'s husband. [I had never before received such an inquiry about any other patient's husband.] While the secretary was leafing through the files for the name of the physician who, to our has most recently treated Mr. J., the telephone rang. She turned pale. It was P.J.'s father from Massachusetts. He inquired whether I had heard anything about his son-in-law (he had no knowledge of any possible police difficulties or anything else about his son-in-law since the death of his daughter) and his grandson. He expressed deep concern that his alcoholic son-in-law would ruin the grandson. When asked what prompted his call at this precise time, he said that two days ago, for the first time since his daughter's death, he and his wife had had the courage to go through P.J.'s mail. They had come upon my letter and noting that it had been opened, they felt P.J. had read it. They were so moved that they decided to phone me at this moment.

Possibly the physician's sympathetic reminiscences about his deceased patient's son, when seeing P.J.'s former home, telepathically inspired the grandfather to read the letter, or vice versa. Other possible telepathic determinants—or incentives—might include the secretary's (and the physician's) acute anxiety—a splitting situation—over the meeting with the detective inspector. This could also have telepathically precipitated the grandfather's decision to call about his grandson. He had to know the possible destructive effects of the drunken father's driving, and so forth, on the youth. Another possibility could be the grandfather's or the physician's latent (telepathic?) awareness of some supposed difficulty of the father with the law; in this way either the father, the son, the law officer, or others could have set in motion the chain of complex telepathically mediated events.

For various possible combinations the common thought-affect meeting ground was similar for the involved parties. One may speculate (as happens in so many telepathic episodes) that if the detective inspector had not come when he did, this happening, or much of it, might never have come to light.

As a postscript, mention should be made of one more unusual related event. Three years after P.J.'s death, I decided, at the last moment, for a lecture on psychiatry and parapsychology, to present in suitably disguised form some of this material as illustrative of synchronicity and telepathy. Although not so directed, the data could not help but portray P.J.'s husband in an unfavorable light. The gasps and sighs of the psychiatrically unsophisticated audience might have suggested how they viewed P.J.'s husband as a villain. Also, perhaps the physician's sympathy for his patient was communicated. At any rate, during a session the next day with a woman patient who had problems superficially similar to P.J.'s (e.g., separation from a husband who, "was driving [her] crazy," tragic effect on children, past hospitalization and treatment elsewhere for psychotic reaction), the physician was surprised to learn of a completely unexpected change in her situation. On the night of my lecture and my sympathetic comments about P.J., the estranged husband of this current patient, in a city 300 miles away, unexpectedly put their children in the car and drove all night to return them to the mother in New Jersey. By his so doing, the patient got her children back without the anticipated major legal hassle. In her session she said: "... 4:00 A.M. the door bell rang—two children on the doorstep—a miracle—unbelievable—[as told by the children] he brooded and stared into the fire for several hours—panicked and suddenly made the decision to bring them down. I was informed he [husband] received it [the papers of the trial] a week ago. I prayed that within twenty-four hours they'd be with me and they were. It was uncanny. I was so grieving. I felt like calling the doctor. Father [a professor] was stunned. Everybody was."

It can be speculated that this surprise development, totally unexpected by the patient and completely out of character for her husband—and presumably not to his best legal interests—might have been precipitated by the woman's distress which was telepathically mediated and affected all members of her family. One might also wonder if the similar tragic, telepathically tracer-laden example of P.J. as presented by me on the same night to the lay audience could have induced a collective (telepathic) displaced influence upon the husband. His scales of decision could have been tipped, provoking a generous action capable of mitigating some of the bitterness and opprobium heaped upon him, by way of P.J.'s husband.

2. THE CHRISTMAS FIRES

As part of a series of psychodynamic telepathic experiments, the following events took place December 1, 1958, and were reported in 1963:[174] "The [sender's picture of a] fire extinguisher was drawn . . . and was perceived [by the receiver] as a red fireman's hat and mound. There was, however, an interim of several hours before the recipient reported her perception, and during that time some interesting events transpired. One hour after making this group of drawings the writer left his office to go Christmas shopping. At approximately 11:45 A.M. he bought a rather expensive fire extinguisher and a can of pine deodorant for his wife. This was extraordinary for him; it had not been his intention to buy these two items, which were hardly suitable for Christmas gifts. He thought it was foolish, but on the other hand he felt compelled to buy them. While driving home he decided to give both presents at once rather than to wrap them and wait until Christmas. As he brought the gifts into the kitchen, he immediately smelled acrid fumes. His wife excitedly told him that in his absence (at approximately 11:45 A.M.) there had been an electrical fire in the deep fat fryer which had burned a hole through the aluminum pot and a stainless steel spoon. There had never been a fire in the house. This combination of controlled experiment and some additional spontaneous telepathic events seemed to raise the question of precognition, an unusual coincidence, or both, and the agent's compulsive telepathic reaction."

Seven years later, and almost to the day, December 9, 1965, I suddenly decided to go downtown to Photo-Cullen to pick up the prints of an illustration for my *Parent-Child Telepathy*,[184] and also a portrait of Joseph Dunninger. Interestingly enough, I had "forgotten" an unusual profile photo of Jacques Romano[181] as a young man, which was also at the store and had been for some time. I was trying to recall what it was that I sought and was missing. While looking at the Dunninger photo, I associated to one of the most impressive things that he once told me during a visit. It concerned a possible precognitive (or telepathic?) dream of his father's about a horrible ship disaster years ago.* An excursion ship caught fire and many lives were lost. Dunninger's father acted on the vivid grim reality of his dream and tried to save lives by warning the people not to take the ship. However, most would not listen to him.†

Possibly, with this grim association of the fire propelling me, I decided on the spur of the moment to go into the Montclair Gallery, an andiron and curio shop, next door. While there I noticed an electric simulated birch log fire. This, I thought, would be fine for the dining room and a surprise Christmas gift for my wife. While in the store I also noticed a $25.00 fire extinguisher on the wall that was quite similar to the one I had bought seven years ago. It brought back the frightening memory of the kitchen fire.

Upon returning home, I left the surprise package of the simulated birch log fire in the car. My wife, Ardis, met me at the door and in a very excited state informed me that our seven-year-old son Eric, while helping his mother in the kitchen, had climbed up on a chair to lift down a tin of matches, and the matches had spontaneously ignited, causing quite a furor. Ardis had grabbed the flaming container from Eric and thrown it into the sink. Eric had been frightened and had run upstairs. We are very strict about matches and the children know it. Eric never plays with matches. This was the second fire since the event seven years ago, and the only one of its kind in the family. The kitchen temperature was 68° F. and there was no ostensible reason for the fire.

Checking with the technical director of the match company, we were told that such fires are "unusual but not impossible." Although the matches cannot be ignited by spontaneous combustion, friction of the white match heads would be possible. However, such a fire had never happened before to us, nor has it since. Furthermore, when an equal number of fresh matches were put in the same tin and violently shaken on numerous occasions, no fire occurred.

Ardis said that had she not actually witnessed Eric's taking the matches from the shelf, she never would have believed his story. If she had not been present to see what happened, the fire could have been much more traumatic to the child; his mother would have been reluctant to accept his account of how the fire began; and both his parents' trust and faith in him and his in them would have been undermined.

Although I had originally intended to hide the electric logs in the cellar

---

*The Slocum disaster.
†The writer thanks Joseph Dunninger for his kindness and permission to include this personal information.

and just say it was a "Christmas present," I abandoned this plan after the splitting effects of the excitement. I followed the 1958 example and showed Ardis the surprise and then installed it at once.

The analogy between the 1958 and 1965 events is striking in the concatenation of happenings: (1) a particular type of situation involving fire (coincidence? telepathy? telekinesis?) and (2) telepathic tracers (telepathic experiments, overdetermined association of famed paragnosts, specific Dunninger anecdote about fire, recall stimulated by the fire extinguisher of events of seven years ago).

3. AN ETHICAL DILEMMA

Dr. E, a director of research for a large electronics corporation, was seen in emergency consultation for dysphonia and overwhelming anxiety. In his first and many subsequent sessions there were patient-physician telepathic episodes. In his 19th session, he reported an experience of several years ago when he was under the care of another physician in a city far away. Correspondence with his previous physician revealed he was hospitalized "in a psychotic state with extreme belligerency and destructive acting out." In his session E recalled that during his previous hospitalization, his physician, who was also chief of the institution's psychiatric research center, used E's superb inventive talents in designing various pieces of electrical apparatus.

With much emotion E described how he had once put his former psychiatrist on the spot by telling him in his psychotherapy that one of his first assistants failed to follow E's advice in reference to some electronic device, with the result that a patient was inadvertently electrocuted.

E wondered how his therapist, the director of the institution, had handled this horrible ethical dilemma with his first assistant. Because of his connections, E would know if the matter was investigated and justice rendered. As he put it, if his therapist couldn't handle this with him, or a member of his staff, how could he treat a patient like E who had so many ethical problems in his past life: would he be just, truthful, and reality-bound? What kind of a man was this therapist?

At the end of the session I became aware that a drama was taking place during the time of this 19th session which was similar to—but a miniature or a caricature of—the patient's previously described grim dilemma. Although we only pieced it all together later, it appeared that after the session, when E went out to his prized foreign sports car (one of the few things in his life that meant something to him at that point), he found his left front fender badly dented and scratched. Although I was already in session with the next patient, E came back to the office to seek information about his damaged car from my secretary. Because of the scheduling of patients at the time of the accident, it was evident that one of three must be responsible for the damage to E's car: (1) the patient F,* just before E's session, (2) patient V, who followed E, or (3) still another one who came for an electroencephalogram during E's hours.

The auto accident was unique, for in the thousands of instances of vehicles coming and going on the property through the years, none had so much as sustained a scratch before E's mishap, nor has one since.

Since no one confessed responsibility, it posed a problem for myself, the therapist. I had to find out who was responsible and see that there was restitution to E for damages. This had to be done tactfully without unnecessarily involving innocent people, revealing their identities, or divulging details about what had happened. It was therapeutically imperative not to introduce situations that could delay or compromise the treatment of other patients with extraneous (reality-bound and also countertransference) problems. Needless to say, to pay for the damage myself would be unethical, unrealistic, and therapeutically contraindicated. An act so lacking in self-respect would have had a deleterious effect on the patient E, and, moreover, my insurance policy did not cover accidents of this sort. It would have been equally destructive had E, the innocent victim, been obliged to pay for the damage himself and thereby compromise or ruin his treatment.

Investigation of the parking area, the position and condition of the cars at the time of the incident and knowledge of the various patients, led to the deduction that the person responsible was most likely the next patient, V, an ex-nun, now college professor. V's problems had never been in the realm of dishonesty. However, when she was tactfully asked about the accident on the telephone, the ethical conflict worsened, for she flatly denied any knowledge of it. When she was gently quizzed about the shade of paint on her rear auto bumper, reported to be similar to the color of the damaged car, she said that this was from a minor accident several months ago (which the physician knew about previously) when her car was rammed in the rear bumper by an auto similar in color to E's. The previous accident had involved an off-duty policeman, with much unpleasantness, threatened legal action, and jeopardy of her insurance.

Fortunately, several hours after the denial V telephoned and sobbingly confessed to the accident. She said she was frightened and afraid to lose her insurance. V was distraught because she had not lied since childhood. In her subsequent treatment she traced the current episode of clumsy childlike lying to several very disturbing childhood experiences with her domineering mother. The patient had never "won any arguments" in her past or current life; she felt she was a "born loser." The car accident was proof of this and

*F was an unusual patient who had many extraordinary psychic experiences in his therapy.[177,179,186]

the crowning blow to a series of recent disappointments. Thus E had his car repaired; the damage was paid for by the therapist who in turn was indemnified by patient V.

Through insightful and just handling of this situation the distinguished researcher E and the ex-nun V made great progress in their treatment. The transferences and countertransferences were strongly polarized for the better. This time E's tossing of an ethical "hot potato" into his physician's lap was turned to a good end. The earlier unresolved conflict of the electrocution and the previous physician was therapeutically nullified. E was given another chance to test out authority (his physician) and reality; the damaged-car episode counteracted the earlier wrong and became a powerful corrective emotional experience for two patients with involved ethical problems. E's faith in another human being (also in himself!) was solidified and many crippling past life experiences were aligned in a new perspective. V's regressive lie in the face of an anxiety-provoking situation was nullified and she worked through "forgotten" experiences of long ago.

4. TELEKINESIS—OR WHAT?

On May 28, 1960, my wife and I were invited to a Memorial Day barbecue. After much debate with my wife, I presented K, our host, with a copy of *Mad Magazine,** which had a cartoon of "Glamorous Stockbrokers." It showed a broker being led away from the courtroom by the police, with flashbulbs exploding. The caption read, "Set up fraudulent brokerage firm." Although we insisted our host read it and pass it around for laughs, he quickly put it under his seat cushion and completely avoided the subject. We had never been to his home before and had only seen him on three other social occasions in the midst of many other people. Never before had we given such material to someone we hardly knew.

On Thursday, June 16, 1960, we were shocked to read in the local newspaper that K had been arrested at 2:00 A.M. for allegedly embezzling $60,000 from a widow. A few days later I unexpectedly met K downtown. He seemed embarrassed and upset. After hearing some of his comments, I said, just to make small talk, "Don't worry, K , the woman is probably a crank, and will commit suicide." I comprehended my completely irresponsible and unqualified statement to a man I hardly knew, and then only as a social acquaintance and not in a professional capacity, only when I read in the newspaper a few days later that the widow had committed suicide. The case was settled shortly afterward.

Six years later, May 22, 1966, at 5:00 P.M., just before my lecture on para-

*No. 56, July, 1960.

psychology for Stewart Thompson's Conference on Corporate Strategy in St. Adele, Quebec, Canada, I was interviewed by P., a reporter for the *Wall Street Journal*. Although he seemed a fine young man, he had a literal mind and I found it impossible to explain to him the psychodynamic aspects of telepathy. His knowledge appeared restricted to card-calling statistical experiments. My inability to explain my researches to him through various examples frustrated me. I thought that if I could not present clearly to this reporter my material from everyday life and my medical practice on how telepathy works between people, my lecture to the businessmen would certainly be a flop.

Finally, feeling completely thwarted and becoming more apprehensive and conflicted over my lecture that was to follow in a few hours, I told P about a possible telekinetic experiment, which, among my many examples, was the *pièce de résistance*. This involved the psychodynamically charged and tracer-laden sudden crashing of paragnost Jacques Romano's oil painting. Also, in disguised form I mentioned the unusual happenings of the patients E and V described above.

Throughout our talk, I silently debated whether to describe the tragicomic "embezzlement" example of K. Although I did not mention this to the reporter, my wife, who was present during the interview, was well aware of my ambivalence. (This I had discussed with her; I did not want to risk the example appearing in the newspapers and receiving undue attention. When I finished preparing my lecture later that night, the typed K example was at the top of my stack of notes; still I was undecided.)

Upon our return home from Canada to New Jersey, we were shocked to find a segment of ceiling, 32 by 37 inches, completely denuded of plaster, with dust around the office reception room, canvas pads on the floor, and the rug saturated with water. The furniture was disarranged and draped. Strangest of all, an oil painting, the only one my father had ever given me, was down. When the plaster had crashed to the floor it had sheared the picture-frame wire.

Upon checking my secretary's messages and seeking an explanation, I noted two things at once: One, the ceiling had collapsed at 5:00 P.M., the time of the frustrating reportorial interview in Canada. There had been a heavy rain in Montclair in the morning; nevertheless, it should be stressed that the ceiling had been in good condition and had never collapsed before, nor has it since. It was a freak accident.

Second, my secretary had left a note stating that on Thursday night—the time of my interview with the report—K had telephoned, asking me to dinner with him. I had not seen him for three years; the last time we had met was at the local hospital while he was under the care of his family physician, and we just exchanged greetings. He had never invited my wife and me out to dinner before (nor has he since) and it was quite unlikely that he had knowledge of my activities. Certainly he knew nothing of my plans to discuss the odd coincidences involving him that he had never been apprised of.

My secretary had also left a verse on my desk:

> *Return you must from this momentous vacation*
> *Only to find to your consternation*
> *Your prediction come true—a culmination!*
> *You will recall your parting threat*
> *To crash a few goblets—from that distant point yet!*
> *So Thursday, at five, I was willing to bet*
> *You'd caused a great crash on the reception room deck*
> *And left your poor secretary a nerve-frazzled wreck!*

One can hypothesize that K's anxiety and turmoil over his alleged embezzlement triggered my wife's and my unusual telepathic response of presenting K with the telltale cartoon. As in numerous examples of parent-child telepathy, secrets are relative.[184] Suppressed and repressed material on the thresholds of consciousness (preconscious) is often uncovered. There may be something to the old adages concerning love at first sight and the truth of first impressions. Also, spontaneous remarks or impressions are often more revealing of one's feelings than carefully deliberated, highly cognitive statements. Truth is, among many things, an emotional reality or telepathic awareness between two people.

My completely out-of-character, offhand remark about the widow's suicide might have been a telepathic awareness of the widow's intention to commit suicide, or of K's unconscious wish for her to do so. Other reasons for this remark as, for example, possible precognition, are impossible to fathom without more information.

Possibly, the anxiety-provoking and splitting episode with the *Wall Street Journal* reporter triggered the decision to choose the Romano painting (telekinetic) example. In reality, however, "my thoughts" could in fact have represented my secretary's associated ideas that were provoked by her anxiety over the office damage in Montclair at the time of my personal frustration in St. Adele. That is, her thought telepathically precipitated my "free choice" from any number of possible examples.[178] It was the particular way, then, that an unexpected happening in nature, the crash of the ceiling, was reacted to and used—unless in some strange manner telekinesis was involved again. My secretary and I, at widely separated places, had at the exact time common purposes in communication that criss-crossed from our respective self interests.

In such a charged, splitting atmosphere of telepathy and events, K might have contributed to the unique cluster and specifically responded over space and time as if to say: "Don't use the example about me. That is private. Look, I'm inviting (bribing) your wife and you to dinner. Be good to me." My secretary's jingle might have been a caricature of my parting (precognitive?) quip before leaving for Canada, that one way or another goblets would explode. Certainly nothing as costly and destructive as the fallen ceiling could ever have been wished for—even at the price of coming close to calling the shots for telekinesis.

SUMMARY

Synchronicity is defined and related to telepathy. Four illustrations are given of how synchronicity and telepathy may happen in life. Understanding of synchronicity and telepathy can give wider dimensions to psychotherapy and show the unique interdependence of people and events.

10
The Telepathic Hypothesis and Genius: A Note on Thomas Alva Edison*

Arousing from a coma a few days before he died, Edison suddenly opened his eyes and gazed "upward into space, his face illuminated with a smile as he said, 'It is very beautiful over there.' "[131] Thomas Alva Edison, benefactor of mankind, genius, died at 3:24 A.M., Sunday, October 18, 1931. In his laboratory office three minutes after his death a large, spring-wound, thirty-day wall clock stopped. Three of Edison's top executives and associates noted that their clocks also stopped at 3:24 A.M. These facts were disclosed in interviews with Norman R. Speiden, close friend of the Edison family. The incident of the stopped laboratory clock and other personal data about Edison were independently supplied by Paul B. Kasakove, who worked closely with Edison for the last 10 years of the inventor's life. Kasakove, a chemist, recalled how he often opened the laboratory at 8 A.M. when Edison arrived and then worked with little heed of the number of hours until 10 P.M., when Edison went home.

In none of these four instances of clock-stopping, each in a different location, was any trickery found nor was an ordinary explanation supplied. John Flanagan, Edison Laboratory night watchman, then approximately aged 70, said that the clock stopped at 3:27 A.M. In a private interview Flanagan also told Edison's son Charles that he did not stop the clock himself. Because of Thomas A. Edison's keen interest in possible communication after death, this was an important point. Although Flanagan was questioned by many people through the years, he never changed his story. Nor did the three exec-

---

*The writer thanks Norman R. Speiden, supervisory museum curator, the guides and the archivist of the Edison National Historic Site, West Orange, New Jersey; and Joseph Dunninger, for their assistance in this study.

utives, also men of truth and character. Unfortunately, no other details were available in any of the four episodes.

Some of Edison's former associates wondered about a possible relationship between the clock-stopping at Edison's death and the words of the popular song, "Grandfather's Clock," which Edison had recorded on both cylinders and discs: "It [the clock] was bought on the morn, of the day he was born, and was always his treasure and pride. But it stopped, short, never to go again, when the old man died." Since Edison's early manhood his employees had called him "The Old Man." To this day there has never been a satisfactory explanation for the clock-stopping.* If, as seems credible, the clocks stopped spontaneously, there must be considered the alternative hypothesis of telekinesis, involving the persons already mentioned. For the clock-stopping to have been coincidence would be most unusual in view of the known facts.

This report explores the relationship between Edison and his views on psychic matters as well as the possibility that his genius might be better understood by application of the telepathic hypothesis.

Despite the spectacular nature of the clock-stopping episode at Edison's death and his documented interest in applying his genius and scientific know-how to various psychic matters, this aspect of his life is either completely omitted or glossed over in some of his excellent biographies.[105,131] Although a genius like Edison presents problems for a biographer, it would seem that a man's beliefs about spiritual values, his soul, or call it what you wish, might be very relevant to an understanding of his character and purpose in life.

A little-known aspect of Edison's career was his long-time interest in telepathy and possible communication with "entities" after death. Although

---

*Two other events involving unexplained clock-stopping, of which the writer has firsthand knowledge, concerned Professor James H. Hyslop, founder of the American Society for Psychical Research, and the paragnost Jacques Romano. According to personal interview material and published data, Miss Gertrude Ogden Tubby noted: "And from the moment of his [Professor Hyslop's] death, when his daughter's watch was stopped—which he later claimed to have affected, when communicating with me [Miss Tubby] through Mrs. Sanders [a medium] before I knew anything of the watch-stopping—to the present time, he has not ceased to make his individuality known and felt in this life." (Tubby, G. O.: *James H. Hyslop—X His Book: A Cross Reference Book,* York, Pa., 1929, p. 35).

When the author was called to Romano's apartment at approximately 2:30 P.M., Sunday, October 14, 1962, to pronounce him dead, it seemed, on circumstantial evidence, that Romano had died close to 8:40 A.M., the time indicated by his stopped pocket watch, which had been removed from his trousers and placed on the living room table. Since the author had witnessed many strange psychic things Romano had done while under a prolonged period of study, he specifically noted Romano's watch before entering the bedroom for the examination necessary for filling out the death certificate. Upon his return to the living room, the author was shocked to see that the watch had spontaneously started running again. When the others in the room, who were far removed from the watch, were questioned about this, they were also very surprised. No one had been near the watch and there was nothing to account for its running again.

only fragments of his diaries and vast correspondence have been catalogued, there are some published references to his interest and experiments in mind reading. Some of these are as early as 1885,[160] when he was 37 years of age, and some are comments at the end of his career, nearly a half-century later. In his unique and often humorous style, Edison even anticipated mass resistance to telepathy which "could stop civilization and everybody would take to the woods. In fifty or a hundred thousand centuries, when mankind has become perfect by evolution, then perhaps this sense could be developed with safety to the state."[160]

Some of Edison's other published statements that might be relevant to his views on telepathy and genius[162] are connected with his theories of entities and swarms.[162] (These theories have some similarities to Jacques Romano's vibration theory of telepathy[230] and Dunninger's opinions.)[25] Edison also made original observations on possible former incarnation[164] and memory, which he compared to a filmstrip that could be scanned for the past, present (and future?).[163]

Deaf* since age 12, Edison commented on his overcompensation for this defect and how this affected his imagination and creative (telepathic?) abilities.[164] Indeed, he refused corrective surgery that was advised for his deafness. It may be surmised that, as in clinical practice with patients who have various physical defects that can be remedied, Edison was not as fearful of failure of surgery as he might have been paradoxically fearful of success. For then the deafness disability that he had used to his creative advantage might no longer exist and operate in his behalf. Deafness isolated him from his fellows and might have, in his case, furthered his powers of concentration and independent thought. For his purposes a liability had been turned into an asset. In such a state of relative sensory deprivation, telepathy might have served as a useful auxiliary means of communication.†

In several places Edison referred to his invention to communicate with the unknown.[166] In one instance he said, "I am hopeful, therefore, that by providing the right kind of instrument, to be operated by this [deceased] personality, we can receive intelligent messages from it in its changed habitation, or environment." While the apparatus was being built, one of Edison's laboratory technicians, Walter W. Dinwiddie, an astronomer, died. Because of previous long discussions on this subject of survival after death, it was hoped that the apparatus could be used for spirit contact.[208]

Although Edison's former associate, Kasakove, did not know the specific

---

*Presumed conduction deafness as diagnosed by ear, nose and throat physician, L. Emerson.[208]
†"We know that senses can be developed, because persons deprived of one sense invariably develop the others to an uncanny degree. There is also reason to suppose that such persons increase their telepathic ability, although they rarely recognize it. It is significant that Thomas Edison, who was quite deaf, had an intense interest in the subject of telepathy."[30]

rationale, he recalled how Edison's roll-top desk was locked by Charles Edison after "the Old Man's death." It was reopened 16 years later on Edison's centennial in the hope that there would be some message from Edison. It seemed likely that Edison had made plans for possible communication after death with some member of his family. However, nothing was found apparently.

Dunninger, who has "about 20 letters" from Edison, and an autographed photograph, told how Edison showed him a machine with which he attempted to contact some "outer sphere—some communication from somewhere, somehow, that wasn't the earth plane—" and how he received undecipherable signals. Edison accepted telepathy and had experiences "where he would concentrate on someone and they would come and see him —or concentrate on doing a thing and it would pass on to the person it was intended for without any verbal communication." During his life Edison had left a secret message with Dunninger, and for many years Dunninger offered $10,000 to whoever could correctly get the message after Edison's death. Although Dunninger received from mediums, interested people, cranks, and so forth, messages purportedly from Edison, no one ever succeeded in obtaining the correct one.[24,*]

Dunninger has also written: "In numerous demonstrations which I gave for him I found that his [Edison's] thought impressions came through clearly."[27] For example, Dunninger describes how he telepathically detected a cigar-burned hole in the tablecloth Edison was thinking of and how this, as well as other experiments, were performed under clinically well-controlled conditions.[28] Dunninger continued: "He was highly impressed with my ability to name a single card chosen from an entire pack in another person's possession. Mr. Edison tested it with a pack of his own cards. I named correct cards ten times in succession.[106,29]

Dunninger has also said: "Edison's mind was constantly progressive. His specialty was that of putting existing discoveries to use through inventing new ways to develop them. Once given a scientific fact, Edison did not care to let it remain idle. I've always found that inventors were interested in the subject of telepathy, perhaps because their minds are naturally telepathic.

---

*Dunninger also had written messages from his friends Houdini and Sir Arthur Conan Doyle. As with Edison, no one has ever succeeded in getting the messages. Edison once said about Dunninger's telepathic abilities, "Never have I witnessed anything as mystifying or as semmingly impossible."

According to Norman R. Speiden, the Edison family never received a message from a purported Thomas Alva Edison that was judged to be genuine or worthy of further study. As a matter of fact, when Speiden questioned each member of Edison's family about this phase of Edison's Research in the spirit world, he received only negative answers.

They themselves receive impressions or gain ideas that seem to come from some outside source."[31],†

Other well-documented sources, such as telegrams, letters and newspaper clippings, testify to Edison's interest in telepathy, and his experiments with the mentalist Professor Bert Reese[133,34] (nee Berthold Reiss). In one letter Edison wrote, "Reese has a sense organ apparently that only appears in prodigies occasionally." In another instance Edison wrote, ". . . it is as you say—or some newly developed sense which at present is rare." Edison studied Reese for several years, and Reese passed all the telepathic tests "with flying colors." In a letter to the *New York Evening Graphic*, July 20, 1926, Edison answered an attack on Reese by one Samri Frikell: "I saw him several times. On each occasion I wrote something on a piece of paper when Reese was not near or when he was in another room. In no single case was one of these papers handled by Reese, and some of them he never even saw; yet he recited correctly the contents of each paper." In response to a letter from Houdini after Reese's death, Edison wrote (August 2, 1926) that Houdini "ought to try to find some theory as to how Reese could produce such results as he showed me."

Unfortunately for research purposes, according to Dunninger and Romano, Reese, a stage performer and showman, mixed some of his telepathic feats with legerdemain which made it more difficult to separate the psychic wheat from the chaff. Romano once reported how he demonstrated before Edison and Luther Burbank one of Professor Reese's magic stunts with a message on a paper that was substituted by sleight of hand.[156] The author, who had seen Romano perform a similar stunt on numerous occasions, agreed with Romano's opinion* that the public is greatly taken in by the part of the stunt which is the trick and ignores the truly amazing part—the telepathy—which is genuine. It should be stressed that Edison gained nothing from his psychic experiments and on the contrary might have had much to lose by his courageous defense of Professor Reese.

It might be conjectured that Edison, the self-made man, who had less than six weeks of formal schooling, was himself a natural paragnost, but that he was unaware of his own telepathic abilities. However, as a genius he could combine the fruits of his own intense concentration with the telepathic im-

---

†Dunninger has invented countless illusions, many of which were used by various outstanding magicians, his good friend Houdini, and himself. Similarly Jacques Romano was a great innovator, and for his livelihood he devised many unusual therapeutic iodine compounds. For years he was a friend and employee of the inventors George Eastman and John Hays Hammond. Finally, the unusual Maine dowser and game warden, Henry Gross, has a very inventive mind in reference to nature-lore observations and in the construction of various animal traps.

*Seymour S. Wanderman, M.D., eminent researcher in his own right as well as a friend of many inventors and scientists including Edison, Einstein, Crile, Chen and so forth; and also Romano's personal physician for 40 years, recalled how Romano on numerous occasions demonstrated his paragnostic feats before Edison as well as other scientists.

pressions that he received from others and synthesize them as his own creative acts and inventions. Although more information along this line would be desirable, during their courtship Edison's first wife once made this cryptically suggestive remark, "Oh, Mr. Edison, I can always tell when you are near me."[105]

Other indirect and anecdotal evidence for Edison's possible paragnostic abilities includes, for example, his keen interest in various aspects of telepathy which could have been a tracer-like indication of his own (unconscious) telepathic talents. Other suggestive personal attributes for a possible telepathic talent are his unusual intuitive ability to select the right man for the right job, his tremendous self-confidence and optimism even in the face of nearly insurmountable opposition from contemporary leading scientists, and his unique talent for "getting answers [in his experiments] by his own sense of when a thing was right or wrong."[208] Edison's unorthodox sleep habits are well known—he would catnap on a desk, lie on a couch for 4 hours, work for 72 hours without sleep, and so forth. These might offer some clues. Also, Edison claimed he never dreamed. It can be speculated that he could have been in a state of altered consciousness—minus state—much of the time, and so in frame of mind accessible to telepathic reception. Edison could be in close touch with his unconscious and the unconscious of his associates—an area where strange ideas as in dreams would not a priori be considered impossible, too fantastic or incongruous with supposedly established facts.

The great inventor's freethinking, open-mindedness and disciplined imagination are indicated by his abiding interest in Thomas Paine, the patriot whose spirited writings sparked the American Revolution, and Paine's biographer, the still-living freethinker, Joseph Lewis. Edison's copy of one of Lewis' books, *The Bible Unmasked,* has many of Edison's penciled annotations. Edison's poorly understood inspiration might have been related to such personality traits as the fact that he could work for long periods of time with great concentration and then comfortably regress to boyhood behavior. Edison might have had ready access to his unconscious where new ideas were hatched free of crippling censorship and authoritative proscriptions. For example, after periods of hard work his laboratory was often transformed into a place of tomfoolery, merriment, pranks, organ and zither music, songs, and even mock prizefights.[132]

There are also hints of his interests in telepathy in his one-time intention to collaborate with a young writer, George Parsons Lathrop, on a "fiction thriller on the style of Jules Verne and H. G. Wells. Amazing inventions never before heard of were going to be introduced." The incomplete manuscript of 1890 contained some of Edison's prophecies, many of which have since been fulfilled.[108]

It is a fact that, although he permitted the backs of his hands to be photographed, Edison never allowed pictures of his palms.[208] He claimed that he did not wish to be bothered by palmists, various cultists, and the like, but it might also be supposed that on a deeper level of consciousness he might have been concerned over the possibility of some palmist-paragnost (?) making a reading that could be too successful and personal. In the life of a genius such as Edison, who enriched all of mankind with countless patents and major discoveries, serendipity might have been telepathy.*

The genius is a bold innovator, one "who bring(s) to society new and original values,"[115] one who has "neither ancestors nor descendants; (he himself) form(s) (his) entire posterity."[116] Among many possible explanations for genius are presumed favorable genetic endowment, a monomania for the problem at hand, high intelligence, appropriate psychopathology, a prepared mind for discovery, and so forth. Despite the explanations, this uniquely creative and inspired condition is still shrouded in mystery.

The telepathic hypothesis might be applicable to the understanding of genius, as is evident from the literature. The paranormal aspects of genius were brilliantly explored in Myers' classical work[137] which emphasized intrapsychic processes and subliminal and supraliminal influences. More recent experimental data[174] indicate that it is often impossible to determine which person was sending or receiving a telepathic impression. This is further complicated when there are additional participants in the experiment or when another person spontaneously and unexpectedly joins in when volleys of thoughts are sent. At such times a complicated crisscrossing effect was observed in the telepathic transactions.

Further clinically corroborative evidence for the telepathic hypothesis and genius has been noted in numerous parent-child[184] and patient-physician telepathic transactions.[177] These complex exchanges of thoughts and emotions in the interpersonal relationships have often unexpectedly involved other people and often transcended the usual person-to-person position. For example, in psychotherapy, spectacular long-distance effects, have been produced, such as a recurrent telepathically induced apparition in a specific

---

*Over the years the writer has occasionally come across Edison's former employees or their close relatives. Although none of these people ever denied him due credit, it seemed odd that many had sour-grapes reactions: they felt that they, or their relatives, did not receive proper recognition for their contributions. Yet when Edison died, few of his former associates made the consistently dazzling array of discoveries that their former chief had. It could be conjectured that Edison might have fortified his own tremendous talents by telepathically picking the minds of his employees which were open to his views, methods, and purposes in the common research endeavor. The resentment some of his employees felt might indicate a dimly perceived awareness of their role in this relationship with Edison. Neither Edison nor his employees seemed to have been conscious of what might have happened. It would seem no accident that Edison repeatedly made one discovery after another. A possible example of this sour-grapes attitude is documented in reference to one of Edison's greatest discoveries, "the Edison effect."[107]

patient and later for this same patient even presumed telekinesis: e.g., at a critical moment in psychotherapy for both patient and physician, an oil painting by paragnost Jacques Romano crashed to the floor.*†

Clinical proof of spontaneously occurring telepathic events has been indicated by (1) the tendency for such episodes to recur nearly predictably when conditions are similar: built-in controls; and (2) under certain conditions, the ability of the psychiatrist to send thoughts telepathically.

In almost all the described instances except the latter, the telepathic episodes were hard to recognize and were usually on the fringes of awareness. The technique of developing awareness is not a simple matter but can be learned by one having an open mind, knowledge of psychopathology, patience, skill and understanding.

By virtue of his comments, which sometimes have glittering telepathic tracer effects, the patient (child or parent) might occasionally have a preconscious awareness of his personal part in the telepathic episode. However, he rarely overtly recognizes the telepathic nature of what has happened. That means, because of various mental mechanisms of the unconscious mind (e.g., repression, displacement, projection, etc.), it is difficult to develop the technique of mental diplopia necessary for recognizing the unmasking a telepathic episode *in statu nascendi*. These problems are illustrated in the following example from everyday life:

December 23, 1965, Thursday, 5:40 P.M. I felt very happy about picking up my wife's friend, Priscilla, at her apartment and bringing her to our home for a pleasant pre-Christmas dinner. As I parked the car before going to the apartment, a thought entered my mind to tell Priscilla about a recent all-night radio show (Long John Nebel) that I had participated in on the subject of telepathy. I suppressed this thought and my mind shifted to the foreign-body thought of writing a parody of the poem "The Night before Christmas" for my secretary. However, I suppressed this idea also, and didn't tell Priscilla since it seemed silly and completely out of context for me. I had never written a poem for my middle-aged secretary and felt on sober reflection that this would be out of place and utter nonsense! No sooner did I "forget" this, pick up Priscilla, and put her in the car, than she, bubbling over with Christmas spirits, said that she wanted to show my wife and me an unusual poem, which she had in her purse, about a teacher's ordeal at school. She said it was a parody on "The Night

---

*With another patient, who seemed to have a talent for telepathy, this same effect occurred when the emotional constellation for patient and physician was again similarly highly charged. This time, however, the picture frame split on the opposite side.
†Other examples from clinical practice of how telepathy might aid discovery and decision making are (a) a gifted biological researcher who in psychotherapy has had much telepathy, (b) a successful real estate broker who through presumed telepathy "stumbled" on one successful venture after another, and (c) a business leader who apparently successfully (unconsciously) uses telepathy in his daily competitive situations.

before Christmas." Priscilla, a middle-aged spinster school-teacher, had never shown me any poems or such personal material in the past. I then told her my thoughts and we traced out our ideas. She had received the poem at noon from a student at her school and she had been thinking about it ever since. Thus it would seem that my inspiration and silly idea was really Priscilla's thought which she had telepathically sent me and which I had translated into terms unique for myself.

The juxtaposed thought of the Long John radio show on telepathy was the tracer that identified the event. This example shows how unconscious telepathic plagiarism might work and how an idea one thinks to be his own can be sent telepathically by someone else and then can be modified and distorted by unconscious mechanisms by the one who perceives it. The synthesis or interpretation depends on various experiential and psychopathological factors.

Although the thought content of this simple example, chosen from countless possible telepathic episodes because of its triteness, has nothing in common with the sublime thoughts of genius, there are certain analogies. It might be supposed that a genius is one who has all the usually recognized attributes of his unique state plus a concentrated intuitive ability by means of which he can telepathically apprehend other people's thoughts as they specifically apply to his work. The genius can successfully integrate his thoughts with telepathic impressions from others. In contrast, the paragnost picks up the ideas of others and recognizes their telepathic origin. He himself, unless he is also a genius, can neither create nor invent to any extent by combining his own abilities with telepathic impressions. He is simply a catalyst who brings the facts together. For the most part, telepathic communication, as in the above example from everyday life, occurs on an unconscious basis without awareness in the minds of the particpants. They become unwitting pawns.

As with Professor Tenhaeff's paragnosts,[214-216] the mentalists, or the psychiatrist sensitized to telepathy, the specific applications of telepathy depend on various background experiences. For example, the psychiatrist can use telepathy as an excellent practical counter-transference psychotherapeutic tool. It follows that much of what passes for empathy, intuition or serendipity might really be telepathy.[85]

Socrates' guiding demon, Joan of Arc's inspired voices, and Swedenborg's celestial communications are classical examples suggestive of the interaction of telepathy and genius. A recent example of discovery occurring independently and approximately at the same time is Charles Darwin's and Alfred Wallace's theory of evolution. It is of interest that as a possible indication of his own unconscious awareness of paragnostic abilities (tracer effect) Wallace later became a spiritist. Another historical example possibly supporting this hypothesis is the independent invention of the telephone by Alexander Graham Bell and Elisha Gray, both of whom filed patents the same day.[106] The credit went to Bell because his patent was filed a few hours ahead of Gray's.

In conclusion the telepathic hypothesis offers intriguing insights into the understanding of genius. Even limited study of the life of Thomas Alva Edison points toward highly suggestive evidence for this point of view.

11
Death of a Parapsychologist
Possible Terminal Telepathy
With Nandor Fodor

Nandor Fodor (1895–1964) was a well-known parapsychologist and psychoanalyst who in his many classical contributions to the literature fruitfully applied the techniques and insights of psychoanalysis to the understanding of psychic phenomena. After four years of occasionally exchanging letters and reprints with Dr. Fodor, we finally met at Montclair, New Jersey, on May 8, 1964, for a very pleasant evening. Fodor struck me as an intensely humane, warm, sensitive man, who was very intuitive. His keen intellect was leavened with radiant kindness and a gentle sense of humor. We were immediately in complete rapport and looked forward "to a great friendship."

The purpose of this paper is (1) to explore a series of possible telepathic dreams and episodes connected with the unexpected death of Dr. Fodor; and (2) to see what telepathic overflow effect there might have been between the writer, a psychiatrist, and his patients from the time Dr. Fodor first appeared in a dream to the time the details of his final illness and death were learned.

Since telepathy has many significant emotional aspects and seems to conform to the mechanisms of the unconscious mind, this report might have some interest because it deals with a man who was a virtuoso in both parapsychology and psychoanalysis. For this reason, it might demonstrate the potentialities as well as the pitfalls of a qualitative, psychodynamic study of telepathy. This report is chiefly concerned with the telepathic components of the reported experience. It does not attempt to delve into the more usually recognized psychoanalytic interpretations. All dreams act as attempted communication at one level or another. They are usually considered occult only when they seemingly transend the psychodynamic mechanisms. For the most part the reported dreams speak for themselves.

I

During our visit in Montclair, New Jersey on May 8, 1964 Dr. Fodor seemed to be in good health. He told me of his various planned research projects, publications, and so forth. But, on Friday, May 15, 1964, he developed an acute cardiac seizure and was transferred from his New York City home to a hospital where he died on Sunday, May 17, 1964. A Masonic funeral service was held on Tuesday, May 19, 1964. Until 11:15 A.M. of that day, the writer knew nothing about what had happened to his new friend.

During our only meeting the writer mentioned a recent, very personal, unusual presumed telepathic dream. Dr. Fodor had been present in the dream's manifest content. This was the first time the writer had ever dreamed of him. The dream, with multiple specific telepathic tracers, vividly and accurately portrayed the unexpected acute mental derangement of a person who was a well-known psychic researcher for many years and well known to both of us.

Also, during our May 8 visit, Fodor gave me two of his books, *New Approaches to Dream Interpretation*[69] and *Mind Over Space*.[65] As I bade him good-bye, he told me he was quite pleased that his publisher did not omit his chapter on the Tetragrammaton (A Personal Analytic Approach to the Problem of Holy Name, Chapter 3, Part III, pp. 206–222) of the dream interpretation book. Because of Fodor's comments, I quickly flipped through the pages of the book and scanned this chapter later the next day. I hoped to go back and read it more carefully later.

II

The following morning, May 9, 1964, at 7:00 A.M., while I was rapidly reading Fodor's *Mind Over Space* my eyes fell upon the footnote on page 217: "When something injurious has insidious designs on the organism, the latter ... awaits motionless and deathly still for what is going to happen. It makes itself resemble and be identical with the surrounding physical world. (Mimicry) ... Every trauma still evokes that old fantasy pattern of camouflage, of disappearing into the universe [quoting Dr. A. M. Meerloo. "Shock—A Psychosomatic Phenomenon," *Journal of Nervous and Mental Diseases,* June, 1950]." Simultaneous with my reading this, my seven-year-old daughter Lisa trotted into my office and jolted me with. "Daddy, what would you do if I were sinking in quicksand?" When I wanted to know why she asked this, she said not to ask her. Lisa seldom or never rises this early, in fact she usually arises only after prodding. At her level, Lisa precisely and horribly expressed what had caught my eye. Perhaps she was reluctant to see her father's rapt attention devoted to something other than herself.[184]

III

On Friday, May 15, 1964, I had a vivid, very personal presumed telepathic dream of a formerly close friend whom I had neither seen nor heard about in six years. The dream was apparently fulfilled when I noticed a pertinent newspaper announcement the next day. Although the details of this experience, like the recent acute derangement dream, are not closely relevant for the purposes of this report, the episode is mentioned because of its possible conection with the preceding and following reported experiences. That is, it is hoped that some day the possible physical-emotional parameters of telepathy will be better understood: e.g., atmospheric conditions, cosmic radiations, etc., and that there will be an explanation for the occurrence or absence of serial telepathic episodes.

IV

Saturday, May 16, 1964, 8:00 A.M., I recorded the following dream and associations: "Four saxaphonists, with Carl Bethel (my aged music teacher), are playing the bass saxaphone: with one loud chord, a blaring fanfare, then I see four muscular white guards called The Four Israelites. I know the magic word; and someone (myself?) swims deep in the ocean, says the word, and the Four Israelites fall over dead, and I recover the precious golden necklace. The fanfare said, 'Pay attention! Something very important is to follow.' And in the dream I almost woke up."

The associations were: "The magic word Shem (as described in Dr. Fodor's article 'A Personal Analytic Approach to the Problem of the Holy Name[68])–I have it! It will uncover the secret of telepathy and provide an answer to Floyd's [a colleague] question: how to find control over telepathy; then we will demonstrate this. The precious golden necklace equals the Golden Fleece. A Mr. Kron [proprietor of a men's clothing store of that name]–the Holy Grail and Parsifal imbued with his sacred mission. Antiquities–Sir Wallace Budge, Egyptologist.

"The Four Israelites stumped me, but then I realized they stood for the meaning of the four-letter word, the Tetragrammaton (JHVH for Jehovah's name). Also, Four Israelites is a reference to the doctor's name, Fodor-four-and what I believe [erroneously] was Dr. Fodor's religion [Hebrew], and the serious [religious] nature of his contributions.

"Mr. Bethel [my brother's and my music teacher], by feeling, was immediately associated with my brother Eric who was killed in action during World War II. In previous dreams my brother had appeared on very rare occasions. On one such occasion he correctly telepathically heralded an approaching death in actual life. Bethel could also have double meaning because of its Biblical definition, which is a house of worship, a hallowed spot or structure, scene of Jacob's vision of the ladder with angels ascending. The saxaphones [the instrument I used to play] were associated to *horns* [a term always used by Mr. Bethel for all brass instruments] and an excellent paper of Dr. Fodor's on precognitive dreams entitled *Through the Gate of Horn.*[66]

The dream had an element of fear and, upon arising, I discussed it with my wife. As usual in such instances, I asked such questions as, Is my mother all right? My father? My sister? and so forth.

At 10 o'clock the same morning of the saxaphone fanfare dream, my wife, who was quite intrigued with it, came to tell me that she had just heard on the telephone from my mother the rather disquieting news that my parents had recently asked friends of theirs the procedure for buying a cemetery plot at the Mount Hebron Protestant cemetary (Upper Montclair, N.J.). My wife and I both immediatey connected this news to my dream. I thought the fanfare symbolized the chilling news (cemetery plot) and my deceased brother might have been warning me. Although the biblical term Mount Hebron symbolized the religious motifs in the dream, it still did not add up properly emotionally. My wife's news made me uncomfortable but for the moment my dream was mentally filed away as deciphered.

V

Three days later, on Tuesday, May 19, 1964, at 7:00 A.M. I awoke having an exhaustingly beautiful dream and wrote as follows: "In the beautiful country of Küemmel [means Hungary in the dream], high, snow-capped mountains, fluorescent lava-like liquids cascading down beautiful, strange rock formations, I walk on other-world-like rocks. I descend at first, then start climbing, and noting unusual foliage, evergreens and cacti. I must follow a trail to avoid quicksand—I'm not sure of myself but this scenery is gorgeous, stupendous.

"At the top there is a beautiful clear lake and there are many people. Unbelievable beauty. Walking is easy and the breathing is invigorating—most unusual dark clouds behind me in rocky valley. Despite the fear, I walk on, in this new mysterious land. My initial reaction on the rocks is whether to go or not to go, loneliness, fear and menace, yet a grand adventure and temptation—a great discovery in uncharted areas!

"This dream symbolizes danger and beauty, ancient yet new, like telepathy—it is there all the time but you may not see it. Here in the dream I have a chance to view this unusual process symbolically. The baby pines and cacti represent beauty in miniature. The softness of the moss underfoot, the purity of the air, represent mescaline synesthesis where the senses are short-circuited between themselves: one feels color, sees sounds, floats, etc.

"I have sensation that my daughter, Lisa is in early part of the dream. I go back for her but then decide to go on ahead because I don't see her. I feel that Lisa has the ability to see ahead—great prevision. The Lake represents tremendous beauty, transquillity, Nirvana, sex, privacy, everything and anything good.

"[The Associations were]: Küemmel, Fodor, Hungary, birth dream, telepathic dream, down to the valley of darkening and up into light. The trees are pubic hair, rebirth, beauty, peace, love and (symbolized) mescaline experience of sublime, great, extraordinary ecstasy on another planet—out in space."

This rather cryptic dream, like the previous one about the saxophone fanfare, was a mystery and not interpreted. Despite all the implicit symbology related to Nandor Fodor and numerous telepathic tracers, the dissociation or failure to correctly synthesize the dream persisted. However the dream was so emotionally moving, unique, and laden with telepathic tracers that it was written down in full.

At 11:00 A.M. my secretary, Mrs. Catherine W. Matthews, came into the laboratory with the shocking news that she had just heard on the telephone from my former secretary, Mrs. Isabel M. Sayre, that Dr. Fodor had dropped dead on Sunday! Mrs. Sayre had read it in the morning newspaper. I had not bought any newspapers for a long time and had no way of knowing of this tragedy. The dreams of May 16 and 19 exploded into immediate understanding, and I showed my dream notes of these dates to Mrs. Matthews. I wrote the following:

"This is a typical birth dream as described in many of Dr. Fodor's papers and books. This is quite new to me personally, as well as very uncommon in my work with patients. Küemmel means sweetness, a precious liqueur (milk), and is supposed to mean Hungary. In the dream I emphasized the return to Hungary, the womb, the land of Dr. Fodor's birth.

"This dream is possibly a telepathic dream from some member or friend of the Fodor family. Could it possibly, in some way, have come from Nandor Fodor himself?"

Almost instantaneously with the shocking impact of this dream about the land of "Küemmel," the dream of the preceding Saturday (the day before Dr. Fodor's sudden and unexpected death) was immediately revealed to my understanding. I wondered if the dream of the saxophone fanfare was a precognitive dream of Dr. Fodor's approaching death and his finding the answer to the meaning of the Holy Name and the secrets of the occult as symbolized by the golden necklace—the Golden Fleece.

VI

Although now aware of Dr. Fodor's death, I still did not know any of the details. Despite my professional awareness of the influence of suggestion, various dream mechanisms and disguises which show the mind's prodigious talent for the dramatization of unconscious conflicts, and so forth, the following dreams of May 20 and 21 seem worthy of inclusion. The possible wisdom of deciding to record these notes was verified by some unusual developments I first learned on May 24 when Dr. Fodor's family supplied the missing links.

On May 20, 1964, Wednesday night, there was a slight rainfall. I slept poorly because I awakened many times during the night thinking that I heard bells ringing, and loud clapping sounds. This was not my wife's experience.

On Thursday, May 21, 1964 at 6:30 A.M., the following dream and associations was recorded:

"At the *Golden Fleece,* a men's clothing store, Mr. Kron, the propietor, and a new assistant by name of Mario were fitting *suits.* They had a beautiful new store wtih most extraordinary furnishings and material. I got a *new* suit of gray English tweed with thin red stripes. While being fitted I heard that Nandor Fodor was widely beloved and had recently got a *new suit,* a most unusual one. Although I had this information in mind I did not see it (or him). I got the notion that he isn't dead but there is something odd. He is different in his *new suit,* a most unusual *new suit.* While leaving the Golden Fleece, I met a patient of mine, Mr. Fords, Pseudonym, who was also called Mario in the dream. He too was getting a *new suit.* He said that he had to leave to consult with a new manager of a nearby hotel (The Beacon Manor), Mr. Joseph Solomon,"

The assocations to this dream were: "friendly, different, new, rebirth dream, patients, Kron, gold, *Golden Fleece,* precious, custom-made for body perfection, contentment." While writing this down, I recalled having seen royal purple shirts with broad black stripes on the shelves of the *Golden Fleece* store in the dream. This symbolized royalty and death.

Mario was identified with my patient Fords, who, while recently on vacation, grew a beard and moustache. This was a surprise development in his treatment. Mario and Fords have some resemblance to the conventional pictures of Jesus [resurrection]. The further associations were, hystolysis and metamorphosis: how a caterpillar changes into a buttefly, the analogy that Dr. Fodor used when discussing materialization as part of a book he was working on.

Fords also symbolized other unusual things, for he had a Christ complex and strangely enough, on three occasions in his therapy,* the physician "spontaneously" appeared to him in presumably telepathic episodes.

At the time of our May 8 meeting, I discussed with Dr. Fodor these recurrent apparitional episodes involving Fords. He commented on the writer's sometimes impish nature and speculated that a clear visual imagery is usually associated with this sort of event. Fords' name has the same first letter and total number of letters as Fodor.

In the dream, the patient Fords was talking to Joseph Solomon, who in fact owns the Beacon Manor (named after a famous old Methodist hotel on the New Jersey coast). The associative significance of the biblical Joseph and Solomon, men of integrity, religion, great knowledge and wisdom, is obvious.

Kron meant crown, golden horn, Golden Fleece, Gate of Horn, precognitive dream, a mythological quest for the secrets of telepathy and all the rewards they would hold: Dr. Fodor's statement (to me on the night of our meeting) that sooner or later science must come to grips with psychic phenomena.

Because of the repeated symbol of the Golden Fleece in the dream series, out of curiosity, I looked up in the dictionary† and was surprised to find under "Order of Golden Fleece" the statement that this was an award of the old Austro-*Hungarian* Empire and that it was reserved only for royalty and the highest nobility: "The Golden Fleece hanging from an enameled flintstone emitting flames."

I wondered if the Golden Fleece could have been a personal symbol of Nandor Fodor, a Hungarian patriot. In our only meeting, Dr. Fodor proudly told me about his speeches and efforts in behalf of Hungarian freedom after World War I. Hungary, Dr. Fodor's native land, symbolized his return, and being reborn—a return to Küemmel—sweetness, the first nourishment. Hungary is also a word play on hungry (for) land of birth . . . Dr. Fodor's rebirth—his refitting in a new suit (histolysis, materialization)—an achievement of the most sublime satisfaction, the award of the Golden Fleece, the award reserved for the greatest accomplishments.

Some of the unusual and repetitive symbolism of this (May 21) dream was clarified on Sunday, May 24, 1966, when the writer visited Mrs. Fodor and her daughter for the first time since Dr. Fodor's death. They told me about many presumably telepathic or precognitive episodes related to Dr. Fodor's death.[70,71] Some of their comments seemed to pertain to the elaborate and

*Since the date of this dream, Fords has perceived presumed telepathically induced apparitions six additional times and on one occasion during a critical exchange, for patient, physician (and in the past life of Jacques Romano) in psychotherapy, and oil painting by the paragnost Jacques Romano crashed to the floor.[77]
†Webster's new International Dictionary, 12th Edition, G. & C. Merriam Co., Springfield, Mass., 1942.

esoteric imagery of my dreams. Although I had experienced many deaths among my family, friends, and colleagues throughout the years, this dream series that seemed to relate to Nandor Fodor, a man I met only once was entirely unique, personal, and compelling.

On the day of the *new suit* and *Golden Fleece* dream, Mrs. Fodor had packed her husband's clothes to send to a relative in England. While doing this and under great strain, she noticed a ten-cent piece that fell from a cabinet to her feet. She felt this was an answer and symbolized the actual worth of the otherwise costly clothes: "What does it matter—this body is but a shell; the suit can be changed. The spiritual is what really counts." She requested her son-in-law, "Take the rubbish to the incinerator," which is something she had never done; and then again she answers herself, "because it is rubbish, only to be burned" referring to the thought of the cremation of the body in contrast to the spirit or soul.

The Golden Fleece motif stressed in my dream series might have been related to the fact that Dr. Fodor was cremated in his beloved Masonic apron and the original one was kept in the lodge. The writer did not know that Dr. Fodor was a Mason nor how much this organization meant to him. Furthermore, the writer knew next to nothing of Masonic ritual and rites; therefore, the final dream of the Fodor series (May 21) might have had some suggestive telepathic components.

It should be stressed that one must be cautious in seeing that the criteria are satisfied before a dream or psychotherapeutic exchange can be considered as possibly telepathic. However, the other side of the coin should not be neglected: telepathic components to dreams or to interpersonal communications must be analyzed for their own intrinsic and special significance if full justice is to be done to the patient. It is just as reprehensible to neglect a priori or shut out of awareness and from analysis the poignant telepathic aspects of interpersonal communications, as to be scientifically lax in applying the telepathic criteria.

VII

Because of the unusual nature of the Fodor series of possible telepathic dreams, it was thought worthwhile to check all the psychotherapeutic and consultation sessions with patients from May 3, 1964, the day preceding the first dream involving Nandor Fodor that later was shown to be telepathic, to Sunday, May 24, 1964, when the writer learned the details of Fodor's death from his family. It was wondered that if there was any telepathic or other form of communication between Nandor Fodor, his family and friends, and the writer, there might be additional clues in the material, free associations, and dreams of these sessions. In a series of psychodynamic drawing experiments it was often noted that presumed telepathic episodes autochthonously bubbled up between participants and nonparticipants (patients) in a way that conformed to life itself. Such episodes "just happen" and they evaded the rigid experimental design as usually understood.

The records for the described period of time revealed that 21 patients were seen for a total of 75 psychotherapeutic hours. It was noted that in 31 of the sessions there were single or multiple telepathic exchanges between patient and physician. The events were qualitatively similar to those described elsewhere.[184,174,177] In eight of these sessions there were presumed telepathic episodes directly pertaining to the Fodor family, or there was material that was indirectly applicable to them.

Although this qualitative approach from reading spontaneous material does not pretend to have any of the highly desirable refinements that can be statistically validated in the laboratory, it needs no apology, for it has certain other values that the laboratory techniques lack. For example, there might be clues about how telepathy works, and how it can span a wide range of interhuman communications. That such episodes are often fragmentations, condensations, and so forth, does not mean that the presence of such implicit difficulties invalidates the episodes. The animal must be seen as he is in life and not in the simpler way one might desire to have him in the laboratory.

In the session of May 11, 1966, in quiet moment, the physician thought of Mrs. Fodor as being artistic or arty, at which point the patient, a schizophrenic woman, responded with a foreign-body thought: "We met A.O., a *decorator,* at a cocktail party."

On May 13, with a patient in collaborative treatment (her son, a schizophrenic, was being treated at a hospital far way), the physician thought of a colleague—who was also a patient and who had had recent heart surgery—when, completely out of her asociational context, the patient blurted "People get heart attacks because of high cholesterol." [Dr. Fodor died of a heart attack]. On May 15, in a moment of silence, the physician thought of his need for examples of precognition, in his collection of psychic material, when this same paitent responded with, "How frail we humans are in this life. We latch on to one human. We have to take the unexpected—how I would feel if you suddenly got sick. It proves you can't hold on to things. We need reserve stamina; we can't put all our eggs in one basket."

On the 5th of May, an ambulatory schizophrenic patient who fancied herself a spiritualistic medium said at one point in her session, "P. V. talks to her deceased mother who tells her of anyone who dies." The writer then thought of Dr. Fodor's wonderful books on dreams and the patient said, "I read every book in the library up there [N.H.]. These are things you don't do at home [N.J.]."

On May 15 (the day of Dr. Fodor's heart attack), Mr. Fords, a patient who has appeared on rare occasions in the physician's dreams, and then almost always under telepathic circumstances, apparently responded to the writer's highly specific thoughts of a "Fodor paper" (he had *read* long ago) describing how he took *mescaline* and did not want to repeat it, ". . . a beautiful experience [like the writer's] but too much *vomiting.*" Immediately after his physician's thought, Fords told of his dream where he was ". . . in the doctor's office and took two *mescaline* pills and one pill for vomiting." In his associations he said how he *read* of hallucinogenic drugs several years ago and how in his dream he was coming across with his head down part of the time, then with his head up, with hope for happiness. The physician's thoughts after his patient's account of the dream were of Nandor Fodor and his birth theories. At that point, for no ostensible reason, there was a loud click in the office.

On May 19, 1964, a woman patient who had much everyday and some spectacular telepathy throughout her therapy* had a telepathic exchange with her physician. In a moment of quiet he thought of sending "the Fodor" telepathic series of dreams to the Indian journal, *Samiksa* (The Indian Psychoanalytical Society), where Fodor had published some of his own far-out articles, [quasi religious, philosophical], and wondered about the *cost* of printing—when the patient said completely out of context, "There is no charge for baptizing but you can *donate* to the minister's vacation fund." She might have picked up at her level the condensation or concept of a deep religious or baptismal (birth of Christ) significance which was fused to the mundane concern of cost. At a later point in the session the writer associated to: "Poor Mrs. Fodor, . . . funeral, Tuesday, when shall I visit and console her?" when the patient said, "He told me a sad thing of a neighbor who has a son who will die in one year."

On May 22 the physician was again with his patient Fords and he mused about the Fodor dream series and the unusual dream (May 21) that involved Fords (Mario), the new suit,and the caterpillar changing into a butterfly. Fords responded to his physician's mental imagery of metamorphosis by saying, "I'd be more comfortable in a cocoon than out of it—switch to a larger place rather than falling back in a shell. I'd rather become a person in my own right!"

It is plausible that most of the aforementioned abrreviated examples of possible patient-physician telepathic episodes illustrate how emotionally

---

*Years later, in a planned experiment for telekinesis and thoughtography with Dunninger, the renowned mentalist, nothing of note had happened. However, at the exact time of this experiment, this patient, far away in her own home and naturally unaware of her physician's researches, had four pictures mysteriously appear on all the tiles of her kitchen.

charged thoughts can be sent or received in psychotherapeutic situations. The examples also demonstrate the difficulties of psychodynamic interpretations, for if these events, as they spontaneously happen in everyday life, have so many variables—all that is human— it is hard to describe convincingly the factors that led up to the presumed telepathic exchange. It is almost impossible to define a cut-off point, which is often quite arbitrary. It might be necessary for literary purposes: viz., space, clarity, and so forth but in fact the psychic situation is usually a continuum. It seemingly has its own laws, and often the telepathic sparks jump the gap and involve many others than those in direct confrontation in a wide array of interpersonal contacts.

On the other hand, a series of spontaneous presumed telepathic episodes might still have much of value. Impure, by comparison with the controlled statistical laboratory data, admittedly contaminated with all the variables that are life, the breakdown of any telepathic psychotherapeutic physician-patient exchange still yields much material, that from the overall viewpoint can be quite compelling. It is hard to see how any laboratory experiment could ever be so emotionally honest and sophisticated that it could approach the necessary, genuine, deep emotions, fine nuances, and sensitivities that are part of a human being's life. The myriad surprises, reality itself, the conscious contacts, and unconscious sinews that exist between people are the stuff that is telepathy.

In conclusion, it would seem that there was some kind of terminal telepathic communication between Nandor Fodor (or some member of his family or a friend) and the writer. It is plausible that Nandor Fodor by virtue of his profound knowledge of parapsychology, psychoanalysis, and his own uniquely sensitive and intuitive personality was well prepared for the possible telepathic communications. The experiences might be unique because they involved two people who met only once in their lives and yet apparently became partners in tragically unforeseen, unplanned, complex, telepathic series of dreams and experiences. One might wonder how much more common episodes of this sort might be if other trained observers in parapsychology and psychoanalysis looked for them. The implications of such events are great and offer endless possibilities for speculation and experimentation.

12
Possible Human-Animal Paranormal Events

Folklore, myths, and legends supply countless examples of the strange affinity between man and animals. Vincent and Margaret Gaddis[87] have recently collected many provocative examples of this. Ivan Sanderson,[168] a well-known biologist, has also noted many such events between a variety of species and man. Although he had handled many wild animals on his TV shows over the years, he jokingly says that he still has his 10 fingers. One very weird case studied by the psychoanalyst-parapsychologist Nandor Fodor,[13] concerned the bizarre poltergeist example of a talking mongoose. In another study he cited and speculated about the amazing animals that materialized in seances[78] witnessed by eminent scientists. In his memoirs the newspaperman Pierre Van Paassen[226] wrote about his personal experiences with a possible poltergeist dog that savagely fought with van Paassen's two German police dogs, one of which dropped dead immediately afterward. Other celebrated controversial man-animal biocommunications include horses that were allegedly telepathic* and could calculate, and of course the not uncommon news stories of dogs and cats (and other pets) who had been abandoned or lost and then returned over great distances and time. The scientist Milan Ryzl[167] has summarized much of the animal parapsychological data. Von Urban,[227] the psychoanalyst, recalled his own turmoil and the bellowing and howling of animals before a major European earthquake in 1895. The research physician Abraham G. Ginsberg,[181] who independently discovered a device similar to radar, recalled how when he was living in the Adirondacks his dog crawled under the bed and stayed there every time his sister, who was very fond of the animal, was operated on by Dr. Will Mayo in Rochester, Minnesota. Lilly,[119] the multifaceted research physician, has studied the

---

*Dunninger investigated several of such cases and never found an example of genuine paranormal ability. He contended that the horses were trained to respond to cues.

intriguing communications between man and dolphins. Keel[113] has recorded many bizarre man-animal interactions that deserve serious consideration.

Although Grad, Cadoret, and Paul,[93] in well-controlled laboratory studies, demonstrated the effects of psychic healing on guinea pigs, there has been little critically analyzed clincial material presented in the medical literature. The telekinetic hypothesis gives clues for a possible modus operandi for placebo effects in the study of drug actions, and it might explain the different results sometimes obtained from identical experiments by various investigators. This is a practical question which should not be overlooked.

Because of the intimate nature of their work, psychiatrists are favorably situated to observe possible telepathy between patients and their pets, as well as to be sensitive to such possibilities in their own lives. For example, Mrs. Krystal[176] and her sons presented convincing evidence of how, when she was traveling in Mexico (pp 11–12) she telepathically (and correctly) learned of her dog's death in Maryland. In a planned experiment with myself (B.E.S.) that was spontaneously derailed, she telepathically picked up many of the segments of a horrible situation where a dog savagely attacked my friend (pp 22–24).

It is of interest that Jacques Romano,[118] the extraordinary nonagenarian paragnost, claimed he was never bitten by a dog, although he was exposed to many dangers in his life.

Pets, mostly dogs and cats, have always played a large role in the personal life of the distinguished telepathist, Joseph Dunninger. Both Romano and Dunninger, interestingly enough, called attention to the possible telepathic affinity between cockroaches and man. For example, if one thought of squashing a certain cockroach in a group of several, *that* specific cockroach would frequently scamper away. The parapsychologist Mrs. Anita Gregory reported[96] some cockroach experiments done by Russians which were based on an earlier study done by an Israeli scientist; and recently Schmidt[171] has reported his investigations using cockroaches.

In a previous report[177] brief mention was made of a woman who had persistent success in winning substantial sums of money at the horse races. I studied her until I was unable to keep up with her fast pace. I did go to the races with her once, however, and was satisfied that she seemed to have some genuine abilities.* Her family physician, who had observed her over the last decade, told me that she was still successful (1972). It is of interest that this woman's whole life seemed to be focused on horse racing, and that this interest, which she shared with her husband, might have been the means of

---

*In a psychodynamically devised clincial experiment that was designed to take advantage of the transference, I gave the woman a small sum of money to place bets that, if successful, would be sufficient to bring to the United States for a visit, the distinguished parapsychologist and expert on proscopy, Prof. W. H. C. Tenhaeff. The experiment flatly failed.

keeping her otherwise precariusly balanced marriage intact. Although her husband approached racing in a scientific, mathematical way, his luck was terrible. But she, at the last moment just before the races started,† would rush to the betting booth, place a small bet, and almost always win. At times, when she departed from her usual custom and told her husband about a race—including the long shots—he would never follow through on her advice, and he would lose. The woman would then be overcome with a near orgy of success.

Among hypotheses for such feats are these: (1) the lady telepathically cognized a crooked race; (2) she exercised true precognition; (3) she had direct communication with the horses and in some obscure way determined who would win from them.

The following examples from research on Joseph Dunninger, from psychiatric practice, and from personal life explore this topic.

Dunninger's Cat O' Four Tales

Dunninger once recalled an event which happened near the turn of the century when he was a child. His older (by four years) brother Louis had become acutely ill with an obscure fever and an oozing discharge from the eyes, nose, and ears. Every day for several weeks between midnight and one o'clock in the morning, Louis would become very frantic, exhibit violent behavior, and "the family had a hard time holding him down. Dr. Steinach, our family physician, and later consultants were unable to make a diagnosis or prescribe a remedy that could relieve the condition."

Dr. Steinach, who knew Mr. and Mrs. Dunninger, Sr., very well, surprised them by asking: "Do you believe in witchcraft? Lou's illness is so bizarre that I wonder if it could be caused by suggestion or a curse. I have read many books about this kind of thing in medieval Scotch-English literature." The doctor was cautious in his statements because he knew this was a way-out position for a physician; and furthermore, neither Mr. nor Mrs. Dun-

---

†Dunninger, unlike his father and brother, was not particularly interested nor knowledgeable about horses or horse racing. However, he went on two occasions. The first time was at Belmont Racetrack when he was accompanied by his wife, an NBC executive, and the latter's girlfriend. The executive wanted to impress his girlfriend by having Dunninger pick the winners. Dunninger was as surprised as anyone when he picked five winners in a row, but no one won any money because Dunninger did not place any bets and his friends did not follow his directions. "Dan T. (executive) said I chose long shots and plugs." The second horse race that he attended was in San Francisco, when he was again accompanied by his wife, who verified this information. He entered the arena and as a stunt wrote his prediction for the big race of the day on a small slate and showed it to the grandstands. He again picked the winner.

The only time the dowing paragnost Henry Gross[176] dabbled in horse racing, he picked both the winner and the loser of the Kentucky Derby (p. 153). Moss and Sands have reported a contolled investigation in picking the winners. (Why Did I Flunk the Horse Test? Parapsychology Review. [No. 5.]:10–12, 1970) ninger believed in the supernatural. Nevertheless, the very day of the physician's statement, the family's white cat disappeared from their home in New York City without apparent reason. The next day, an employee of Dunninger's father, a Mrs. Ellit, who also knew the brothers and who had originally given them the white cat as a present, surprised the family by returning the cat. Mrs. Ellit lived on the lower East Side, more than a mile away from the Dunninger factory. She said, "The cat came into my house last night; it must have escaped."

Joseph Dunninger commented: "This event made my mother and father very suspicious, for on the night that the white cat disappeared my mother saw several cats sitting on the window sill of Lou's room. Although the window was closed, my father had to get the broom and chase them away. The following morning, when Mrs. Ellit brought the white cat back, my mother accused her of bewitching the cat and of cursing Lou. My father fired her.

"My parents knew that Mrs. Ellit was a vindictive woman who felt she was given less sewing than the other German and Italian women who worked in my father's factory. Mother was infuriated. She picked up a pair of shears and said if Lou didn't improve she'd kill the woman. Mrs. Ellit took the white cat away and from that night on Lou gradually improved until he was better. We never told him the story because it would upset him."

The Dunninger family had numerous cats and dogs as pets through the years but they never had cats on the window sill, as happened that night. "When Dr. Steinach heard of the strange events, he suggested that if we ever saw Mrs. Ellit again and she touched Lou or one of us, Mother should strike her. One day Mother met Mrs. Ellit by chance on the street and when the lady touched Lou, Mother hit her on the hand. Although Dr. Steinach didn't believe in the supernatural he had an interest in the occult. My parents just accepted the doctor's explanation and that was that."

Many years later, when Louis was twenty-one years old, he died on December 21, of tuberculous pneumonia. Joseph Dunninger recalled: "The night before Lou died he yelled to me to come into his room and screamed, 'Look at the window. Get the cats away. They're bothering me. They'll kill me. I can't sleep!' There were no cats. His room, and mine which was next door, was high up, and cats couldn't climb up the side of our brownstone building. This was the first time Lou ever mentioned any cats. Nothing like this had happened before."

Another related event to these cat experiences occurred in October 1933, about 31 years after Louis' death, when Joseph Dunninger, with the New York *Journal American* staffwriter Joe Cowen and columnist Louis Sobel, wrote a series of articles on Dunninger's investigations of spiritualistic mediums.

One day they purchased a Harlem newspaper and read ads about mediums and fortunetellers. They chose one name and immediately dropped in unannounced. Among several items, this otherwise unprepossessing tall, thin Negro medium told them was that Dunninger had a brother who had died as a young man and that his death had something to do with cats. Furthermore, she described a particular type of high collar that bothered Louis in life, so much that he couldn't wear it. Dunninger was quite taken aback: "I wasn't thinking of this: if anything I expected to have a laughable reading and to hear only nonsense. But what she said was all true." His brother never liked high collars and preferred a winged collar. Also, when Louis died, the undertaker tried unsuccessfully to dress him with a high collar. The undertaken called Joseph Dunninger for instructions, and he was told to substitute a winged collar. Only Dunninger knew this.

The last major family cat experience might have happened when Joseph Dunninger's mother was in the twilight of her life. Once she went away for a few days. Her cat, Mimi, who was accustomed to lying contentedly at the foot of her bed and purring, became very upset—apparently at being abandoned— meowed incessantly, and refused food. Only when Joseph Dunninger summoned his mother and she returned, did Mimi settle down again. This happy state persisted until Mrs. Dunninger's death.* Then, contrary to expectations based on the previous experience with Mimi, the cat surprisingly enought jumped up on her mistress's bed, looked around, "as if someone was there, purred, and assumed her serene previous adjustment." This continued until she died several years later and was interred with her former mistress.

The accounts of cat episodes which were always similar, were related to me by Joseph Dunninger on many occasions through the years. They were buttressed with appropriate scrapbook newspaper clippings and independent corroboration by Mrs. Joseph Dunninger and Joseph Dunninger's late older brother Max.

The Bat

My wife and I took my "summertime bachelor" colleague, Dr. Brewster Breeden, to dinner for the first time. I knew that part of his military service

---

*Throughout her son's career; Mrs. Dunninger, Sr., used to look out the open window of their apartment, with a shawl over her shoulders, waiting for him to come home late at night. The shawl was then neatly folded and placed on a chair by the window. The night before Mrs. Dunninger's death her son returned from a performance that also featured the soprano Jessica Dragonet. "I noted that Mother was very ill and her shawl was crumpled on the floor. I took her to bed and she died the following day of pneumonia. It was very odd that the formerly crumpled shawl on the floor was now neatly folded and placed on a chair. I could not think of any acceptable explanation for this. I am also superstitious about the 6 of spades which I had dropped that night during my performance. Anytime I encounter that card it seems that I'm in trouble."

had been in Japan so I told him about a fascinating article in *Science,* that I had read earlier in the day. It was about the U.S. plans for using bats to which incendiary bombs were attached as a secret weapon against Japan during World War II. This was a focal point in our discussion. After my wife and I had returned home from dinner and had retired, we were awakened at 1:30 A.M., hearing a strange noise—first a pummeling against the screen and then odd sounds all around the bedroom. When I turned on the light, I found that a bat, by some freak accident had crashed through the screen and was flying around the room. This happened on July 23, 1960; it had never happened before nor has it since. One wonders about a possible communication, coincidence, synchronicity, or precognition.

The Squirrel

A middle-aged woman was visiting her sister in a nursing home. It was the ninth anniversary of the sister's severe hemiplegia and motor aphasia. Although the sister could comprehend sufficiently to successfully manage her investments, she had to be fed, dressed, pushed around in a wheelchair, and attended constantly. The visitor, who was an animal lover, noted that her sister was concerned over a newspaper article she had read a week before about numerous animals in the South that were killed on the highways because of the drought. On the way home the woman went into a florist shop that she seldom patronized and among many items bought a stuffed toy squirrel as a surprise present for her sister. She later learned that at this time, many miles away, the nursing home attendant had wheeled the sister outdoors where she had a shocking experience: a squirrel jumped into her lap and ran up her arm and lay on the back of her neck—apparently the animal was tame. When the nurse swatted the animal with a newspaper, it jumped down, ran up the nurse's leg and bit her. The police were called, and they shot the animal.

The squirrel's head was examined by the Board of Health for rabies, but no disease was found. Was this coincidence? Or, could this unique experience of the disabled sister with the squirrel have telepathically prompted the sympathetic woman (who was an animal lover) to buy the toy squirrel at that exact time (there were other choices) as an unusual telepathically occasioned means, as described elsewhere[184] of reassuring the sister that the animal was really harmless and should not have been shot? Or, did the kind thought of buying the stuffed animal in some way cause an interaction between the disabled sister and the squirrel who took a shortlived liking to her? A possible telesomatic exhange (Case six) involving this woman and her family is reported elsewhere.[180]

The Robin

Lester Riley, a middle-aged handyman-gardener of old Scots-Irish stock was standing by his truck in the backyard of my New Jersey house telling me about the trip he had to make to Virginia the coming weekend to see his 90-year-old mother, who was ailing and might be dying. While he was describing his mother's health, we were startled to see a bird (a robin) fall from the sky, crash onto the hood of his truck, and skid onto the ground. It gasped and died. Neither of us had ever had an experience like this before nor have we since, although I had on rare occasions seen birds crash into the window when the lights were on in the office. It was a cloudy, cool day, and there was no apparent reason for this strange happening. I immediately looked at Mr. Riley and said "It's very odd, but I guess you'd better go at once." Although I was not superstitious, this statement was foolish and out of place for me. When I next saw Mr. Riley, a week later, he said that because of the weird coincidence, he left immediately for Virginia instead of three days later, as was his original plan. He arrived just before his mother died. When he told his brothers and sisters about the bird experience, they were astounded. They all vividly remembered how 25 years before, their father who was in poor health since an auto accident three years previously, told them how he saw two bluebirds flying out of a window and interpreted that as an omen of *his* death—which happened three days later. Mr. Riley was so disturbed over these dovetailing coincidences involving his parents that he discussed them with his minister.

Such an event as this may be the folklore origin of the common parlance, "to get the bird."*

The Eunuch Cat

A young housewife, who had chronic anxiety hysteria and who had been adopted as a baby, had many telepathic events in her life and treatment. On November 8, 1966, she came to her session and told about an odd event with her seven-month-old male cat. She and her husband had planned to leave for an Atlantic City vacation late one night, but had to postpone their trip until

---

*Once, at the railroad station at Colombo, Ceylon, in the early thirties, Dunninger met ". . . a tall, swarthy gentlemen in flowing robes. He spoke good English, had long hair, and a saintly face. He asked: 'You look like a professional man or an artist, are you.' 'No, I'm a magician. I am here to see what you fellows can do.' The Indian then said, 'I'll give you a demonstration.' He then whistled softly, like a steaming teakettle that could scarcely be heard, and shortly the sky was swaming with hundreds of blackbirds. They settled on the ground, all around him, and stayed until he whistled again, when they all flew off and the sky was black with them. Another amazing stunt was performed by a fakir and Dunninger recorded it on movie film. "He had a container of hundreds of beads which he threw on the ground. He also had a threaded needle and a blackbird rapidly strung all of the beads."

early the next morning because their cat, who was to be altered in their absence, had suddenly run away.

The cat, who was outside and therefore did not see them pack their suitcases or make preparations, had never run away before. They searched for him in vain. When they got up early the next morning, they still could not find the cat. Finally they received a telephone call from a neighbor who said the cat was in their backyard. The cat refused to be coaxed home, however, and ran away again. In anger, the woman asked her husband's sister who worked for a veterinarian and was familiar with animals, to have the cat castrated while they were on vacation. When they returned four days later, they found the cat meowing and shivering in their parked auto in the garage. The husband's sister said that when she came to the house on the morning they left, to take the cat to the vertinarian for castration, he attacked her, ripped her sweater, and scratched her whenever she tried to get into the car. So she left the cat and went home. The cat had no food or water for this period of time.

One can wonder if this usually docile cat sensed the separation from his masters, as well as from his generative organs.

As a built-in control[177] sequel to this experience, in a session at 2:15 P.M. on February 2, 1970, this woman patient, who also had endometriosis and tried to become pregnant for a long time, asked me (B.E.S.) about spaying my cat. She recalled the aforementioned example how her cat was finally spayed, and then said that she had just returned from an appointment with her gynecologist who advised her on the eventual need for a bilateral oophorectomy.

Prior to this patient's session I wondered when my paper on Edison[178] and Dunninger would be out. In truth, during the session my mind occasionally drifted to this personal matter, and during this interplay of polarized material involving the previous possible telepathic cat experience, the patient's discussing the castration of my cat (displaced unconscious wish for her phsyician who was not paying proper attention?) and herself, plus my thoughts of Dunninger, Joseph Dunninger telephoned me about another weird story concerning his cat, who was just spayed! Touché.

As a backdrop, it should be mentioned that this patient, whose husband's family had once been patients of my father, had one striking thing in common with the outstanding paranormal event in Joseph Dunninger's early life. During our session on October 2, 1969 she talked about the fiftieth anniversay of the Slocum disaster (celebrated one year previously) in which her father-in-law's mother and sister and several other relatives perished. Ever since that session, I wondered about the odd coincidence of this event that associatively linked me through her to Joseph Dunninger. From the thousands of patients and myriad hours of psychotherapy, I had never come across this specific associative link before. One of Dunninger's most vivid childhood memories concerned his father's prophetic dream of the Slocum disaster which occurred June 15, 1904. Dunninger and his two older brothers were going on an annual outing up the Hudson River on the steamer, "General Slocum," until their father following his prophetic nightmare, forbade them. He ran around the neighborhood and kept 30 to 40 other children from going. The "General Slocum" caught fire, and in the concatenation of horrrible mishaps and errors 1031 lives were lost. It was the greatest ship disaster in the United States.

The last part of the patient's session was concerned with her dream of an airplane crash, which she associated to a recent Swiss-air disaster in which 40 people were killed by Arab terrorists, who claimed they planted a bomb because of suspected Israelis on the plane. Although the patient's session was over and she did not elaborate on her dream, I inwardly smiled at this capstone of the fusillade of associative telepathy, because in all of his career and worldwide travels, Dunninger had never flown* until very recently. Very few people knew of this fact and virtually no one knew of Dunninger's past telepathic and precognitive experiences that may have accounted for his fear. It was no wonder that Joseph Dunninger made one of his infrequent calls to my office during this session of criss-crossing telepathically *a trois* when one considers the matrix of polarized associations.

At first glance it might be hard to follow these reported complex interactions and the psychic nexus, but this is the essence of telepathy and the associations are simple and more easily grasped if the telepathic hypothesis is used. Once one hears Chopin's "Nocturne," one does not choose "Chopsticks." As the therapist calls on his (and his patient's) reservoir of experiences, he finds telepathy a useful tool in treatment. This example is in accordance with what happens in the physician-patient relationship in psychotherapy or Professor Tenhaeff's[214,216] observation that the paragnost continually rediscovers himself in his consultants. The sensitized areas seemingly reverberate ad infinitum. In a related vein, Joost A. M. Meerloo has written: "... in the psychic world, the new time contains an older one. In the sequence of mental events, later moments include earlier ones."[129]

---

*Dunninger recalled: "Whit White, an advertising man and a friend, would call me up every time he flew because he knew about my experiences. I'd advise him. I never told him not to go and he never had an accident. Once I stopped Dan Tuthill, formerly a vice president of NBC and later my manager, and got him drunk to keep him from flying to San Francisco. The plane he was to have taken came down. Another time I tore up either the tickets or reservations of an insurance agent for a specific plane flight—this man was a neighbor and we bought our house from his relative. That plane too, crashed. He then called me and thanked me for saving his life. He had confidence in what I had to say." This type of experience and its relation to the psychic nexus is discussed elsewhere.[186]

The Monkey

A senior premedical student in psychotherapy, who was working on a monkey project with a psychiatrist, came into his session to report a possible telepathic episode between a juvenile male rhesus monkey and himself. The patient had just finished a seven-month period of controlled observation—totaling 232 hours—and he and his mentor were preparing to kill the monkeys in order to section their brains. Four of the seven monkeys had undergone midline thalamotomies to study the effects of that lesion on their social behavior. In no previous sessions did the patient note any unusual exhanges between the seven monkeys and himself. This was also his experience from more than 40 hours of observation of a colleague's monkeys (four had dorsal lateral frontal lobotomies; four were untreated). However, now he noted: "We have a chain hanging from the ceiling of the enclosure, which the monkeys either held in their hand and walked around in bipedal fashion, or climbed up and down when playing with the others; or they would mouth the chain. I always wondered why they did not swing on it. While I was thinking about this, Nelson, who was an operated monkey, suddenly grabbed the chain and swung like Tarzan. Nelson, the third of a group of seven, was shy. He was different from all the other monkeys in that he was the only one who would look me in the eye. I felt close to him. The next day when I entered the room to complete my observations, I wondered about the previous day's performance. Nelson swung like Tarzan for the second time!"

It might be wondered if the patient was upset and split with the forthcoming sacrifice of the monkey which was symbolic of the patient's past social and academic school performance. Perhaps he sent his thoughts to Nelson, who of the seven was closest to him. Possibly the monkey had some awareness of the significance of what would shortly follow and reacted by telepathically complying with the researcher's wish. The repeat performance might have supported this view because, although this thought was not foremost in the researcher's mind, both he and the monkey were sensitized to this behavioral communication. Although the data in this case is insufficient, it would be of interest to keep the psi hypothesis in mind in a variety of experiments with animals who have undergone various neuroanatomical and other (e.g. bilateral adrenalectomy) extirpation procedures.

This patient has had many telepathic episodes in this therapy, including telepathically detecting Christian names on occasion, his physician's unannounced pending short trip out of the country, and one episode of spectacular tracer-laden overdetermined episode of telekinesis with built-in controls and involving an exploding can of carbonated soft drink.

The Myna Bird

A referring physician, Dr. L, whom I have known for more than 30 years, invited me to his home to meet a middle-aged couple who were also his patients and neighbors. It developed that I had seen the wife's father years ago in electroencephalographic consultation and I had known the husband, who was the manager of an automobile agency that I had dealings with off and on for many years. He told me the following story, which was confirmed by all present. Although anecdotal, the veracity of the informants was impeccable.

"Walter was my father's and my father-in-law's good friend, and he also was my sister's father-in-law. Walter was an inventor who lived in Florida, and he was a former patient of Dr. L. Walter was an alcoholic, and at such times he could be very mean. On a number of occasions he jokingly told his son, daughter, my mother-in-law, and others, 'When I die, I'm coming back as a myna bird.' No one knew why he said this since none of us ever had a myna bird or an unusual experience with one. It was just his dumb joke. This stuck in my mother-in-law's mind, and when Walter died in Florida a few years later, my parents attended his funeral. Following the services they returned from the interment and sat down in my parents' patio to have a drink. They were all amazed to see a myna bird in a tree in the back yard. My mother-in-law shouted, 'That's Walter!' The bird stayed there for one week and then flew away. This was in Florida, and it should be noted that these birds are not native to that state, and these people had not had this type of experience before.

"Then a few days later the myna bird turned up at my brother Rolf's house. The bird followed Rolf on his rounds—he has an advertising agency and travels all over Palm Beach. Where ever Rolf would go, there was the bird. Finally, the bird disappeared and they didn't see him again until my father died eight months later, on his birthday, January 14, 1969. Remember that Walter and my father were also good friends, and that Walter joked how he would return as a myna bird.

"I flew to Florida from New Jersey to make arrangments for my father's funeral. Throughout the whole service in the funeral home Mother and all other members of the family saw the myna bird in the window—that is, before they took my father to the cemetery. After the service we drove to the cemetery and there was the myna bird sitting in a tree, looking out at the grave. Walter was buried only two graves away from my father's. Three days later the myna bird was again in my mother's backyard where she saw him for the last time.

"However, the finale occurred just this winter (February 1972), four years after my father's death. For three weeks we had a myna bird fly to our backyard in the morning and spend the day with us, take off, and then come back the next day. I fed it suet, apples, and even bought 25 pounds of sunflower seeds. I'd go out and say, 'Hello, Pop!' The myna bird wasn't afraid of us, but he wouldn't come and perch on our hands. My wife called the Turtle Back Zoo—they had a few reports of the bird—and they sent an expert over to capture him, but the bird eluded him. Our home is in a wooded suburban New Jersey area and there has been snow and ice. Finally it must have gotten too cold for the bird and he took off. It is odd that this incident happened at the approximate time of my father's birthday, which was also the anniversary of his death."

Addendum

On June 7, 1972, while at the annual Associated Physicians' Banquet, Dr. L and his guest, the automobile agency manager, called me over to their table. The manager wanted to tell me the latest development: "The oddest thing happened two Saturdays ago when my mother returned from Florida to New Jersey. While she visited my family in our backyard, there, again, was the myna bird in a tree. We hadn't seen him since February, or after this visit with Mother. My wife was so upset that she wouldn't talk about it." The manager then repeated his strange story to several curious physician friends at the table. He looked in vain for an explanation.

The next time I met the manager was at the annual banquet, one year later. He seemed perplexed as he related the most recent development: "On the anniversay of Father's death, Mother and I flew to Florida where we joined my brother and drove to the cemetery. There, on the branch of a tree overhanging the grave, was the myna bird."

Comment

Examples of these strange, spontaneously occurring paranormal events between man and beast could be greatly expanded. The exact nature of the events makes coincidence and chance an unlikely explanation. What can the link be between man and his pets, and between man and sometimes exotic wild animals? Could similar interactions from ancient times have been the source of the worldwide greatly embellished legends, myths, and superstitions of dragons, monsters, witch's cats, etc? How might possible man-beast paranormal events tie in with the many documented accounts of UFOs[15] (flying saucers) whose presence has often been heralded by animals such as barking dogs, clucking chickens, stampeding cattle? John A. Keel[113] has shown how many UFO experiences often have associated paranormal activities, including telepathy, poltergeists, precognition, etc. Could the key to an understanding of psychic matters be found in the mystery of ufology, or vice versa? Are there other dimensions to the life spectrum so that when the man-beast sensitivies are attuned to a common resonance these strange communications can take place? What might be the common physical modalities for such esoteric biocommunications? Are they, as it seems, outside the electro-magnetic spectrum and comprise some untapped source of energy? What might be the man-beast neuroanatomical and physiological substrates? Could animals be telepathically summoned, hallucinated, teleported, or ma-terialized when the man-beast needs and other factors are spontaneously ful-filled?

Eisenbud[52] has posed an intriguing exploratory generalization which he terms the *"principle of confluence,* according to which 'psi'—some basic psi manifestation that is, not just telepathy or PK, for example—is, like other great process-abstractions in nature (e.g., electromagnetic, or, queer as this sounds, "the unconscious') an integral component in *all* events (change of state of definable systems, let us say) and as such represented in some mea-sure as a determinate of the final, common pathways of these events."

The study of human-animal paranormal events should be vigorously pur-sued. If such disparate data exists, it should be used and not swept under the rug. The clues for the solution of the riddle are there.

Acknowledgment

Thanks go to the human (and animal) participants mentioned and unnamed in this study. Particular appreciation is expressed to Joseph Dunninger, the eminent telepathist, who most generously recalled personal incidents from his life, and more than 60-year career, and gave permission for these events to be recorded in a medical journal.

13
Telepathic Humoresque*

Humor can act as a safety valve. Humor sometimes prevents catastrophic detonations of unchecked hostility. It can tide us over rough spots and help make life bearable. It is one of the highest psychic functions and the sine qua non of the civilized man. Humor has its role in sexuality. Used tactfully and sparingly, humor can be an adjuvant in psychotherapy.[69,145] Bergler's excellent monograph[6] reviews theories on the role of humor and wit in psychic development and in interpersonal relationships. There are many examples showing how humor is intimately related to the unconscious and how it is similar to dreams and mental mechanisms. Humor tells us about the individual: how he sees himself, how he believes others see him, and how he actually is.

The extraordinary paragnost Jacques Romano,[181] who knew Mark Twain, once commented that many of Mark Twain's humorous writings were really a defense against his being overwhelmed by melancholy. Incidentally, Mark Twain himself had many telepathic experiences.[33] In my studies of such gifted paragnosts as Gerard Croiset, Joseph Dunninger,[24,25] Henry Gross,[176] and Jacques Romano, I noted that they all had a keen sense of humor. These sensitive, energetic, supremely self-confident gentlemen of proven psychic accomplishments all had delightful repertoires of humorous experiences and jokes, which seemed to provide them with a necessary respite from the serious, demanding nature of their work. Some of their most ridiculous examples also involved presumed telepathy.

For example, Thomas A. Edison once challenged Dunninger to tell him what was concealed under his dinner plate, and Dunninger promptly told Edison that it was hiding a hole in Mrs. Edison's new tablecloth—that Mr. Edison had burned the night before with one of his cigars.[25,24] On another occasion Dunninger walked into a restaurant with a friend and called the

*Presented at the 125th Annual Meeting of the American Psychiatric Association, Dallas, Texas, May 2, 1972, at a panel, "Science and Psi: Transcultural Trends," sponsored by the APA Task Force on Transcultural Psychiatry.

waitress over and told her to think of her name and birthday. Dunninger was shocked to have the unperturbed waitress respond: "What are you telling me that for? I know that!"

The purpose of this report is to show how telepathy and the paranormal (which is deeply rooted in the unconscious) might be allied to humor. Telepathic interaction and transactions are personal and truthful. By unmasking the unconscious and "telling it as it is" they reveal in sharp relief the realities and dynamics of interpersonal relations. The telepathic hypothesis in many instances makes an otherwise inexplicable communication intelligible and often humorous. Eisenbud has given examples involving humor and telepathy.[53,50] His documented researches of "thoughtography"[51] also provide a rich load of weird and tragicomic examples. Perhaps such techniques and insights could illuminate reported humorous classical paranormal events.[152] Let us look at three categories illustrating the role of what appeared to be telepathy in (1) humorous situations from early parent-child episodes; (2) physician-patient psychotherapeutic relationships; and (3) strictly personal anecdotes obtained from patients and my own life.

Humor in Parent-Child Telepathy[184]

In more than 1520 possible parent-child telepathic episodes in my family, there were many examples of telepathy and humor* where the child frequently pre-empted his parent's attention by (1) uncovering his parent's jealously guarded secrets; (2) supplying the forgotten "key" word to a joke; (3) complementing his parent's suppressed critical attitudes; (4) supplying captions to his parent's mentally envisioned or actually seen cartoons; or (5) in slapstick fashion acting out his parent's specific suppressed fantasies in socially forbidden areas of sex, aggression, or body image. As in involuntary humor, telepathy gave added dimension to the unexpected—but always the naked truth.

The contagion and hypersuggestibility of humor among children is self-evident. The credulous child, who looks upon his parents as omnipotent and omniscient, offers a fertile soil for telepathic reactions. Compared to adult-to-adult presumed telepathic examples, the parent-child telepathic dynamics are simple and unsophisticated. Many of the later parent-child telepathic episodes resemble adult-to-adult exchanges and so tragicomic and revealing that they cannot be published.

---

*For example, see episodes 69, 538, 612, 793, 1116, 1210, 1269, 1297, 1324, and 1505.

Example 1. (No. 612, May 4, 1966)

While the family and I were having dinner, I meditated about the afternoon's consultation. It concerned a woman who had just gotten off welfare with her husband and seven children. The lady told me how her husband had once seen a welfare psychiatrist who had advised him to get a job. The husband ridiculed his psychiatrist and warned his wife (my patient) not to seek consultation with myself. When the patient was leaving my office she critically commented on my supposed treatment of a friend of hers, whom I had seen once in consultation but had not in fact treated. In my moments of silent deliberation at the dinner table, I reflected on the irony of my patient's husband who, by his wife's own words, sat around for six months and did nothing but look at television and the like, and used her as a baby machine. He was a free loader and society (including myself) was forced to support his biological delinquency, and in addition I, a worker, had to suffer this loafer's insults.

While preoccupied with these frustrations my seven-year-old son Eric broke in with: "Dad, if you weren't a doctor, and if you didn't have a job, would you watch TV?" I rushed to my desk to write down the episode, and when I returned, Ardis, my wife, said that Eric had repeated his question twice more. Eric was on the right track and he knew it.

Eric was ambivalent toward me because of my earlier reluctance to immediately drop everything and go purchase for him a new baseball mitt, when he already had three of my old ones, plus his own which he could learn to use better before getting a new one. Eric's question dramatically transposed my anger into laughter at myself. His realism compounded my irony and brought me back to earth: viz., if the patient's and my roles were reversed, and I was unemployed, would I have been any different, or less shiftless than her husband? Eric was my philosopher, ally and critic. His query to me went to the heart of the matter and exploited my help by shoving me into a more generous state of mind. My annoyance at his importunities over the baseball mitt was analogous to my being used and outslicked by a not-so-helpless as would appear, critical welfare patient.

Example 2. (No. 1269, February 22, 1969)

Ardis, Lisa age 12, and I were having lunch. Lisa was talking to her mother and there was a quiet interlude when I sneaked a look at my *Modern Medicine* (Feb. 10, 1969, p. 231) and noticed a cartoon where a shapely woman nurse was shaking medicine. While the male patients ogled her a male doctor said, "Uh, better let me shake the medicine." At that, Lisa, who could not see what I was reading said, "Ann's (girlfriend) cat is so fat (pregnant) she can't walk straight." Naturally I wouldn't discuss an off-color cartoon with Lisa, and Lisa's comment was totally out of context, unless the telepathic hypothesis was considered. She merely exposed my secret voyeuristic pleasure and humorously transposed my reaction to her needs of the moment.

Example 3. (No. 779, February 17, 1967)

One day when Eric was nine, Ardis went with him into a stationery store to buy an evening paper. Eric went to the back of the store to look at magazines while Ardis, in the front, looked among the papers for the *New York Daily News*. A few weeks previously while at Lincoln Center in New York City with her girl friend, Ardis had been interviewed by John Stapleton, the Inquiring Fotographer from the *Daily News,* who took her picture and said that it would shortly appear in his column. This was a secret she had kept from the whole family. She was embarrassed about the subject because she felt the reporter asked a silly question, and perhaps also she felt the picture would be uncomplimentary. While she was preoccupied with her surreptitious examination of the paper, Eric ran from the back of the store and thrust a magazine in his mother's face, saying, "Here is your picture, Mom"—a picture of a woman who was half beautiful and half ugly. Eric had not done anything like this before and his unexpected action could not have been more perfectly timed to embarrass his mother by divulging her secret, as if to say on an unconscious level that his mother could not fool him. The picture Eric showed might have reflected his mother's ambivalence concerning the article she had yet to see.

Ardis had added reason to be concerned and embarrassed about her husband's possible reponse. Later on, when a friend sent her the clipping I swallowed my tongue as I read the question: "Should women shoulder most of the blame for the decline of chivalry?" and the last sentence of Ardis' answer: "Children don't see chivalry at home, so they don't practice it." Ardis' girl friend, who is single, was kinder to the male sex with her answer: "You can't fault men for being less chivalrous: They're so intent and preoccupied with business."

Humor In Psychotherapeutic Relationships

During the course of psychotherapy many patients spontaneously report humorous situations that might best be explained by telepathy. The examples are analogous to the parent-child telepathic episodes but of course are more complex. The examples often pertain to emotionally loaded secrets, eroticism, hostility, and embarrassment.

Example 4.

In the course of the psychotherapy of a young woman referred by a surgeon, she mentioned how attracted she was to him and how occasionally she could not resist the impulse to telephone him at late hours and chat. The woman did not know what the surgeon confided when I saw him: On the rare occasions when she mustered the courage to phone him, he was, on one of the still rarer occasions in his life, cohabiting with his wife, from whom he had been estranged. When I offered the surgeon the telesomatic hypothesis, he blushed and said, "Why, of course!" This type of example is not unusual, and was mentioned by Stekel.[47] I have other examples where a colleague was incorrectly convinced that he was being framed by Cupid because almost every random time he came to visit me the woman who interested him came, on no notice, to visit my wife. The colleague was being telepathically garnisheed.

Example 5.

A young college man was arrested for indecent exposure. Of this he was very ashamed; it was his most jealously guarded secret—or so he thought. One day several weeks after his arrest he happened to meet one of his old high school friends. This was his first contact with someone from his past in a long time, and he was very concerned about his secret although he knew that it was impossible that his friend or anyone else should know. However, his friend opened the conversation by saying: "Do you know they passed a new law in New Jersey that automobiles cannot be driven without hubcaps because their nuts would be exposed?"

Example 6.

A middle-aged, rather hot-headed, phobic patient had a problem with her domineering, heavy-drinking husband. They kept it secret that their child was adopted because her husband was sterile. The patient felt cheated because of this. Her husband was very sensitive about his problem, and his wife found it hard to restrain herself from reminding him of his "masculine deficiency." One hot summer day the husband and wife had to entertain a prominent visitor and his wife from India. This was an auspicious dinner engagement and if carried out successfully could mean a promotion for her husband. The patient thought she would ingratiate herself with her guests by offering them for dessert a choice of homemade American pumpkin pie or cherry pie. When she presented the desserts the esteemed dinner guests started snickering. The patient's husband, who ordinarily preferred pumpkin pie, had chosen the cherry pie. The guests from India stated in jest that they appreciated their hostess's thoughtfulness but they, like her husband, could not take the pumpkin pie because in their part of India it was a superstition that pumpkins were a cause of sterility. The patient's departure from her usual culinary routine—serving pumpkin pie in the summer—unwittingly made her the hit of the evening. She downgraded her downtrodden husband in more ways than she might ever have bargained for.

Example 7.

A young businessman who had many phobias had avoided most social contact for years. One day in the course of his treatment, he said,

> I'm a born loser, Last night I went to my first cocktail party in years. I knew only the hostess, whom I met a few weeks ago. The party was on the 39th floor of a Manhattan apartment building. Of 50 people in the room I picked out one and started to talk to her. To make small talk, which is difficult, I said,"Those who read the *Reader's Digest* are idiots." She said that she worked for the *Reader's Digest*. I was flustered and didn't know what to say, so I continued, "I hope you are not in the editorial department." And she said, "Yes."

This example of foot-in-mouth telepathy might illustrate a common event in the psychic-dynamics of everyday life.

Example 8.

Late one Sunday night I checked my appointment book for the next day and to my horror discovered an error. Mr. S, a fragile schizophrenic, had been scheduled for 7:00 in the morning by my secretary, but she had also unthinkably scheduled Professor B for 7:30. To avoid a conflict and to make the simplest adjustment in this case, I tried to contact Professor B, to ask him to come at 8:00, a half hour later than usual. Since I couldn't reach B on the telephone, I had to ask S to come at 6:30. When Professor B came at 7:30, he said:

> I set the alarm for 7:30 instead of 6:30. It's a funny thing. This is the only time I've done this in two years of therapy. I had a dream of coming to your office a half hour later than usual.

Furthermore, the professor identified his dream as being telepathic. Yet despite this urgent message, he decided that he should still come at 7:30. Thus in his dreams and conscious associations he correctly divined the situation and my confusion and made the suitable adjustments. He even identified the telepathic nature of the event. Some of his telesomatic experiences are described elsewhere.[180]

Example 9.

Mr. J was invited to a formal banquet and went to the store he had used in the past to rent a tuxedo. Although the suit was wrapped in heavy paper, he was uneasy about it. When he got home, despite his wife's joshing him for "superstition," he insisted on unwrapping the suit then, and not a few hours before the banquet. His fears were confirmed when he discovered that one trouser leg was eight inches longer than the other. His hunch came in the nick of time and saved the day.

Example 10.

Mrs. O, a housewife in her thirties had ambulatory schizophrenia and symptomatic alcoholism. Prior to my seeing her, she had had intensive hospitalization. Among her problems she was unable to care for herself and love her only child. During the course of treatment, it seemed that gentle humor could sometimes help unlock iron barriers to communications. Once, during an advanced session, when the patient had returned from a short vacation, she was quiet at first and then in the interlude, I (B.E.S.) had the autochthonous and impish impulse to conjure up the mental cartoon of another patient, a tall Amazon, who in my mind's eye was wearing a high, broad-brimmed hat and was sitting in a motion picture theater along side her pip-squeak husband and behind a row of teen-aged girls with huge broad-brimmed hats.

Hardly had this mental cartoon flashed into mind, than a second ridiculous situation occurred to me of people eating sandwishes of Italian bread stuffed with celery and cellophane. While thinking of the first cartoon, the patient said with a smile, "There was a saying at the hotel that the only thing to fear was fear itself." What could have been better satire than the ridiculous situation of the pip-squeak husband with his immense wife sitting behind the teen-aged girls with huge hats? He dared not protest to the girls who obstructed his view lest he offend his similarly bedecked wife. In her life situation my patient was up against it and she was afraid to take a stand. She was petrified by the fear of fear itself. My cartoon hope for her of the battle-ax wife with the pip-squeak husband—that she become strong—was well reacted to.

Scarcely had the cartoons obliged with this first possibly telepathic caption, than she gave what could have been a suitable caption for my second mental picture of people noisily gnawing at the indigestible Italian bread sandwich: "Great One, let me not judge another until I have walked in his moccasins for two weeks." It could have meant that this shy woman who was lacking in self-confidence, was overtaxed with the care of an infant son, and under her husband's thumb, wouldn't dare comment on the absurdity of people eating sandwiches which sounded great but which were without nutritive value and could even be dangerous—because in her helplessness she was in a desperate situation and unable to complain. She would have difficulty in swallowing such food as I had my psychotherapeutic problems with her. And her unconscious sarcasm "Great One," might have been an ambivalent feeling toward her physician, husband, or other surrogates, that could also be viewed as a placation and warning not to play tricks (e.g., conjure cartoons, induce unwanted laughing, or disturb the forces that prevented her from caring for her child), lest the situation be turned about and a joke be played on the perpetrator.

The physician-patient possibly telepathic pictographic-caption exchanges might have signaled the patient's dim recognition of the fluidity of our relationship rather than an inflexible, fear-ridden interaction. And the possible telepathic exchanges might have also portrayed the patient's improving ability to cope with the give and take nuances of the transference and her developing new skills in other interpersonal relationships. In over 90 psychotherapeutic sessions there were more than 22 possible telepathic episodes and there was also presumed telepathy (as confirmed by phone calls) from her to me (in New Jersey) when she was living in Vermont, Connecticut, and Florida.

Strictly Personal

These possibly telepathic episodes of everyday life comprise husband-and-wife and adult-to-adult exchanges. The events are the most poignant and intimate. Brill[8] once wrote that analysing a patient's "favorite joke" was an excellent way of understanding him. He had many hilarious examples, but when people in the audience would ask him what *his* favorite joke was, he dodged their questions by saying he would give only his second-best joke. And so it is with what follows.

Example 11.

On the way to Don's Drive In, for lunch, Mrs. A shared a recent embarrassing secret with my wife. As a surprise for her husband, Mrs. A had bought a half-gallon of Gruning's ice cream. Mr. A, because he has heart disease, had been on a strict diet and the only vice he permitted himself was a rare treat of his favorite Gruning's ice cream—a flagrant violation of the rules. As Mrs. A pulled into her driveway, her attention was diverted from the ice cream which she had placed on the back seat of her husband's new sports car, to ladders on the side of her house. At first she thought they were burglars and jumped out of the car to investigate. When she learned that the ladders belonged to her trusted roofers she was relieved. However, in the pandemonium she completely forgot about the ice cream until the next morning when she drove her young daughter to school. It was then that she noted her husband's favorite ice cream had melted into a sticky mess all over the back seat, down the sides of the car and onto the carpeting. She struggled to dislodge and remove the seat, lift up the carpet and scrub the interior.

Later that day, she was alarmed when her husband surprised her by coming home early. Noticing the seat out of his car, he put it back and casually asked Mrs. A what had happened. He took it for granted that she must have spilled some milk when shopping for groceries. She said nothing, the subject was changed, and her husband didn't learn of his wife's embarrassing secret.

Perhaps Mrs. A felt relieved after telling her friend, my wife, about this incident, for they laughed together when they noticed a sign at the drive-in cash register counter stating that if a star appeared on the sales slip you were entitled to a free half-gallon of ice cream. Needless to say, Mrs. A's laughter turned into a double gulp, when she won! This was the first time she had had such luck. It can be wondered if her recent unique overdetermined experience with her husband's ice cream, about which she felt much shame and guilt, were factors that played a role in the possible psi solution—the magic replacement of the lost ice cream by "chance" and thereby securing her absolution from embarrassment—a humorous compensation for her horrible revelation.

It can also be speculated that the deeper implications of innocently wronging her husband (e.g., buying him the forbidden ice cream, "forgetting it," and soiling the upholstery of his expensive new car), might have jolted her psychic equilibrium. When confronted by the "lucky star" sales slip and her good luck, the absurdity of her underlying ambivalent feelings were transformed into laughter which she shared with my wife, who was aware of some of the underlying currents and thus informed me.

Example 12.

During my studies of Joseph Dunninger, he once mentioned how he heard about Mrs. Marie L. D'Alessio of New Jersey, who told him of her experience with a phantom telephone call. Coming from Dunninger, one of the world's foremost telepathists, who had seen almost everything—legitimate and otherwise—in his investigations of psychic phenomena for more than 60 years, such a statement naturally made me curious. Dunninger would not be easily fooled with well-intended but unconsciously spurious examples, outright fraud, nonsense, and the like.

We we interviewed Mrs. D'Alessio, she confirmed her weird phantom-telephone-call experience. She told me that many years ago she dreamed that a girlhood friend of hers, Lorna, sank into a pool of blood. Because this was similar to past dreams that symbolized something tragic, she told her husband, who suggested that she call her friend, whom she hadn't seen in a long time and who lived many miles away. The husband overheard her learn that Lorna had gone into the hospital the previous week but, "Because of a cold they sent me home, and I'm going in tomorrow." Mrs. D'Alessio went on, I said I'd like to visit her, and she said she preferred that I didn't because she would contact me. When I didn't receive any call or Christmas card, I thought something was funny. I tried calling her, and not receiving any response I phoned a neighbor, who said that Lorna had died. I thought Lorna must have died in November [the time of the dream-prompted call]. The neighbor said that Lorna's husband was still away in Florida and that he would come and see me when he returned. When he visited us, he said that everything I told him was true except one one thing—that I must have been mistaken about when I spoke to Lorna, because she had died on May 20.

While listening to Mrs. D'Alessio's account of the grim phantom-telephone commentary, I wondered if she had any humorous telepathic examples. She might have picked up my thoughts, for she laughed and gave me an amusing, possibly telepathic experience pertaining to her son, Arthur, who was in college in Georgia, more than 800 miles away. Mrs. D'Alessio said she dreamed

> that our son Arthur was upset because he couldn't find a key. I woke up my husband and told him. He said, "What did you wake me up for?"—I always do that—and he added, "Well, what could it be?" So the next morning I phoned Arthur, although I always hesitated calling him, because he didn't like it; he wanted to be a man and show that he was on his own. However, Arthur laughed and said that at the time of my dream he had been taking a shower and the boys in the fraternity house had locked him out of his room and taken the key. He had to sleep on a couch in the hallway wrapped in a towel.

When I returned home from my visit to Dunninger, I dictated my notes of Mrs. D'Alessio's examples. I wondered about the weird, witnessed, alleged voice-after-death situation. In my mind this grim event seesawed with the more palatable locked-out-of-the-room situation, which was easier to understand. I told my secretary and members of my family about them. The locked-out-of-the-room example was similar to other reported humorous examples where a mother telepathically tuned in on her sons when they were away at college.[176]

While still chuckling over the missing-key example and thereby denying the fascinating but frustrating case of the phantom voice, I retired to my bedroom and closed the French doors. Since my wife had acute influenza, she was sleeping in a different room. When I awoke next morning, I had to dress in a hurry in order to see an early patient. I was shocked to discover that the doors to my bedroom were locked. Try as hard as I could, the custom-made gold-plated latch was immovable. Although we had lived in this house for 16 years, this had never happened before. I naturally thought my wife had played a trick on me and was carried away by the funny example I told her about before retiring. However, I was puzzled about how she could lock the doors when there was no key. I still felt that she must have done something and that it was in bad taste, since I was pressed for time. Finally, in desperation I phoned from the private line in the bedroom to the office phone, located in another part of the house, and my wife came to the rescue and opened the doors by releasing the top and bottom latches of the companion door. We both had a hearty laugh, for she was not responsible for this incident. To discover the difficulty and satisfy my curiosity, I removed the lock, which my wife took to a locksmith. When he opened it, he commented that one of the pieces of the mechanism had slipped down and jammed. We laughed again but couldn't help wondering how this bizarre coincidence could happen. It seemed that for indulging myself in the unfortunate plight of another I received the horse laugh on myself and thereby could not possibly deny the weird phantom-voice example and the difficulties in formulating an explanation.

Example 13.

This highly personal example might be familiar to anyone who has had contact with the service—the Internal Revenue Service. Once, my wife and I were having our annual income tax checked by a particularly redoubtable gentleman. Although he had little need to prove to us his expertise in mathematical prodigies, he insisted on demonstrating his skills. At the conclusion of our session he graciously accepted my invitation for lunch. While he and I dissolved some of our tensions in a nearby restaurant, my wife, who was home alone, noted that the agent had left some papers in plain view, scattered on the desk. Although it undoubtedly was wrong, she could not resist the temptation to glance at the top papers, which were reports by a previous IRS examiner. When the agent and I returned to complete the task, he entered the room first and sat next to my wife. When I walked into the room, I don't know what madness seized me—for it could only have been that—but I put my hand to my chest, my hat to my heart, and started coughing. The agent blanched and in a very short while excused himself, saying he could readily finish the rest of the job in his office. Our ordeal was over. As soon as the agent left, my wife could hardly contain her laughter, for she told me the contents of the visually purloined former agent's notes. They were to the effect that the former agent was trying to justify to his supervisor my low income in previous years by stating that "The doctor, a psychiatrist, does not work as hard as the general practitioner who sees many more patients, because he has had pulmonary tuberculosis."

Possibly my wife had telepathically sent me the necessary information in this uncomfortable situation, which I had unconsciously acted out in our behalf, with a near catastrophic effect on the IRS agent's psyche. If I had known what my wife knew, I could never have played such a ham role. My secret, which was the agent's also, had boomeranged to my benefit. As a postscript it might be added that the agent and I are both well and my wife and I even received a small refund that year.

Comments

What have all these examples in common? Why might they be funny? What purpose does presumed telepathy serve in humor or vice versa? And how might telepathically tinged humor differ from other humor?

From these examples and others, it would seem that most of the telepathically mediated humorous events occurred under keyed-up, or crisis, circumstances. One person was trying to suppress or repress a secret or information that would be embarrassing to him, while another person was unwittingly revealing the information. For both persons the telepathic data symbolized an important part of their lives or their body image in relation to the other. Usually at the height of the polarized emotions there was a telepathic crisis-cross between the two persons, and the forbidden or forgotten material suddenly exploded to the surface. Depending on the psychodynamics, this forbidden material telepathically catalyzed the data and usually signaled a change in the interpersonal relationships. Or perhaps it was analogous to Ehrenwald's discription of *kairos* and the existential shift.[41] The whole process was, of course, unconscious: a secret was divined or a situation uncovered without either person being aware of what he had actually stumbled upon.

Telepathy in humor might be like some of the intuitive flashes of the genious or poet[178] and be akin to the folklore axioms of "love at first sight" or "first impressions are correct," for telepathy short-circuits social amenities, penetrates hypocrisy, and exposes redundant diplomacy. It can strike like lightning, have the pull of a magnet, and go to the heart of the matter. By catching us off guard, it arouses our curiosity and has the ring of the uncanny. By being able to combine the sublime and the ridiculous, it is akin to the unexpected or incongruous responses that are often seen in humor. The unconscious, which does not know the difference between fact and fantasy, magic and reality, provides the woof and warp of telepathy and humor. A situation which can be grimly suitable for shuddering or weeping can also paradoxically evoke laughter. Better to laugh than to cry.

Telepathy can serve a useful purpose in preparing us for emergencies and maintaining homeostasis. Like much ordinary humor, telepathically mediated or occasioned humor might not be funny to its participants at the time but may indeed be so to outside observers. Later, when the participants have recovered from their bewilderment, they too can laugh. The observers' amusement is similar to the mirth of an audience who watches a previously hypnotized subject carry out posthypnotic commands while offering ridiculous rationalizations for his actions. Such a situation is familiar to the astonished audiences who gleefully witness the fireworks between telepathic gladiators such as Dunninger or Romano and their willing or unwilling subjects.

As one cannot tell the same joke twice to an audience and get the same laughter the second time, telepathic events, like involuntary humor, must "tell it as it is" and be uncontrived.

Both telepathy and humor are often highly inventive and creative. Telepathy, occurring in a crises, almost always dovetails the needs of both parties. Telepathy is a two-way street. It is similar to jokes with a snappy punch line. The analysis of humorous telepathic events reveals sender-receiver roles similar to those in a comedy team such as Laurel and Hardy, where there is a buffoon and a straight man. One is as necessary as the other. Although some of the data in this study suggest the telepathically mediated humor might have a regressive survival function, some might also be interpreted as having a progressive function, reaching out into new directions and trying to establish a more stable equilibrium.

Highly successful laboratory ESP experiments are notoriously difficult to repeat. There might be good physiological and psychopathological reasons for this. Eisenbud has remarked that in such studies any success at all is unusual, since the experiments seem to be designed to ensure failure.[54] Like involuntary humor, telepathy in the psychotherapeutic relationship is the quintessence of spontaneity and improvisation in the subtle nuances of ever-shifting and changing interpersonal relationships. By its very nature it is hard to confine. Complex humorous events, particularly the presumed telepathic ones, are stripped of much of their glamour and mirth when reduced to print.

Both telepathy and humor might have Scheherazade-like effects. The Oriental heroine Scheherazade could only save herself from being strangled at the orders of her husband the Sultan by telling him a new story every night. Her 1001 Arabian tales had to be fascinating, creative, and spontaneous if she was to survive. In order to hold the Sultan's rapt attention, she undoubtedly had to be able to understand her own resistance to the unusual telepathic-like situations in order to be able to penetrate the Sultan's defenses. It was a transference-countertransference situation—a problem of understanding resistances with her life at stake.[126,50] Thus, like Scheherazade's precarious predicament, telepathy and humor fundamentally have their serious aspects; yet paradoxically when they surface they often appear to be trivial, insignificant, or coincidental.

Possibly a deeper exploration of the subject of telepathy and humor would yield many clues about this relatively neglected but important means of human communication.

III: PSI AND THE LIFE CYCLE

14

The Seven Ages of Man: A Potpourri of Psi*

PART I

Introduction

Psi happens throughout the entire life cycle—from birth until the end, and for all that anyone knows, maybe before and beyond. Although many people are aware of the extensive laboratory statistical studies of ESP and of the existence of many spontaneous case reports of telepathy, often replete with weighty documentation, affidavits, and the like, they may not be so well acquainted with the no less respectable and well-studied psychiatric or psychodynamic investigations of telepathy by such pioneers as Eisenbud,[50] Ehrenwald,[37] Fodor,[67] Meerloo,[126] Stevenson,[210] Tenhaeff,[217] Ullman,[225] and others.[21] The speculations about the psychopathological and physiological significance of psi in everyday life illuminate all of psychical research and, if confirmed, offer a renaissance for mankind, no less notable than the first historic reawakening.

During my psychiatric training I noted occasional telepathic exchanges with patients during psychotherapy. Because of this, as well as some personal presumed past psychic events in my family, and other experiences in treating patients, I wondered if telepathy could have practical, everyday significance in our lives and if it could be a contributing factor in various behavioral and psychosomatic reactions. Were spontaneous telepathic and other psychic events isolated occurrences or were they perhaps not uncom-

---

*Paper presented at American Society of Psychic Research Symposium, Parapsychology: Today's Implications—Tomorrow's Applications? Section on Psychiatry, May 18, 1974, Barbizon-Plaza Hotel, New York City.

mon and of intense significance? How does one go about answering these questions?

In the course of my initial psychiatric interviews of patients, for the past 18 years or so, I have asked them about possible psychic events in their lives: "Have you ever had unusual events in your life—so strange yet true that you wondered about them and what they could be?" As a result, I have obtained all kinds of anecdotal psychic, and at times UFO, material. This data, whatever its validity, often seemed to have a direct influence on the lives of these patients. The clinical "facts" told me that it was not right to ignore such material. I gradually came to realize that one could not fully understand a patient without taking account of this psychic material—genuine or spurious.

Psychiatric studies over the past 50 years have revealed how telepathy is related to the subconscious mind with all its propensities for symbolization, distortion, displacement, condensation, and other mental mechanisms. The dream and altered states of consciousness can also be ideal vehicles for telepathy. These pioneering researches spelled out clear-cut psychodynamic criteria[39] for the recognition of telepathy: (1) the unique, actual or close symbolic meaning of the thoughts of two or more people happening at the same time without the aid of the usually recognized senses; (2) the "tracer thought" or word that is an allusion to the psychic nature of the event; and (3) the tendency for the telepathic event to recur when the psychodynamic constellations are similar—so called built-in controls.[177]

During my extended psychiatric investigation of Jacques Romano,[181] my wife Ardis and I noted the increased frequency and quality of telepathic events and other psychic phenomena in our family. We found that following highly exciting and interesting sessions with Romano there were clusters of psychic events within the family, between our friends and ourselves, and in my practice. The next step was to start keeping records of all possible telepathic events involving our children, Lisa, and later Eric, and ourselves,[184] and concomitantly through the years, physician-patient exchanges.

The latter technique included making entries on 3 x 5 file cards of any presumed clinically creditable psi events for the patients, obtained during their initial consultations, as well as the session number for any presumed psi episodes between the patient and physician (B.E.S.) in those instances where the patient continued with psychotherapy. Thus, from December, 1955, to December 1973, 3764 patients were seen in consultation, and in 3077 instances there were examples of psi or one or more physician-patient telepathic exchanges. This does not include numerous presumed telepathic-physician-patient exchanges that happened outside the psychotherapeutic sessions, or of course, the wax and wane pattern of psi in one's personal life.

In numerous instances there were telepathic dreams. During the same period of time I collected 61 personal and physician-patient possible telekinetic episodes. There were 77 possible telepathic death experiences. Fortunately, none of the latter were then current physician-patient experiences—that is, patients, under treatment or who had previously received intensive therapy. However, these examples did include some deaths of patients whom I had seen previously in consultation, but where my advice was not followed, and cases of suicidal attempts. By such record-keeping, the physician is in a position to learn much about the psychic-dynamics of the paranormal (and also about himself).

Other psi data included 35 instances of possible precognition, 33 telesomatic reactions, and 22 human-animal possible paranormal episodes. Out-of-the-body experiences were rare, but there were several instances of induced apparitions or telepathic hallucinations which were reported elsewhere.[177,186,185] There were no instances of levitation, materialization, or histories for reincarnation, unless one discounted the telepathic hypothesis, as in one interesting anecdotal example.[176] The unreported psi examples are similar to those in the literature, and, if anything, the totals for the various categories of episodes are conservative and understate the actual figures, since there is much cross-filing. Many examples are "missed" because it becomes a tedious process to record countless data, and some episodes are just too personal. Therefore, the total numbers are only an approximation of what happens frequently and to all people, I would guess, allowing for differences in personality, biological factors, interests, motivations and special talents. The psi ability is there at the beginning—but the awareness for any particular psi talent must be developed.

Psi awareness might also have been expedited by the intensive study of other gifted paragnosts, including Henry Gross,[176] Joseph Dunninger[23] and, for a short time during an American visit, Gerard Croiset of Holland. At this point it might be helpful to mention an example of an occupational control, where the people involved might presumably have an interest or proclivity for psi by virtue of their professional calling (doctrinal compliance).[40] From April, 1959, to July, 1970, I saw 32 postulants for the ministry in consultation for the Episcopal Diocese of Newark. My overall impression was that in no cases was there any increased incidence (or interest) for psi beyond that which occurred in my general patient population. This impression also held for clergy who were seen in consultation or therapy.

For the patients, most of their psi events were telepathic. There were no striking occupational, age, sex, or religious correlations. If anything, the more intelligent patients seemed to have a better interpersonal awareness for telepathy. The underlying personality factors, states of consciousness, physiological, and pharmacological aspects (e.g., effects of tranquilizers, psychotropics, and patients who had been under the influence of alcohol, marijuana, LSD, mescaline, etc.)—the substrates for psi—were entirely in accord with other published observations.

By recording and annotating all possible psi, I not only defined, refined, and possibly sharpened my own awareness of it and ability for it, but I also learned how telepathy seemed to relate to everyday life, to psychopathology, and to the use of our other senses. By not omitting suspected events, I minimized the element of coincidence. In these ways it was seen how telepathic episodes, recorded over the years, had certain psychodynamic and psychophysiological features in common. This conclusion is similar to Professor Tenhaeff's observation of how the gifted paragnost (for example, Gerard Croiset) will, in highly significant ways, repeatedly discover himself in his clients through his psychic abilities. Paragnosts frequently have their skills developed in certain directions that harmonize with specific experiences in their past lives. Thus, Joseph Dunninger has performed "incredible" feats in his 60-year career which, when analyzed, are usually variations on his genius for apprehending specific numbers or letters. In other respects however, as in his personal life, Dunninger is as mystified as anyone else at the diversity of spontaneous psi. Psi examples with young children, who have a limited vocabulary and nonexistent or rudimentary reading ability, are usually simpler and less sophisticated than are the complex and often more intricate adult-to-adult examples. With growth and maturation, parent-child telepathic episodes do not disappear, but take on an adult configuration—often of a psychic or telepathic nexus, where it is difficult to define the beginning or end of an event extending through time.

It is stressed that the possible psi recorded here differs from the classical method, where the experiences are usually derived from disparate numbers of people with the usual affidavits and the like. In contrast to that method, this study might have the advantage of a common denominator, namely, one person presenting his possible psi experiences with many people: patients, family, and friends.

At an earlier stage of my experiences many of the psi events had an element of a personal thrill, but as time went on this feeling diminished, and although the episodes still happened, they were more mechanical. I became more analytical. Psi seemed to fuel a real need; a change; a novelty or challenge. For example, if there was one "good" physician-patient possible telepathic exchange, I could usually look forward to another or several episodes during the session—the confirmatory built-in controls. By going over the material collected through the year,* It is often hard to believe that these events

---

*By so doing, it is a common occurrence to receive telephone calls from patients from the past for appointments, etc. In such instances, the severity of their situation can often merit a gener-

really happened, but they did—and they do just happen. However, as has been shown, they were always part of an intense, highly meaningful, unconscious exchange. It often happened that the failures—where one might have anticipated "success" and there were none—were almost more enigmatic: for example, why one particular death could be missed, and another one apprehended; or the ever pressing question of how does psi elude conscious control? Thus, it is imperative that all possible psi events be recorded immediately after they happen, or even while happening, if one is trying to develop an expanded awareness as well as for reasons of accuracy. In such cases, the element of dissociation is often so strong and persistent years afterward, that if I were asked to write a detailed account of 10 to 20 good telepathic examples without resorting to files of typed accounts, I'd probably fail the task. What holds for remembering life events in general is even more formidable with psi. It is all too easy for the mind to censor and filter out telepathic material. It takes work and emotional honesty to expand one's awareness, to record the events as they happened, and perhaps in many cases to learn most of all, from the technical failures that might otherwise be considered parapsychological successes.

For this reason a study of recorded psi examples ("telepathic analysis"), when scrutinized over the years, is quite revealing for hitherto unsuspected dimensions in the physician-patient relationship. I would guess that a review of such exchanges could be as meaningful as a personal psychoanalysis. It takes courage to write down exactly what happened, the people involved, circumstances, and the feelings. All the psi data I have collected* fully confirmed the observations of Eisenbud[50] and Meerloo,[126,128] who have shown how understanding resistance to psi can be a key factor in developing the ability within oneself. One must be able to see oneself as others do and, unfortunately, this means not as one would always like.

PART II

PSI and the life cycle can perhaps best be illustrated with an assortment of examples, roughly divided according to Shakespeare's "seven ages of man" (*As You Like It,* Act II, Scene 7, Line 137).

I. "At first the infant, mewling and
puking in the nurse's arms"

---

ous telepathic discount, since I "know" that their response is as much telepathic (pertaining to the physician—unconscious doctrinal compliance[40] as autochthonous.
*It should be stated that, for the sake of brevity, "obvious" explanations, including less obvious subliminal factors, have been omitted from the case reports.

Case 1. In the Beginning

Barbara, a healthy newborn, was brought home by her proud parents two weeks ago. Mrs. Love, a mother for the first time, had had many previous telepathic experiences and came from a family where psi was accepted as an everyday event. When being interviewed she said: "I always walk in when something has happened. The other day the baby was choking and gagging. The milk was coming out of her nose. Bill (husband) and I were in the living room taking down the Christmas tree and Barbara was in the bedroom with the door partially closed, so that we wouldn't disturb her. We live in a ranch house and we couldn't hear anything. We didn't intend to go in and possibly disturb her. I usually don't go in when she's sleeping—it's usually 3½ to 4 hours—and Barbara had already been fast asleep for one hour. But I just felt I had to go in and check her. I had a hunch. It happens a lot. I think she's OK, and I don't want to be overcautious, and I say, 'No, she's all right.' But, I still go in. On another occasion, I kept getting the feeling that something was happening and I started walking around. I felt that I better go in. We both went to her room and she had the blanket completely over her face. If something went wrong with her, I'd know it, because I've done it so often. When I'm in there, I say, 'Gee, I'm surprised to be in here now.' I just feel this—that I should be there (compulsion)."

Possibly this simple experience could be the type of telepathic event that transcends and merges with subliminal stimulation. Could this episode, where the young mother heeded her infant's needs be the prototype of crisis telepathy which alerts us and prepares us for danger and which aids survival and which will happen again and again throughout life?

Case 2. Mother's Secret

Early in her psychotherapy for depression, a young mother once reported: "I was having breakfast with Tina, my three-year-old and Frieda, our mother's helper. I was thinking about how depressed I was and that I did not want to upset my husband, for he had so much unhappiness in his previous marriage, due to the fact that his first wife was an alcoholic. While I was thinking of this first wife, whom I never knew, Tina, who was eating her breakfast, suddenly said, "Look, I'm a ghost." I replied, somewhat automatically, "Caspar, the friendly ghost? (her favorite TV cartoon)" She said: "No, Sybil!" Sybil was the name of my husband's first wife! To my knowledge Tina had never used the name or heard it before. Frieda questioned her by asking: "Susan? Sandy? etc." But Tina was insistent on Sybil.

Can the child pick up sensitive areas from her parents and then amaze them by correctly synthesizing them, as in this instance with the forbidden name; and if so, how often and how significant a clue is this to the child's emotional development?

This patient did well with minimal assistance and managed to cope successfully with the death of her husband, caring for a newborn, and, a few years later, remarriage. However, because of some difficulties in the second marriage, she was seen again, and once during treatment she reported the following incident with Tina, then age seven: "Alex (husband) put on the TV program 'Open Heart,' and my stomach became upset. I didn't tell him to turn it off, but afterward I told him about how the surgeon had operated on Walter [deceased husband] from 7:00 A.M. until 8:00 P.M., and that the program brought everything back to my mind. During this, Tina walked in her sleep, came downstairs, and said, "Mommy, I need you. I never want to lose you!" Tina was fully aware of my being upset as I sat there reliving how I didn't want to lose Walter (first husband). I hugged Tina and she finally woke up. Her room is upstairs at the other end of the house and she couldn't know what was going on. When she was fully awake, we went upstairs together. The haze lifted and her eyes cleared when she said: "Is Daddy (Alex) still watching the news?"

The mother continued: "Many times when I'm upset, Tina and Betty May (other daughter, age four) pick up what is closely correlated. Somehow Tina would awaken and become disturbed because I was disturbed."

Many sessions later the patient related a dream: "I was a mass murderer, going to an analyst and I said, 'You have to help me before I kill more people.' It was a dream, and I knew it, but I couldn't wake up until Betty May came to my room and woke me up saying: 'Mommy, there is someone trying to get in my bedroom door.' " This patient had many similar experiences with both her daughters by her first, deceased husband, who was also well known to me as was their home. It might be wondered how often the underlying (unconscious) events in life that are brushed aside actually determine our decisions and behavior.

Case 3. "All is Not Well that Doesn't Begin Well."

The middle-aged mother recalled how her teenage schizophrenic son would scream out horribly and inconsolably when he was a baby. At those times she and her husband would be in their bedroom, and the father who was an alcoholic, would be berating his infant son. The mother was puzzled because the baby's room was down the corridor and out of range of hearing. She was sure that her son was telepathically aware of the father's hatred for him.

She cited other instances, where, for example, she planned trips to another city as a surprise, or to visit someone and scrupulously kept the information to herself; yet her son would blurt out what she thought was a secret. She herself wondered if this process was related to her son's problems.

Perhaps these early examples are not unlike the undue heightened sensitivity that the schizophrenic has for heteropsychic stimuli and perhaps becomes a missing link or the nucleus for later paranoidal ideation. Some split schizophrenics in their sessions demonstrate telepathic fireworks. It is a shame that this data has for the most part been so overlooked. It could be a most significant piece to that varied and complex syndrome.

II. "And then the whining school boy"

Case 4. Like Father, Like Son

(Parent-Child Telepathy Series, #866, August 26, 1967, Saturday, 11:00 A.M.). I was working at my desk and had just read on page 26 in *The Return of Russell Colvin* by John Spargo (Bennington Historical Museum and Art Gallery, 1945): "Chief Justice Dudley Chase presided. He was a jurist of eminent and acknowledged ability. A graduate of Dartmouth College, he was 48 years old at the time of the trial." I thought this historic reference to a crime involving a spurious telepathic dream would be useful for my projected paper on "Crime and Telepathy." This "heirloom" reference had been lent to me by my father's dear friend, an old Vermont Yankee, Mr. Arthur H. Kehoe. In the past Mr. Kehoe had told me about his meetings with Thomas A. Edison, and I had written a paper on Edison and the telepathic hypothesis for genius. I next wondered if Daniel Webster (a famous Dartmouth alumnus), of the Dartmouth College case, was connected with this notorious murder case, having to do with a false (from a legal point of view) psychic dream. At that moment, my son Eric, age eight, came into the room and said, "I thought Dartmouth was built in 1944—but this penny [in his hand] is 1946—remember when you had a penny that said when you were born? When Eric was asked what his statement had to do with Dartmouth, he became flustered and said he didn't know. Eric picked up the central theme of (1) Dartmouth, with overdetermined telepathic tracers (psychic dream, Kehoe's letter, Edison paper, projected paper on telepathy and crime) and also the specifically sensitized area of (2) a birthday (the age, in this case, of the justice, a mature man at the time of the famous trial; and his father's birth date). Eric also delved into the past: the founding of Dartmouth—and the 1820 Colvin case. Eric was in positive rapport with his father.

How much love of the past and of tradition can be traced to such simple roots as this example, in which a young boy seemingly picks the thoughts out of his father's brain and almost succeeds in correctly synthesizing them?

By collecting many similar cases, it is easy to see the possible role of telepathy in acquiring values for good or evil, various prejudices—or simply thoughts for the learning experience. This example also shows the mechanism of the unconscious mind and telepathy, in which the person involved is totally unaware of his role and offers a flimsy excuse, not unlike a post-hypnotic-command rationalization. One amusing everyday example of this mental mechanism is when a waitress in a restaurant, properly "tuned in," is given a verbal food order, but then brings the "incorrect" but telepathically correct—unconsciously wished-for—item. When asked about her "error," the waitress will offer all sorts of excuses except the real one (for a similar experience see Case #22).

This episode might also illustrate the hypothesis of doctrinal compliance, a concept developed by Dr. Jan Ehrenwald,[40] the father of parent-child telepathy research.[42] In this example the child (or patient) tried to supply evidence supporting his father's emotionally charged psychic viewpoint. But isn't this what motivates many people in their pet explanations for various effects—be it in psychic research, political outlook and inlook, or even the suggested reasoning behind the choice of a favorite brand of canned ham? You might be able to find what you're looking for if you try hard enough, but this does not explain away the many successful, repeated telepathic bull's-eyes of a series of several specific thoughts, names, and other data that are recorded over a period of years.

Case 5. She Reads Me Well

(*Parent-Child Telepathy,* series #793, March 13, 1967, Monday, 6:00 P.M.). I had finished dinner and was reading with intense interest in *The World of Ted Serios* (William Morrow & Co., Inc., New York, 1967), by Jule Eisenbud, M.D., the following sentence on page 108: "There is no doubt that a clever machinist or an instrument maker could contrive a means, not only of arranging somehow for a single and prepared image to be produced upon freshly inserted film, but also doing it with several images without having to reload the mechanism, or having any grossly detectable way to alter the outside arrangements of this trick camera." While I was reading this rather long, obtuse statement, Lisa, age 10 (at my desk), started singing, "My baby has hanky-panky." Her song of frivolity distracted my attention from this long complex sentence that defined a clever means of possibly committing fraud. Lisa's song was out of context unless telepathy was considered. Dr. Eisenbud's excellent book is also a powerful psychic tracer. Complex ideas might sometimes be better understood or the underlying meaning seen through by the most direct type of communication—telepathy. Examples like this might also give clues about learning, reading disorders, etc., not just the acquisition of knowledge (intellect) but ways of grasping underlying intentions—emotional learning.

III. "The lover"

Stekel, as noted by Eisenbud,[47] observed that telepathy is often a *via regia* for love and sex. Unfortunately this excellent clue has not been as actively followed up as it might have been. There are amusing cases of lovers meeting under the strangest conditions, unless the telepathic hypothesis be invoked; cases of possible telepathic apprehension of unfaithfulness causing presumed telesomatic reactions[180] in one instance and acute anxiety in another, and examples of sexual deviations that might have been telepathically extended.

This is a robust age, when the acme of physiological function yields many spectacular examples in which the libido and telepathy synchronize. There are instances of coitus being interrupted (telepathically?) by importunate phone calls from a jealous, unrequited lover,[193] and there is the example of a patient who had an infertility problem (azoospermia) where it seemed that on the infrequent occasions of cohabitation, as advised by his physician, the patient received embarrassing phone calls from his mother.

Case 6. Lovebirds

The last time I saw R. H. he and his rejected girl friend phoned my office within minutes of each other. However, three weeks later R. H. came to my home on a surprise visit—and his former girl friend, who lived miles away and knew nothing of these unplanned developments, made a "spur-of-the-moment decision" for an overlapping visit. These examples happened so often that my wife and I had a hard time convincing R. H. that he was not being "framed" by well-intentioned but unwanted matchmakers. Perhaps it was his, or his girl friend's, ambivalence, or the telepathic mischief-making of his friends that was being exploited.

Case 7. An Old Flame

L. L. was at a reunion banquet with classmates whom he had not seen in years. After a few cocktails he confided to an old friend about his girl friend, whom they both knew years ago, and he wondered how she was doing. L. L. still had affection for his ex-girl friend but was circumspect about it since at the time of his relationship his wife was very ill. Shortly afterward L. L. was surprised to receive a letter from his old flame, postmarked Japan. The dates of his fond clandestine reminiscing and his former girl friend's writing about herself coincided. She answered his question. There was no other ostensible reason for her writing. Old flames never die, they just fade away—or do they?

Case 8. That Old Feeling

F. O. had recently returned after three weeks at a psychiatric hospital because of homosexual panic that was precipitated by his failure to hear from a young man whom he had befriended and for whom he had arranged studies abroad. F. O. was upset because the night before he left for the hospital, he had visited his friend's parents, and hardly had he walked into the house when his friend's parents received a phone call from Europe. His friend, then in Europe for one month, had no way of knowing what had happened to F. O. nor had he called his parents before. The telepathic hypothesis might have become more plausible when this event was repeated under similar circumstances several weeks later. F. O. was quite perplexed on both occasions and said several times, "What a strange coincidence!"

Case 9. "Unwanted" Invitations

M. T., a young man with bisexual conflicts, was shocked after a very disquieting dinner conversation with his family on "the modern subject of homosexuality." This topic had never been discussed in his parent's home and it precipitated considerable anxiety for M. T. Later that night, when M. T. returned to his bachelor's apartment (in New Jersey), he was shocked to receive a telephone call from Maryland, from a former male paramour whom he had been thinking about during the dinner conversation, when he had been fearful that his parents and brother would learn his secret. He had not seen this paramour in years, but he was now inviting M. T. to go to Washington. The next two "unwanted" invitations occurred at widely separate times and under slightly different psychodynamic circumstances: (1) the same former male paramour phoned when the patient had made arrangements for a date with a lady whom he had recently met and who was from the same city as the former male paramour. The patient was worried lest the paramour find out about his date, yet there was no way for him to do so. Thus, this former male paramour responded to the patient twice under specific polarized situations where the patient was thinking of him, and touching on areas of an unresolved, unconscious conflict. (2) Another occasion took place one evening after a heated psychotherapeutic session, where the patient lambasted a prestigious former college teacher and would-be male paramour who attempted to seduce and blackmail him. The teacher of long ago phoned from California to try to arrange a "meeting" in New York. Although upset, the patient was relieved when he spontaneously recognized a thread of meaningful relationships in these, as well as other, examples via the telepathic hypothesis. He stood steadfast and was on the road to a soul-relieving improvement.

PART III

As might be surmised, Eros is a vigorous age of life that also provides a vertible three-ring circus for psychic-dynamics in other areas. In addition to the possible role of telepathy in sex, at this time there are exciting telesomatic reactions,[180,191] the telepathy of everyday life and its role in psychopathological states, as seen in psychotherapy. Perhaps an example of its possible influence in crime,[68] or acting out, might be mentioned.

The following case might apply to many instances of antisocial behavior and crime—that is, examples where there might be a presumed telepathic precipitation of acting out. This aspect of telepathy has also been neglected in the literature. There are many examples on the other side of the coin where both supposed seers and ordinary people have reputedly successfully detected telepathically the machinations of plotters or assassins and then "predicted" what subsequently happened. But, what is not discussed is the possible "telepathology" of such people, whereby they might have unconsciously taken advantage of potential criminals with whom they had close relationships and possible telepathic controls, and then precipitated dangerous hair-trigger impulses on those who had poor ego control.

From this type of situation and other examples it can be supposed that some adults in certain unique relationships could conceivably precipitate antisocial behavior on the part of others and through telepathic means. There is also the reverse situation, where some adults have an amazing ability to avoid danger although they are repeatedly exposed to situations and instances where still other people at this robust age of life "attract" dangers and become prey to all sorts of difficulties. Although one cannot rule out subliminal factors,, they might well operate with the telepathic factors (or hypothesis), as in the example of a patient who repeatedly was involved with *frotteurs*.

Case 10. Escape

A middle-aged woman recalled possible telepathic examples with her teenage schizophrenic son. Once, during her treatment in New Jersey, I learned how shocked she was over the morning newspaper's headline of a "Russian roulette" murder. She was acutely fearful that her son, who was then hospitalized in Florida, would "commit a horrible crime like his best friend had just done (who murdered his brother)—there but for the grace of God goes Billy." Billy might have picked up his mother's horror that he would lose control of himself and do something "wrong" as his friend had done; for, at the time of the mother's panic over him, he escaped from the mental hospital where he had been doing well for an extended period of time. In a phone call to me, the hospital confirmed this unexpected and ticklish situation, for they took great pride in the care they gave their patients and it was a long time since anyone had escaped from the closed and locked division. Could this mother have telepathically sent her sudden fear that something horrible would happen to her son and in this way have given him the impetus for losing control of himself and escaping?

Case 11. The Wedding Gift

Mr. F. E. in the concluding session of his long-term treatment, referred to some of the extraordinary possible paranormal events that happened in his sessions (even though he didn't fully know of his physician's role): the recurrent apparitions of his physician,[177] the crashing of the Jacques Romano oil painting; the Venetian blinds rattling; and some amusing and not-so-amusing episodes of possible precognition. The patient concluded his treatment by symbolically giving me a bottle of tranquilizers which I had prescribed for him on an emergency Sunday session at the beginning of his treatment and which he had never used. His symptoms had long since subsided. He was happy that he had made progress and was now going to be married.

The following excerpt from his thank-you note for my wedding gift indicates the extent of the telepathic transference which may have been a factor in his successful treatment:

"My warm thanks for the Mark Cross pen and pencil set. This is the gift I selected for my best man and ushers, and I reluctantly decided not to treat myself to a set. I was completely surprised and delighted by both gifts."

This superficially trivial episode, when considered apart from his other possible paranormal events, would appear insignificant. However, when considered as a part of the whole—the psychic nexus—it is a different matter. Just as dreams have a serial connotation, in the treatment situation, so do telepathic events. The surprising crisscrossing choice of gifts—his for his best man and ushers, and mine for him—was an excellent finale to our relationship. His personal physician informed me that the patient has continued to do well in the ensuing years.

IV. "Then a soldier"

Case 12. The Cameo

One Sunday, my aunt was visiting in New Jersey and wore the cameo gem I had had made to order by C. W. of Wyoming many years ago. This was the first agate that I had found and it was cut by a paraplegic whom I had never met but had heard about. I thought, while admiring the stone, "How beautiful. It's a shame about C. W. I wonder if he is still alive, or dead with uremia [a complication of paraplegia]. Such a nice man." When I remarked to my wife about the gem, I secretly wondered why she never wore her cameo. As the first gemstone I had given her, the cameo had special sentimental value to me. It was not surprising, therefore, that three days later I received a letter from Mrs. C. W. dated at the time of my comments to my wife. Mrs. C. W. wrote: "In refiling in C. W.'s cabinet we ran across an item that seemed to be yours, and we are enclosing it. My goodness, things can really get pushed back, back to 1955! C. W. was very sick at Christmas; in fact, he was hospitalized with a reaction to the Digitoxin and a bladder infection flare-up. He hasn't been too well since July but is beginning to show signs of a gain, for which we are thankful."

This case might illustrate how a telepathic response to a sympathic feeling —caring—as catalyzed by the cameo and propelled by covert criticism of my wife, who did not wear her gem except rarely, brought forth the answer to my question about C. W. There are countless examples of how telepathy in everyday life involves people and the exchange of unique gifts, acts of kindness. And of course—the other side of the coin—there are instances where trouble is either telepathically apprehended or fomented . . . and all without an awareness.

Case 13. Double Take at the Look-Alikes

At 3:00 P.M., I went upstairs to the laboratory to see Franklin Hart III (pseudonym), a patient who was referred for an electroencephalogram. Mr. Hart was a huge fellow, who strikingly resembled a patient by the name of Herman Whyte (pseudonym) whom I had seen once, in emergency, 18 months ago, when I committed him from the police station to the state hospital. I remembered Mr. Whyte well, for he was in an acute schizophrenic excitement and he tore his cell apart. At the time, his psychiatrist from northern New Jersey told me on the phone how dangerous and homicidal Mr. Whyte was. The police and I were caused much unpleasantness at the time because of the patient's threats.

When I gazed at my current look-alike patient, Mr. Hart, the thought flashed through my mind: "Amazing! Isn't it good that he is not Mr. Whyte?!"

At 5:00 P.M., when I returned from the hospital emergency room on another matter, my office doorbell rang. My secretary went to handle the call, and it was Mr. Whyte! He had come to my office for the first time! He asked for a statement concerning our encounter of more than a year ago. Fortunately, my secretary remembered my warning about this patient which was reinforced by the shock of seeing the lookalike; and, furthermore, she knew about this kind of situation from having typed these not infrequent possible telepathic examples, so that she was then able to handle this patient firmly and diplomatically.

The whole thing didn't seem to hang together unless telepathy was considered: for example, my surprise at Mr. Whyte's "double" suddenly resuscitated the past danger, which might have been telepathically apprehended by Mr. Whyte, who exploited the current situation in his own behalf in an attempt to "right" the previous impression, as if to say, "Look, I'm all right now: don't be afraid."

There are many examples like this. Perhaps telepathic pseudoreminiscence is akin to some forms of *deja vu,* in which the sudden shock when confronted with a "look-alike" or some other strong associative "error" is enough to telepathically trigger hitherto odd and unexplainable encounters.

Case 14. Burying the Hatchet

While at the supermarket, I debated whether to buy a sea conch, saw off the end, and thus fashion a Polynesian horn similar to a conch horn which was given to my by my greatuncle. Dr. H, a colleague, had always admired the heirloom horn, which I once said I would give him, but because of differences between us the matter was dropped. However, the supermarket incident signaled a change in our relationship. Within an hour of my buying the conch and recalling the unfulfilled promise of long ago to Dr. H, he phoned to invite my wife and me out to dinner. I gave him the heirloom horn, and since I hadn't seen or heard from him in a long time, the only rational way to account for his (and my) changed attitude was telepathy. His invitation might have symbolized the burying of the hatchet, which was reciprocated by my giving him the trivial but coveted gift.

Case 15. Telepathic Upstaging

Psychotherapy is a two-way street. Although attention is properly focused on the patient and his difficulties, there are times when events in the physician's life can erupt and interrupt and cause possible telepathic fireworks in the treatment situation.

Such was the case with Arnold Duke, a bachelor businessman, who after several weeks of doxepin and psychotherapy for a neurotic depressive reaction, was starting to come alive. Since it is axiomatic that confidentiality be maintained, I chose this example because it would reveal little specific material about the patient but would expose trivia involving myself.

The session was presaged by a cluster of possible telepathic experiences including a possible telepathic dream the night before, the telepathic apprehension of a letter from Holland, and a few everyday telepathic experiences with an earlier patient. However, immediately before Mr. Duke arrived, I received an unexpected call from Washington, D.C., from Mike Waters, of National Public Radio, who wanted to do an interview on my book, *Parent-Child Telepathy*. Since the book had been published several years ago, and, if anything, I avoided any publicity since I had many other things to do and did not want to be involved in rearguard discussion, I was caught off guard and surprised. Mr. Waters and I had a stimulating talk, and I agreed to an interview at a later time. Just before I was to begin with Mr. Duke, I received another long-distance call, this time from CBC in Toronto, requesting a radio interview for 3:00 P.M. that day. I assumed that Toronto was informed by Mr. Waters, but this might not have been the case. If so, it was either coincidence or possible telepathy.

In any event, because of my commitment to Mr. Duke, this telephone interview was postponed until after his session. I was further upset because my daughter, who had been ill, had an appointment to see her doctor in a city some distance away, on the following morning at 8:00 A.M.—and I had to gather and prepare her reports. Thus, in this keyed-up, alert, and energetic frame of mind, the session with Mr. Duke began. The patient, who had been relatively nonproductive in his previous sessions, opened up after my scurrying for background thoughts on the pending radio interview.

[B. E. S.: The book that won't die: *Parent-Child Telepathy*—the interview with Toronto very shortly; what will happen?] The patient perked up with: "I used to get turned on to things, be it a *book*. [B. E. S.: My studies on telepathy . . . some of my recent telepathic papers are coming out at last. I've had requests for 'Geriatric Telepathy'—oddly, more from Canada than from elsewhere, even one today]. The patient spoke up: "Up until this [illness] started I was a voracious reader. I didn't listen to—or hear interview programs—I learn more [by reading]. They're ten-buck books. I must read! I go out and get the book and read it." When I asked the patient, "Why do you tell me this now?" he answered: "I was getting off on another subject; I don't know why I tell you, I was just getting my diary out, to get the name of the book and the author's name. I always hear this (radio) program coming here." [B. E. S.: Like polluting the *water*, the mainstream is contaminated with telepathy.] Patient: "It's like on *Watergate*. It affects everything it touches. It squeezes into every crevice and crack." [B. E. S.: Some are interested in the odd facts of nature—Mr. *Waters* of National Public *Radio* in Washington—Mystery Hill in New Hampshire—I'd like to cram that onto the radio show, and do a good turn.] Patient: "The principle you have on radio shows is that everything happens for the best. Is this true? Chickens that go nowhere. What was meant to be is meant to be, but can we help to stop a third world war before it starts?" [B. E. S.: (an oath)—I'll never write another book—never!] Patient: *"I'll never write* the great American saga. To do something creative—these people must live it and have a high level of self-satisfaction." [B. E. S.: I made an error in talking to the man in Canada. In the rush and pressures, I didn't mention the co-author, Dr. Ruggieri, of *You CAN Raise Decent Children:* another forgotten book. He's a good pediatrician, neighbor, and past physician for my children, and roommate from our bachelor days at the Mayo Clinic.] Patient: "Take the guy who is married and has a sick *child.* Mother says I had years just thinking of myself, not a wife and kids—a problem-free existence."

[B. E. S.: Little does he know that he is picking my thoughts out of mid-air. His depression has lifted, and he is sort of smiling and dissociated in the whole session.] Patient: "Funny, it's 'much ado about nothing' today. If I ever gave any subject as much thought as I gave this, I'd be a worldwide expert. I'd have powers of concentration. Funny, on that boat Saturday—a beautiful day—why isn't it all right with the world? The days are now sunny and no longer gray." [B. E. S.: I'll turn off the airconditioner—too much noise.] Patient: "Nice and cool in here, Doctor. It's terribly muggy out."

Thus, it can be seen how the patient upstaged, and complemented, my thoughts in a volley of possible telepathic crisscrossing. As he came out of the depression with a bang, he acted like a patient who is under the influence of posthypnotic suggestion. He was saying all this almost as if he were having a conversation with me, although my thoughts were silent, as my notes (made at the time) show. He was dissociated and unaware, yet perhaps there was a hazy indication of his dim awareness of what was happening.

These events occurred when the needs of both of us were served, and there was a keyed-up, splitting atmosphere with powerful tracers and the necessity to produce. The patient had not had any previous spectacular telepathic episodes, just the run-of-the-mill, but this was *his* day. This was also prognostically a sign of his ability to respond and communicate. This happens even in some so-called near-hopeless cases—some schizophrenics for example, and when this happens it shows that the patients, by using this means of communication and trying to hang on, are demonstrating a source of untapped ego strength. Another example of volleys of possible exchanges[188] in psychotherapy but involving an older-aged patient is recorded elsewhere.

PART IV

V. "Then the justice"

Case 16. Baked Fish

Mrs. S. E. invited my wife and me to her home for dinner. The lady lived in a neighboring town, and although we had not met before, she had helped me by phoning me some crucial documentation in a newspaper article which she had and which I needed for a particular study. We went to her home reluctantly because of my pressing schedule—I could have thanked her more easily some other way. "If she would only answer my questions over the telephone with a simple 'yes' or 'no'." Furthermore, when we arrived for the dinner, it was a formal occasion and she served baked fish, which I detest. At the conclusion of the evening, Mrs. S.E. read aloud every word of the news clipping instead of letting me peruse the long-awaited information for critical points.

Courtesy dictated that we invite Mrs. S. E. to our home for dinner (which would not be fish!), but this had to be delayed because of my already-mentioned busy schedule. After much hemming and hawing and admitting that Mrs. S. E. seemed to be a woman of strong will with a lot to say—I decided on the spur of the moment to go through with it once and for all and to invite her to our home Friday night. When my wife telephoned, Mrs. S.E. was almost overcome because, she said: "I've received four invitations from people for this Friday!" Apparently others, besides me, had divined her secret: Friday was her birthday; and she could not come!

Polarized areas—whether of intense ambivalence, controversy, poorly repressed subjects, areas of joy or sensitivity (like a birthday or an anniversary)—are significant factors in psychopathology; and such times of heightened effect are also conducive to psi: the Rumpelstiltskin effect. Jacques Romano and Joseph Dunninger were excellent at divining holidays.

Case 17. Telephone Telepathy

I awoke at 4:00 A.M. from a vivid dream that involved a patient at the new St. Barnabas Medical Center. The patient was being presented to a conference, and two other physicians were questioning me. The odd feature was that the woman had a skin lesion on the forehead. It either was or was not lupus erythemotosus—a dread condition. They were just about to ask me about it and I had to justify my position when I awoke. Later, my wife said that at that time she was also having a dream: "About being examined by a physician."

The phone rang. I told my wife, "It's the office phone. It is probably Mr. Walker in reference to his wife. Just wait, the answering service will be calling on the private unlisted number." And that is exactly what happened. Mrs. Walker was a woman in her fifties, who had a skin lesion, as in my dream, and who had given me reason for concern as she had a severe involutional depressive reaction. Perhaps she had signaled through her husband via my (and my wife's) possible telepathic dream, at a crucial time. Arrangements were made for her admission to the Carrier Clinic where she received a course of electrotonic treatment and recovered.

The night after this dream, I had been talking to my father, also a physician, on the telephone and had omitted telling him about the experience of the night before since my patient lived a few blocks from my father's home and was known to my father. Although technically my father had no right to know about this patient's situation, there might have been some quasi-ethical and practical reasons for him to know since the case was a difficult one and I was very concerned about this woman and didn't want any slipups should another emergency arise. I had hardly hung up and was still in a quandary about whether I had done the right thing, when the phone rang. It was Mr. Walker, who allayed all my anxieties (although he was phoning to allay his own) about his wife and told me about her successful admission to the hospital.

These two examples, as well as countless other instances of possible telephone telepathy are similar to Bendit's concept of metasensory perception (M.S.P.),[5] where someone perceives physical events where he has no right to perceive them.

Case 18. A Hot Potato

Bartholomew A. Ruggieri, M.D., my friend and hardworking neighbor pediatrician, wrote this memo: "On the afternoon of Sunday, June 2, 1968, I went up to my room to nap. I slept fitfully, from about 2:30 P.M. to 5–5:30 P.M. During this time I dreamed that I was at an upper story window facing Avenue B and Sixth Street in New York City, and saw a "parade" of mourners approaching as pictured (diagram drawn by Dr. R). It was more a mass of mourners than a parade. They carried a banner with a phrase with a religious connotation and ending with the words: '. . . KENNEDY ASSASSINATION.' I know the area very well, having lived my youth there, but to my knowledge I have never lived on Avenue B. I awoke, vividly recalling all the words on the banner, felt I should get up and write them down, but did not do so. I lay in bed and, after a period of drowsiness, again fell asleep. Somehow, in my mind I associated this to the imminent assassination of Robert Kennedy (Bobby). The Avenue B would support this. The same evening (6/2/68) sitting at my desk at 9:30 P.M., I phoned Dr. B. E. Schwarz, described the dream, and said I felt Bobby Kennedy would be assassinated on the 6th of June. Note 'Sixth' Street: June is the 6th month.

"At 12:30 A.M., 6/5/68, my wife and I finally turned off our portable radio as we lay in bed listening to the early returns of the elections. Though I usually fall asleep quickly, that night I tossed about in bed for what appeared to be a long period of time, half drowsy and half awake, thinking I had a full day's work the next day, and I had better fall asleep, feeling perhaps the room was too warm, and wondering why I couldn't fall asleep.

"At 5:50 A.M., the same morning (6/5/68), my house phone rang. It was Dr. B. E. Schwarz telling me my 'dream' had come true. That I should turn on the radio, as Bobby Kennedy had been shot. I told my wife. We turned on the radio, and one of the first statements we heard was that, as Kennedy was being moved away from the scene of the shooting, a rosary had been placed in his hands. My wife started crying softly at this tragedy to this family man, and the tragedy of continued violence in our nation. I then told my wife of my dream for the first time. Dr. Schwarz informed me later that he told his own wife of my dream on the evening of 6/2/68. Note: Dr. Schwarz goes to bed early and I'd never call him at that hour unless it were urgent."

In an addendum written later that day (6/5/68) between 9 and 10 A.M., Dr. Ruggieri wrote: "I had a feeling it [death] would occur immediately after the primary elections, but since they were on 6/4/68, I couldn't see how the death could occur on 6/6/68. I felt I had to be wrong on the date, 6/6/68, and yet I distinctly recall it was on Sixth Street that the dream event had occurred." (Though he was shot on the 5th, Bobby Kennedy died on the 6th.)

A copy of Dr. Ruggieri's dream was hurriedly sent to Jule Eisenbud, M.D., on 6/5/68, as the family and I were preparing to go to Niagara Falls with Joseph Dunninger for the dedication of the Houdini-Dunninger Museum.* My own reaction, as dictated at the time, completely coincided with Dr. Ruggieri's statement. When my wife answered the phone and ". . . she told me it was Bart, I was annoyed and said unless it was important, she shouldn't bother me since I seldom look at television and this was one of the rare Sunday nights that I wasn't asleep at this hour, and I didn't want to be bothered. However, I went to the phone and Bart told me the dream, which was simple, and exactly as recorded. I was quite annoyed and had the subjective reaction that he was tossing me a hot potato. However, I told him I'd

*Parent-Child Telepathy, series No. 1106, "On June 6, 1968, Thursday, 9:28 A.M., we (Schwarz family) were at the Cavalier Motel in Niagara Falls. I thought of immediately sending Dr. Ruggieri a card, postmarked June 6, because of his remarkable prophecy on the assassination of R. F. K. for this date. At that, Lisa (age 11), who was walking with me in front of the Houdini-Dunninger Museum, said, 'Daddy, it is officially opened June 6th—today!' Lisa (might have) picked up my preoccupation with this significant date but from her point of view."

be his witness and relayed the message of the dream to my wife. It sounded ridiculous because of the political circumstances, and, in a sense, for many people Kennedy polarized violent emotions and an assassination at some time would not be unlikely. The part that stuck in my mind as odd was the emphasis on the sixth, which meant the sixth month and the sixth day. This was the only time in our association (since 1951 in Rochester, Minnesota) that Bart ever told me of such a situation. Although he had recorded telepathic feats in a paper and has a keen awareness for such events, this time was different. He was compelled to phone me. He did not talk about patients or anything else. The call was solely because of this horrible dream."

Other possible precognitive examples for Dr. Ruggieri include his winning, on one occasion, a handsome radio phonograph, and at another time from the same pharmaceutical house, a set of children's books for guessing the correct amount of dosages of a certain drug to be sold in a given period of time.

Another outstanding event, which was not recorded, but which I distinctly remember, was connected with an oil painting Dr. Ruggieri made of a nude model, who from her facial expression appeared to be very hostile. After one painting class Dr. Ruggieri told several people in an off-hand way that the model would not be coming back any more "because she would be in an auto accident," even though she was supposed to be present for additional sessions. His statement was borne out when the model was involved in an auto accident, which terminated her assignment. What the moral is eludes me: viz., (1) don't be a hostile nude model for Dr. Ruggieri; (2) he's a good friend to have; (3) the concept of coincidence makes life much simpler and more comfortable, etc.

It would not be quite proper to speculate on the possible psychic dynamics of Dr. Ruggieri's dream of the Kennedy assassination. However, it would seem, in view of his past experiences, that he has some ability in this regard. Also, perhaps like multitudes, he was fascinated by RFK, a charismatic figure, and perhaps, for his own ambivalent reasons, might have telepathically tuned in on the assassin. It is impossible to explain the exact prediction of the date of death. But if it isn't all coincidence, it might be related to Dr. Ruggieri's shrewd guess as a physician skilled in pathalogical anatomy and to his great interest in numbers (he took many courses in advanced mathematics). His proven past precision in predicting numbers further supports the genuineness of this, rather than coincidence. What is coincidence, anyway?

As mentioned earlier, it is impossible to tell when events that are yet to take place and are being formulated are also being telepathically apprehended by others, as by Dr. Ruggieri, or in fact, if such events are triggered off in people with a propensity to act out violently.

Case 19. Professor Francesco Basili

Signor G, an operatic impresario, came without an appointment. Although I had not met him before, I knew from the "grapevine" that he incorrectly thought I had been treating his late wife. When the Signor entered my reception room, he spoke most admiringly of two mahogany chairs. With grand gestures he said he had never seen anything else like them. He was the only patient in all these years, or since, to make such a fuss over the chairs. It is odd, because of the many items and other furniture in the reception room these chairs are notable for only one reason: they were supposedly used by Enrico Caruso. The former owner of the chairs told me this. It can be conjectured that, under the strained circumstances of our meeting, Signor G telepathically unlocked this unique memory, which, with clarification of the aforementioned misinformation, formed a sturdy bridge for the ensuing consultation. Perhaps some objects are telepathically endowed for sentimental or highly charged unconscious reasons, and then become suitable for crisscrossing or spontaneous psi (psychometry?), as in this experience.

Years later, when preparing a lecture for Quebec City, I dashed over to my neighbor Dr. Ruggieri's house to check his Encyclopedia Britannica for the facts about Prof. Francesco Basili of the Conservatorio di Milano. This man was remembered solely for flunking an 18-year-old bumpkin, for having no musical ability. While I was going to Dr. Ruggieri's, my peripheral thought was that it's a shame I couldn't ethically contact Signor G, who would undoubtedly know about Basili. The next morning my secretary told me that Signor G, at the approximate time of my query, had phoned (call taken by the answering service) for an appointment.

Later, when I asked Signor G about Professor Basili, he told me that the Conservatory had since been renamed for the teenage bumpkin—Giuseppi Verdi! It can be conjectured that Signor G's needs crisscrossed with mine. Because the physician's needs were stressed and pressed by circumstances, as well as to a lesser extent from the material in Signor G's session, it seemed likely that the acuity of his problem was less than he professed. His problem could be minimized by a generous telepathic discount. This opinion was borne out in our session as well as in many similar cases involving other people. There were later examples of telephone telepathy between the Signor and myself: he from different parts of the United States and Europe, and I, in my office in New Jersey.

PART V

Case 20. Epilepsy and the Psychic Nexus

The following previously reported example[191] was abridged for editorial purposes; and in so doing the main parapsychological points—the psychic nexus were omitted. Although it is at times no less tedious for the writer than it is for the reader of such a report, it would seem necessary to break the ice and to give, in some instances at least, (e.g. for a parapsychology pioneer) a fuller presentation of the psychic nexus.[182,183,186] Telepathy is most often part of a continuum. It is laminated and cuts across space and time barriers. It is not easily caged or controlled. If the chief episode is seen as only the top layer, a deeper understanding is thwarted and much of value is lost.

At 10:00 A.M., August 17, 1967, I received a letter from Henry A. Davidson, M.D., Superintendent of Essex County Overbrook Hospital,* inviting me to give a lecture to the psychiatric staff on electroencephalography, October 9, 1967. Dr. Davidson's invitation was welcome because I now had a legitimate excuse to write him and also to thank him in his other capacity (editor of the *Journal of the Medical Society of New Jersey*) for accepting my controversial paper on telesomatic reactions,[180] which had been submitted months previously. My real reason for writing Dr. Davidson, however, was to add to my pending telesomatic paper my friend Dr. Ruggieri's published reference[157] of a case of possible telepathically precipitated temporal lobe epilepsy. Having also studied this particular patient, I was quite excited about some of the intriguing psi potentialities. Until now I had avoided writing Dr. Davidson with my request for listing Dr. Ruggieri's reference because I feared "rocking the boat," and having my telesomatic paper (which Dr. Davidson had accepted) rejected. In other studies on telepathy throughout the years, my papers were frequently at the altar, even at the stage of galley proofs, but then were rejected for one seemingly flimsy reason or another. However, with regard to the pending telesomatic reactions study, experience and discretion won out, and I omitted this point—the pressing reason for my communication. It was better, I felt, to hold off until later and then contact the administrative editor.

Because the morning's consultation was late, I immediately wrote my lecture-acceptance letter to Dr. Davidson and then began preparations for my October lecture by searching my subject card index file under "brain syndromes and abnormal EEGs." Of the 57 patients whose names were written on the card, the name of one patient with temporal lobe epilepsy was illegible. My secretary searched all her files and even worked backward from the symptoms, but she could not discover this particular EEG record. We were both perplexed, trying to decipher my handwriting and to recall the patient's name: who was she, why was she in the files?

The following morning, August 18, 1967, at 10:55 A.M., I went to the fourth-floor EEG record files and pulled out several pertinent tracings for the October lecture. However, my mind still revolved around the mystery re-

---

*Now Essex County Hospital Center.

cord of the patient with temporal lobe epilepsy. When I went downstairs to my secretary's office, I found she was shocked because she had just had a telephone call from a Mrs. Tray (pseudonym), the mystery name and patient we were looking for. I asked my secretary whom she was talking about, because I still couldn't remember Mrs. Tray, whom I had seen only once in consultation, on April 26, 1967. My secretary reported that the patient called because yesterday—at the exact time that I received Dr. Davidson's lecture invitation and all the associative telepathic "tracer" thoughts about this specific patient (whose name was illegible) and also my half-secret emotionally polarized thoughts of Dr. Ruggieri's case of possibly telepathically precipitated temporal lobe epilepsy—Mrs. Tray suddenly had a seizure. The seizure was identical to her previous ones: (1) the day before Thanksgiving, 1966; (2) early February, 1967; and (3) April 21, 1967. She said: "an odd feeling, a flashback, voices—an awful feeling of someone being in the background—the refrigerator looked like a toy—burning from the stomach—felt weak afterward and fell asleep all day. I never had anything so weird happen to me in all my life." These attacks were witnessed by the patient's daughter, who told me of her mother's pallor and who said she feared her mother was having a stroke. Aside from one episode of transitory lightheadedness, this was the first seizure she had had since April 21, 1967. Therefore, Mrs. Tray's phone call dovetailed with my searching for her record (the nonexistent EEG), and her seizure the day before matched precisely the original search for her record. Mrs. Tray told my secretary the exact time of her seizure because it coincided with her planned shopping schedule.

When Mrs. Tray telephoned my office, my secretary asked: "Did Doctor call you?" and then she thought, "Now, why did I say that? The doctor had no reason to call this lady." My secretary further reported: "And as I listened to her, she seemed to be defensive about not having paid her bill. This puzzled me as I had not sent her any follow-up notice other than the usual monthly statements. When I asked the patient why she had not gotten in touch with us earlier, she asserted that she had been taking care of her daughter's children and had no way of earning any money to pay her bills. When I hung up the phone, I fully realized why this name was familiar to me —it was the one that I could not find in the EEG records. Even at this time, I did not know that this lady had been told to have an EEG but that she had never had it—until the doctor refreshed my memory." My secretary made a note of this communication immediately after the call—as is her custom.

Because of the unusual order of events, arrangements were made for a free electroencephalogram, which was taken and showed a minimal dysrhythmia, generalized, bisylvian, maximal left. During hyperventilation, the patient developed paroxysms from all electrodes and medium voltage synchronous sylvian discharges, maximal in amplitude from the left in comparison with the right. These discharges persisted after overbreathing and were symptomatically related to: "I'm getting sick to my stomach." Neurological examination revealed the central nervous system to be objectively intact. Nonspecific hypnotic regression activation[200] had no electrographic changes or clinical evidence suggestive of her seizures.

It was an odd coincidence that this example of a possible telepathically precipitated seizure developed the way it did, since my secret thoughts about the lecture for the October meeting were that it would be boring to go over routine EEG material when I would rather discuss my more personal and exciting telepathic researches, including the recently published possibly telepathically induced temporal lobe epilepsy case. Thus, this woman's seizure was made to order for my purposes as well as her own. With my free EEG and additional study, she received the attention that she needed and had neglected, and I had my curiosity whetted for her intriguing EEG and clinical evidence for temporal lobe epilepsy with a possible telepathic precipitation. There were mutliple determinants: deadlines, strong motivations, powerful specific telepathic tracers: viz., reference to a case of possible telesomatic temporal lobe epilepsy, and a mutual curiosity for both patient and physician. Unless one prefers to consider the whole complex series of pinpointed, tracer-laden events as a concatenation of coincidences, it would appear plausible that our curiosity and anxiety actually precipitated the patient's seizure, rather than the reverse, where my secretary and I telepathically received the patient's distress.

Unfortunately, it was not possible to undertake Metrazol activation and prove the diagnosis or have a detailed follow-up of this patient. It should be noted, however, that a seizure of a conversion etiology would be unlikely, occurring in a 53-year-old divorcee for the first time in her life, with no previous history for conversion reactions. The patient, who was of English ancestry and a high school graduate, used neither drugs nor alcohol. Although space limitations preclude further speculation of psychodynamics, mention of other possible psychic events in her life might be germane since the patient might have had a telepathically precipitated seizure.

The patient recalled an alleged telepathic dream she had about her maternal uncle's (physician) automobile accident in California, while she was in New Jersey. "We knew nothing until I had the dream. We got a telegram a week later (which confirmed the truth of the dream)." Another experience involved her father's attack of acute cholecystitis while on a train to Toronto: "I dreamt that he was very ill and was giving his watch and belongings to my brother (a Texas lawyer)—we later learned that my father was hospitalized and critically ill (at the time of my dream)." The patient had no awareness of the events involving her seizure and my office. Nor did she ever have any knowledge of my psychiatric-psychic researches.

My last formal contact with the Tray family occurred on October 4, 1967. The day before, I had penned a postscript in my letter to Dr. F. Russell Sandford, Mrs. Tray's referring physician, specifically inquiring about her in reference to possible presentation in my coming lecture on October 9. Although Dr. Sandford had no contact with her (or her family) since the time of the original EEG studies, Mrs. Tray's daughter then phoned my office to ask what should be done because her "Mother was upset with babysitting." The timing and implied sensitivity to this superficially trivial event for the Tray family involving Dr. Sandford and myself would appear to be unique, but not at all uncommon, if such records are kept on patients.

It is of interest that over an extended period of time the referring physician, Dr. Sandford, has had seven presumed telepathic associative episodes with me in reference to this patient and her telepathic tracer-laden experience. For example, just before leaving for my lecture at Overbrook Hospital (2:00 P.M., Monday, October 9, 1967), when I was still debating whether or not to use this possible telesomatic-seizure example involving Dr. Davidson, the Superintendent, and jeopardizing (in my mind at least) the acceptance of my paper on telesomatic reactions, Dr. Sandford called in reference to another EEG patient. He had no knowledge of my turmoil at that point and my irresolution as to whether to be a fool and risk discussing the possible telesomatic seizure case involving the Superintendent (and Dr. Sandford) who might, very rightly, decide to reject my paper, or simply to let matters rest. Dr. Sandford's infrequent, if not only, subsequent calls (April 8 and 29, 1968) also occurred under near-identical circumstances.

For instance, on April 29, 1968, when answering a letter from a hospital in Florida that had a patient whom Dr. Sandford had referred to me for initial consultation, my thoughts drifted to Mrs. Tray, the most interesting case of all involving Dr. Sandford and myself. In an hour he phoned to refer, according to my notes, "the first EEG in any capacity since the last telepathic communication at the time I lectured at Overbrook." Also, my memorandum stated: "I went through my desk and found a stack of notes pertaining to the Tray-Sandford telesomatic case and thought to myself, isn't it strange that every time I think of her like this [as a possible tracer or quasi-conditioned response] either she or Dr. Sandford calls. I had been keyed up and primed for telepathy since my visit with Professor Dunninger [the famed telepathist] yesterday."

To further show how telepathic associations are specific, can work in all directions, and are really part of a psychic nexus: on October 28, 1968, Monday, 3:00 P.M., my secretary informed me that Dr. Sandford had called to refer an EEG recheck on a patient of several years ago. This was the first we had heard from Dr. Sandford since April 29. My notes stated: "It is of interest that I had again debated, and had just checked the telepathic cards* on Mrs. Tray and telesomatic telepathy."

It has been noted that some patients with bizarre seizures and accompanying electroencephalographic stigmata could have the seizure turned off and on by a nonspecific hypnotic technique.[200] In many of these cases, experienced physicians in neurology, neurosurgery, and psychiatry, working in the EEG laboratory, refused to believe their eyes. The seizures had to be non-specifically and hypnotically induced several times before they would accept such evidence. They were then convinced that the seizures were "genuine" on the basis of the history and borderline EEG evidence. Thus, it can be difficult in borderline cases to establish the exact nature of the seizure. One would wonder how many seizures: conversion reactions, borderline, and "organic" including the intriguing reflex epilepsies[7] could be telepathically induced. One must first consider the hypothesis—neither a priori to accept nor reject it—and then test it.

Because there is evidence that seizures sometimes can be precipitated by emotional stress,[98] it is quite plausible that in the Tray example turmoil was telepathically mediated or suggested and caused a seizure. With a good subject: viz., seizures precipitated by emotional factors or possibly patients with

---

*It would be folly to omit related data even though the linkage is obscure and tenuous at best. Although my contacts with this highly respected physician have been minimal through the years, there is, in this example (and many others with different physicians) and associated events, almost always a suggestive telepathic core, as confirmed by checking actual records. For example, one of my earliest contacts with Dr. Sandford concerned his knowledge of an alleged bizarre haunted house in his neighborhood that involved a former patient of his. I had once seen this patient's wife in hospital consultation for another physician, and years afterward, when I learned of the haunted house episode from her husband, I investigated the earlier alleged condition. The patient's husband said that their physician at the time (Dr. Sandford) knew of some of the odd events. Furthermore, this patient documented the haunting by recalling that he had asked an Episcopal priest to exorcise the "ghost." While I was wrestling with the proper way to approach the priest and avoid asking leading questions, the priest, who was a total stranger to me and lived in a town far way, phoned to refer his acutely ill son. Having had this good fortune drop into my lap, I thought I could then bring up the question of the haunted house. The priest, without knowing my underlying research purposes, vividly recalled the alleged events. However, he said that he took no stock of them at the time and dismissed it all with the quip: "I told them they didn't need a priest to exorcise, but a psychiatrist to treat!" Perhaps many of the clues to telepathy or synchonicity will be discovered by studying such records as these, kept over the years, involving many people, and finding a recurring psychodynamic pattern—a psychic nexus—of analogous events. It is of interest that almost always these events happen without the awareness of the people involved, and yet they are seemingly caught in a similar psychic force field. As reported elsewhere,[186] there is actually no cutoff point, and I suspect that many spontaneous cases for paranormal events described in the literature might suffer from the grievous omission of much associative data. This is not unusual when one considers how alien such concepts are to our usual mode of thinking and how tedious it can become in following the zigzagging path of events in time, person, and substance, as in the Tray case. Of course, it makes more difficult reading for the uninitiated; and superficially it can become so complex that it is easier to reject a priori any such material or viewpoint as being bizarre than to consider the intriguing and quite explainable hypothesis of telepathy.

reflex epilepsy (i.e., light-sensitive, auditory, musicogenic), some intriguing clinical telepathic experiments could be contrived, using a variety of tailormade activating techniques.

PART VI

VI: "Then the Sixth Age"

Case 21. "Goodbye, Mother"

Mr. R. E. recalled how his father, in Canada, advanced in years and in a deteriorated state of health, had an uncertain prognosis for life. Mr. R. E. who had flown all over the world on business, had gone to Northern Ireland. Although he had been there many times previously, he decided while there this time to look up his place of birth. He did not ask the police, tourist officials, or others for help, but managed to find his old home and take a snapshot of it to send to his mother. Shortly after this, he heard via telegram from Canada that his mother, who was in apparent good health and much younger than the father, had died at the time he was photographing his birthplace.

This is a beautiful, almost classical psi experience, and is not rare: viz., automatic motor behavior*—a compulsion that is quite inexplicable unless considering the telepathic hypothesis. To my mind it is scientifically unusual only when such emotionally moving events as this are either omitted or not fully considered when recording a patient's history and planning his treatment.

Case 22. To Order or Not to Order

My son and I were having dinner at Willie's Diner in Bloomfield. Our waitress was fat, slovenly, slow, and apparently stupid. It seemed to take forever to receive service. My thought was, "How nice an iced tea might be now, but she is too dumb to realize that I would ask for saccharin, and she would give me sugar and then there would be an argument." My son, who was looking

---

*Could these examples of telepathically mediated motor reactions be related to the American physiologist anatomist G. E. Coghill's findings that (1) "the motor nerve system or the so-called proprioceptive system was developed aeons before the sensory nervous apparatus evolved which eventually culminated in the brain of animal and man and finally in man's consciousness" and (2) this primeval nervous proprioceptive system possesses "mentation, this mentation in terms of movement. But movement occurs neither in space alone nor in time alone. It represents both space and time and to the psycho-organismal individual it is space time" (quoted in Psychic Phenomena—How Far Are They Natural? by Ruth Borchard, Ph.D., in *The American Dowser*, Vol. 13 (No. 13): 96–101, August, 1973).

straight ahead over the counter and obviously unaware of my critical thoughts, might have sensed my disapproval of the waitress, as much as his own appraisal of her conduct, for he said: "What a grouchy waitress." Coincidental with our thoughts, the woman came up to the counter and asked: "You want the iced tea?" I was amazed because although I had said nothing of the sort, and we hadn't been served, it was exactly my thought!

Needless to say, this trivial possible example with a new waitress might illustrate the art of human relations: viz., in this case the wisdom of holding one's sharp tongue and practicing patience. When we were through with our dinner, the waitress had perked up, was courteous and helpful.

Case 23. The Manager

One August 11, I was visiting with my Green Pond neighbors Eric and Craig Van Tatenhove, and because of Eric's skill in winning lotteries and similar events, I told him about a weird telepathic experience I had had with a ouija board years ago. At that time, although I have no ability in automatic writing or skill with the ouija board, I had taken a rare fling at it with Mrs. Pat Schutte, whose husband Walter I knew quite well. They had come East on a visit, having moved to the West some years ago. Pat had no previous experience with the ouija board. In any event, the board said that "George Baum would come in two days." Mr. Baum was the manager of the house behind us in Montclair, and he had left town years earlier for retirement in La Crosse, Wisconsin. This was a most ridiculous prediction, or at least it seemed so earlier—until Mr. Baum showed up as prophesied.

After telling my neighbor about this experience, two days later I received a postal card from George Baum, postmarked August 10th. This was the first message we had from him, other than Christmas cards, since he had left Montclair. He wrote that he was staying at the Plankington House of Milwaukee. He confused my recommendation with the Northernaire Hotel which we had been told about by Walter Schuette's father, many years ago. Oddly, after leaving New Jersey he became manager of Plankington (Division of Swift Meat Company) of Milwaukee. Because of the chronology, it is possible the card from George Baum with the odd garbled message (unless considering the parapsychological hypothesis) precipitated my decision to tell Eric about the incident of long ago.

Although I never heard of Plankington House, and George Baum had never heard of Walter Schuette, George picked up the name of the place where Mr. Schuette, Sr., was the manager and not the recommended place Mr. Schuette, Sr., had originally told us about—The Northernaire, where my wife and I had our honeymoon. George's link to me was strong since the time of our initial meeting. It was after a blizzard when the roads were blocked. He was alone in his house and thought he was having a heart attack, until I skied to his home and rendered first aid.

While this possible psi example has an imperfection in the timing by the aforementioned criteria, it should not be discarded too quickly because it could be conjectured that many telepathic impressions are received like a gentle tapping on the mind, to be acted upon not immediately but a short while later. It might be analogous to a typhoid vaccination, where there is no immediate effect, but within 24 hours there can be local swelling, tenderness, redness, and a systemic reaction of fever and chills. Yet, the end events can be traced back to the initial injection.

VII. "Last Scene of All"

Case 24. A Dream Come All Too True

The night my wife and I returned from a visit to Prof. J. B. Rhine at Duke University, I dreamed: "Someone had an arm around my shoulder, [he was V. V.] the father of a boyhood friend I had not seen in many years. This particular friend lives in South Carolina. In the dream, as we walked across the room, the father kept stumbling holding his hand to his heart, and coughing. Finally he collapsed and could not be revived. The next part of the dream was a party, where I saw a girl from years ago, whom I remembered only as the wife of Mr. Pasteur (pseudonym) who swam around Lake Mohawk, and died of heart failure (rheumatic valvular disease)." It was a particularly vivid dream; and upon arising I wrote it down and told my wife that Mr. V. V. was either dying or dead, that I would like to visit the family; but, on the other hand, one could never be sure of these things, and I didn't want to make a fool out of myself.

The following morning, at 11:00 A.M., my mother phoned to say that Mr. V. V. had died; his son later phoned me also, confirming the details. Mr. V. V.'s death was caused by chronic, congestive heart failure and a complication of hypertension for many years. It was my impression that the dream might have been telepathic from Mr. V. V.'s son, who was my boyhood friend. I hadn't seen the son in quite a while, nor had I seen Mr. V. V. for seven years. Mrs. V. V., Sr., said that several people wanted to visit her at the time of the death without any apparent reason. While associating to Mr. Pasteur, my father's former patient who died of acute congestive failure (or subacute bacterial endocarditis) years ago, I received a phone call from a Mrs. Pasteur (a pseudonym), the mother of a patient we had seen for an EEG several months ago. She telephoned to ask about her bill and because of concern over her son's possible military service.

Polarized feelings, as in this instance, and in others, can sometimes, almost at the moment of thinking of the name, evoke either the party that is being thought of, or another person of the same surname or odd first name, or similar unique associative links. The dimensions and mechanisms of memory, space, visualized letters, spoken words, etc., can be fruitfully explored in this area.

Case 25. "Light—More Light!"

Mrs. B. F. was an 81-year-old widow who wore thick lenses for aphakia (cataract operations), and had a florid paranoid reaction. The patient's daughter had informed me earlier that her brother, Lester, was killed in World War II, but this is what the patient said: "He (deceased son) is a graduate of Maine University. In the Mountain Division. Notice of his death April 3, 1944, and heard nothing from him. Can't come back to life—belonged to FBI since a child, really joined at age 18, was taken into the mountains of Italy. He was really killed, but he came out of it . . ." At this point the floor lamp beside my desk lit up by an intensity of one-third. There are three bulbs at the base, and a large central bulb, which was not turned on. No one touched the lamp, and there was no change in the line voltage in the house, as far as I could tell by later checking and by asking questions. Even if there were a slight increase in voltage, it should not have accounted for an extra light to go on, since the bulbs were all firmly screwed into the sockets; and examination afterward disclosed no simple reason for this. The extra illumination was odd, because it happened so fast, and it was definite. It was "unreal!" The patient continued: "He came out of it. Found in a hospital just outside of Alaska in the Aleutians. Mentally bad but recovered physically but didn't know where he was. In the FBI since—another back injury—now I hear a voice in my head saying, don't tell you [doctor] this. I just heard someone in my daughter's room saying tell him anything you want to, etc."

This example is a fact, in so far as it was observed and written down *in statu nascendi;* and although it did not make sense and I didn't want to "believe" it, it happened. Since it touches on similar very sensitive areas in my own life—my younger brother's death in World War II—it is the kind of situation that is suitable for telepathic sending or receiving in physician-patient or other interpersonal relationships. It might be that psychiatric study of spiritualist ministers, some of whom are seemingly successful in these types of situations, would disclose that they are unusually sensitized to the subject of death because of specific traumatic events early in their lives. This hypothesis is plausible when one considers how certain paragnosts have their own specialized skills: e.g., finding missing children, solving sex crimes, finding missing money, etc. Possibly some psychiatrists can develop their skills along similar lines to be of practical and theoretical value to their work.

Case 26. End of the Cycle

Part 1. On Sunday, May 3, 1964, Mrs. N. phoned to say that our friend Miss Bathe (pseudonym), age 86, formerly an executive secretary who had a lifelong interest in psychical research, had had a slight speech disturbance and was sent to the hospital by Dr. E, her osteopath. While there her speech improved and she was to be discharged the following day. Mrs. N wondered if I would look in on Miss Bathe when she returned home to take care of herself, as she had all these years.

Upon arising at 7:00 A.M. on Monday morning, I wrote down a vivid dream: "Going to meet Dr. Nandor Fodor. He's quiet and talks to me through Dr. Ted Anderson (Essex County Overbrook Hospital psychiatrist), a seance ensues, and everything seems phony because it was so outlandish and I know it must be a trick. I see a materialization cloud that is real and I ask, 'What is it?' A man's head and neck are clearly seen, but the rest of the body is represented by a white cloud. Then I see a Negro achondroplastic dwarf with a long genital. He has a hobbling gait. Dr. Fodor's wife, who is present, is tall and thin, with black hair and hazel eyes. She has two daughters who look like her. I ask, what is the meaning of this strange and unusual man (the dwarf)? Dr. Fodor said something important has happened."

When I awoke I recorded the dream. My most immediate association pertained to a recent patient by the name of Mr. Baffle, an intense fundamentalist, who had a unilateral orchidectomy. I gave the matter no further thought until later that morning when Mrs. N phoned (8:40 A.M., Monday, May 4, 1964) to leave word that Miss Bathe would not be coming home, since late last night at the hospital she had suddenly "become crazy, climbed out of bed, exposed herself by taking off her 'Johnny,' ran around the hall, and had become incontinent." Mrs. N had just learned of this from the osteopath who had completed his morning rounds at the hospital and knew nothing prior to this.

The news came as a bombshell, because with it there was an almost immediate recognition of the interpretation of the dream. Dr. Fodor, the famous psychic researcher and psychoanalyst, was the chief psychic tracer to the dream.[179] As a nonmedical psychoanalyst, yet a member of the healing arts, he was equated with Dr. E, the osteopath, one who is related to the healing arts but who is not a physician. The necessity to talk to him through Dr. Anderson, the Overbrook Hospital psychiatrist, symbolized the necessity for me to make out formal commitment papers for Miss Bathe to Overbrook, for she was obviously psychotic, or "crazy." The head-and-neck materialization, which was a man, represented Miss Bathe, who in her advanced age was hirsute. Also, it might have been a particularly appropriate symbol for her because that was all that was recognizable as she allegedly lay in bed laced in a white camisole (as I learned later that evening). The materialization motif had personal significance because through the years I always asked Miss Bathe, half jestingly if she had uncovered any materialization medium yet. I had searched high and low for this form of psychic phenomena but in vain. Miss Bathe, the leading subject as well as a tracer, was like Dr. Fodor, both of whom symbolized a lifetime of psychical research. My "materialization" quip was an impish but personal form of communication with Miss Bathe. This also tagged the dream as psychic. The Negro achondroplastic dwarf also supplied multiple and immediate interpretations. First, the constitution of the dwarf resembled elderly Miss Bathe's short, roly-poly, hunched shape, and, in particular, her hopping gait. The Negro with the long genital was associated to Miss Bathe's exposure and frenzy, which would be most unusual under ordinary circumstances for this very modest and orderly woman. The dwarf's color symbolized her incontinence. The brown genital brought to mind another highly personal communication, for on visits through the years I would bring Miss Bathe cigars. She was the only woman I knew (this was before women's lib) who was an inveterate cigar smoker. Also these rapid-fire dream associations symbolized Miss Bathe's masculine protest, her physical makeup, and penchant for salty comments.

Mrs. Fodor, in the dream, was immediately associated to Mrs. N, one of Miss Bathe's medium protégés who had helped her on many occasions, and who in fact, had brought her to the hospital and telephoned me. The two teenage daughters might correspond to an actual fact: Mrs. N had two teenage sons. The associated Mr. Baffle, my recent patient who had had a unilateral orchidectomy, had the first two letters of Miss Bathe's name and, in fact, two syllables. He was a graduate of a fundamentalist religious college and symbolized to me strong opinions (as Miss Bathe might have had in reference to spirit survival); and his organic sexual (as well as his psychosexual) deficiency was equated with the sexual confusion in reference to Miss Bathe, as well as the displacement from above to below—from the head (brain) to the genital (sex)—Miss Bathe's loss of mind.

When I saw Miss Bathe at the hospital later that evening, my examination of the record and discussion with the nurses and aides who were on duty the night before confirmed all the aforementioned facts of the episode of nocturnal delirium that were symbolized in my dream. I found that Miss Bathe was completely disoriented, unable to recognize me, and muttering gibberish. She had an acute brain syndrome with psychosis. Arrangements were made for her transfer (commitment) to Overbrook mental hospital.

This presumed telepathic dream was explained to Dr. Nandor Fodor, whom I was honored to meet for the first time four days later when he and Mrs. Fodor came to our home to visit.[179]

Although only the possible telepathic aspects of the dream are touched upon here, they reveal how in such cases the mechanisms of symbolization, distortion, displacement, condensation, dramatization, etc., are similar in their function to nontelepathic dreams. Among the hypotheses to be considered for such a dream are: (1) did Miss Bathe in her delirious phase summon me? (2) Did I reach out, because of the previous warning, and telepathically observe her plight? (3) Was my dream derived from the hospital attendants or from Miss Bathe's medium friends, who in turn might have telepathically discovered her plight and were as yet unconscious of their knowledge?

In experiments,[174] it has been shown that many people can unconsciously pick up telepathic data yet be unaware of their roles and unable to synthesize the fragments or to identify the sources of their information. Yet such presumed telepathic percepts that operate beyond awareness are almost always overlooked as powerful factors in determining the actions and behavior of everyday life. A final hypothesis, which Miss Bathe might have offered herself, is the spiritist viewpoint: did her discarnate friends summon the physician, or others, as a means of protecting her?

Part 2. The final scene had yet to be played. About two years later, on the night of July 13–14, 1966, I had a horrible nightmare, which concerned the deaths of (1) my mother's 90-year-old, white-haired foster aunt; (2) of my mother's own sister, who was my blond maiden aunt; and (3) my strawberry blonde wife. In the dream, Ardis (my wife) was dead but returned as an apparition. I asked her if she could change the hands of the clock as proof that she survived. She obliged by changing the hands from 10 minutes before 9 to 20 minutes after 9. This action seemed to be significant. The dream was tagged telepathic because of the tracers of the apparition, the resurrection (materialization), and the changing of the clock hands.

At 5:00 P.M. (July 14), my wife called me in Montclair from our summer cottage in Green Pond to say that Lisa, our daughter, then age 10, had a horrible nightmare (Parent-Child Telepathy Series, #642) in which there was a fire and the aged white-haired community club superintendent and his wife (parental surrogates?) had perished. I was partially relieved from the haunting horrors of my dream when Ardis told me about Lisa's dream and some additional disturbing news from my father. She had withheld this from me until now, because of some pressing matters that I had to attend to and because she did not want to upset me. Perhaps that accounted for my half-knowledge telepathically of what had happened and my "killing her off" and subsequent resurrection, with proof that it was really all right (the materialized Ardis changed the hands of the clock) and that she was handling matters (in reality a thorny situation had suddenly developed).

Lisa's nightmare of the deaths of the elderly white-haired superintendent and his wife might have been a condensation of my overdetermined dream deaths of an elderly maiden foster aunt, actual maiden aunt—which were perhaps also surrogate symbols for the elderly aunt-like, maiden lady, the white-haired Miss Bathe. My dream death of fair-haired Ardis with her materialization-resurrection episode and her changing-the-clock-hands motif (about which more will be said later), might have pertained to other near-specific symbols for Miss Bathe. Ardis, might have been the clue to Lisa's participation, in addition to the aforementioned possible reason for dream choice: my initial annoyance (death) and appreciation (materialization) over the way she handled upsetting news. Further data suggesting how psychically polarized Miss Bathe was for Lisa and for me can be found in Examples 38, 46, and 146 of *Parent-Child Telepathy*.[184]

PART VIII

Although the interpretations, as far as they went, eased matters, they were still unsatisfactory and labeled with multiple tracers; and, furthermore, the dream seemed to stand apart from the dreamer. It said, "Pay attention." I was compelled to depart from customary politeness and told my colleague, Dr. Floyd Farrant, this dream later that night during dinner. It should be noted that in death dreams—as in this particular one—that out of respect, I would not tell my wife all aspects, particularly the grim part involving herself. In any event, Dr. Farrant crystallized matters, when, trying to be helpful, he asked: "Miss Bathe died, didn't she?" Taken aback because of his obvious interpretation and my gross dissociation from the painful event, I told him that I hadn't seen or heard about Miss Bathe in a long time. Although Dr. Farrant knew of her, he had never met her. Neither he nor I had discussed Miss Bathe since her hospitalization. I visited her at Christmas and Easter. She had been hospitalized since her commitment with a chronic brain syndrome, and, until near the end, her condition was unchanged.

The truth came out four days after Dr. Farrant's inquiry.* Mrs. N. phoned to say that her mentor, Miss Bathe, had taken an unexpected turn for the worse on Wednesday, when my dream was nearly synthesized by Dr. Farrant's question. She was put in an oxygen tent and had died Sunday at approximately 8:30 A.M. (July 17, 1966). This data was shortly confirmed by telephone interviews of Miss Bathe's physician and the ward nurse. They reported that there was no acute change in Miss Bathe's condition until the night of the dream.

At the approximate time of Miss Bathe's death, I took an old, battered

---

*The dissociation or resistance to such traumatic material (death) is a much overlooked aspect. The manifest dream content, or the nearly synthesized preconscious material, is so threatening, or revealing, that the dreamer is reluctant to tell anyone; and yet he is compelled to tell someone, even at the risk of embarrassment, ridicule, etc. Obviously, I was not in the habit of telling Dr. Farrant, or anyone else, my dreams. But a possible "hot potato" telepathic dream violates propriety and is almost diagnostic.

book *Lights and Shadows of Spiritualism* (G. W. Carleton Co., New York, 1877), by D. D. Home, from our lake cottage library shelf intending to bring it home to study, which I later did. This book is an account of Home's extraordinary physical mediumship. This was one of seven books at the cottage, and I had not read it before. Oddly enough, this book had special meaning for me, since it was given to me by the late Les Egbert's son several months previously, and Mr. Egbert, Sr. had originally received it from his friend of many years' standing, Miss Bathe. The cover of the book had an eye in the center of a six-pointed star, which pertained to the most touching and personal part of the book. It was about the survival of a little child.

Immediately after putting the book aside, I went upstairs to wake the children for Sunday School. I was startled by a loud sound that my wife heard also. Being accustomed to noting such odd events, we looked at the clock and noted that of 20 postal cards on the kitchen bulletin board, a particular card—the only one of possible telepathic significance—had fallen off the bulletin board.† A note was made of this event because of the odd circumstance. I wondered what event the card falling could symbolize (it was not tacked but held in place by tacks). The card, in fact, was sent to Lisa by Mrs. Cora Matteson, who was then in Holland translating Professor Tenhaeff's *Telepathy and Clairvoyance*.[217] Of course this event was still not synthesized nor correlated with Wednesday night's nightmare nor Dr. Farrant's correct interpretation on Thursday night, which I had "forgotten." Only with the news of Miss Bathe's death did the pieces fall into place.

One evening, exactly a week after our dinner and Dr. Farrant's prescient interpretation of my dream, he wanted to experiment with his possible psi talents. We discussed this and other instances relating to Miss Bathe. The telltale main feature of the possible telepathic apprehension of Miss Bathe's sudden deterioration was my dissociation—as in many death dreams—from the obvious, yet which my friend could pick up and not myself; the tracer, the overdetermined symbols of Miss Bathe, and our highly personal jocose communications in happier years in reference to the dream materialization and clock stopping.

The latter point was a highly personal and significant tracer that a spiritist like Miss Bathe might have called evidential. For in her life Miss Bathe had

---

†At approximately 2:00 P.M., 11/5/60, I was reading a book on spiritualist tricks on loan to me from Miss Bathe's library. I wondered how she was doing and about her many examples of fraud in the psychic field, when I was interrupted by a loud crash, like plaster falling from the ceiling. To say the least, it startled me; I got up, searched, but could find no cause. The doors were closed and I was home alone. Later, my wife received a call from Mrs. N. stating that Miss Bathe had a fall about that time and sustained a Pott's fracture. I immediately went to the hospital and found this to be the case. I was also introduced to the Rev. F. A., a leading spiritualist minister friend and protege of Miss Bathe, who happened to be on one of his infrequent visits to her. These events, if records are kept, might all have certain psychodynamic similarities, which are touched upon elsewhere.[179,182,186]

told me on many occasions how at the moment of her former illustrious employer's death his daughter's watch had stopped—"which he later claimed to have effected when communicating with me [Miss Bathe] through Mrs. Sanders [a medium] before I knew anything of the watch stopping. To the present time he has not ceased to make his individuality known and felt in this life."[178] As a matter of fact I had sent this reference in addition to a presumed personal telepathic dream (Case 21) and a possible telekinetic event to Dr. J. B. Rhine (letter, June 4, 1962).

However, at the time of trying to tie these various happenings and associations together, the more spectacular example of watch stopping in Miss Bathe's career continued to elude me. I remembered it in a general way, but no matter how hard I tried I could not remember the precise reference. I sought this information after her death in order to add a personal footnote on clock stopping and starting (Jacques Romano's death) in a study that included "four instances of clock stopping, each in a different location," at the time of Thomas A. Edison's death.[178]

While Mrs. N. (and through her, Miss Bathe's other friends) knew of Miss Bathe's clock example that was more spectacular than that which she published herself, no one could produce the exact reference. Matters remained that way until one day several months later when I received the Journal that had my article which included the clock-stopping incident. In the same mail delivery I received an unanticipated surprise from Mrs. N. It was the missing links to the puzzle: an article "When the Clocks Stood Still. Did Two Famous 'Ghost Hunters' Signal From the Grave that They were still Alive?" by Waynwright Evans, *American Weekly*, 6/13/54, Western Edition, San Francisco. Thus, the clock element which I unsuccessfully struggled to clearly recall off-and-on all this time, was one of the most amazing events in Miss Bathe's career and might have tied into the peculiar element of the dream apparition of my wife changing the hands of the clock—an unusual event in my dreams to say the least—on the night of Miss Bathe's sudden turn for the worse. I do not know what the dream time meant unless it could have been the time of Miss Bathe's failure, or, possibly, the more exact time of her death instead of the given time of 8:30 A.M. Unfortunately, it was impossible to check it out further. Who knows?

Anticlimax. At the conclusion of Dr. Farrant's and my discussion of the Bathe material he went home and I, left alone in the house, turned off the foyer lamp by a pull chain switch, and went upstairs. I shouted out, half-boisterously: "Miss Bathe, if you are around in any shape or form, make yourself manifest!" I had hardly walked up a flight of stairs when the light went on spontaneously! Quite shocked, to say the least, I examined the switch in the lamp (etc.) but could discover nothing to account for the peculiar event. This had not happened previously with this lamp nor has it happened since.

This final example, like some previous ones, points out the difficulty of making clear to the reader what is so personal and self-evident to the experient. There might be more to be learned from what seems a failure in interpretation but what in other respects is a parapsychological success, than in more obvious successes. The psychic nexus is a zigzagging path that cuts across time and space and involves many people.

Although at times the psychic nexus might seem more complex than the plot of an Italian opera, it is quite simple when each segment of the concatenation of spontaneous events is analyzed and finally linked together to form the larger whole. What is reported here has been much boiled down. The psychic nexus is actually much more extensive. If one is interested, in additional aspects of this particular telepathic nexus—which has been going on for years—there are other related events.[179,182,186] This nexus, which takes in many families and age groups is really, when reduced to its essentials, not much different from the early easy-to-understand parent-child examples. Life begins with the vital dependency of the infant on his mother, and the earliest fears are those of separation. The problem goes on in one form or another throughout all of life until the final separation.

Now that we have had a possible telepathic purview of the seven ages of man, and who knows, maybe even beyond, it might be appropriate, since we began a preceding case with a quotation of Goethe's last words, to close with some of his verse which Miss Bathe once sent me and which might have characterized her own life quest and could be inspiring to other explorers along the psi cycle:

"What e'er you can or dream you can,
Begin it!
Boldness has genius, power and magic
In it."

15

UFO Contactee Stella Lansing: Possible Medical Implications of Her Motion Picture Experiments†

For several years I have studied Mrs. Stella Lansing,[187,194] a unique UFO contactee. In addition to claiming many bizarre alleged first-hand UFO and UFO-related experiences, Mrs. Lansing, unlike many other contactees, has the distinction of having taken more than 500 color regular-8 and super-8 motion picture rolls of peculiar artifacts, many of which appear to be flying saucers. These studies include controlled clinical experiments done in the field in Massachusetts where Mrs. Lansing lives, in the field in New Jersey, in my office, and at the laboratory of the National Institute for Rehabilitation and Engineering (NIRE, Pompton Lakes, N.J.). These various films, made with different cameras, have yielded the same variety of objective data and in some cases spectacular associated psi—including presumed telekinetic —effects. Some successful experiments and field trips used infrared film, video and audio tapes.

The purpose of this report is to present some recent filmic experimental data and to discuss some theoretical and possible clinical applications for psychosomatic medicine.

1. EXPERIMENTAL PROCEDURES AND PSYCHODYNAMIC SETTING

On the afternoon of September 4, 1974, Mrs. Lansing with Ivor Grattan-Guinness, Ph.D., Principal Lecturer in Mathematics at Middlesex Polytech-

†Presented at the 26th Annual Meeting A.S.P.D.M., September 21, 1975.

267

nic, Enfield, England, and Consultant for *Flying Saucer Review,* his wife and I drove to the home of telepathist Joseph Dunninger, near the George Washington Bridge, N. J. Mrs. Lansing, using her Canon II motion picture camera with super-8 Kodachrome II film, sat in the back seat, away from the driver and next to Mrs. Grattan-Guinness. Professor Grattan-Guinness sat next to me in front. Mrs. Lansing had previously exposed some film footage in Massachusetts and on her trip to New Jersey. Grattan-Guinness used my Eumig Viennette 3 super-8 motion picture camera, loaded with fresh Kodachrome II film. Every time Mrs. Lansing (as is her custom) had an impulse to film the scenery, "UFOs" (?), or what not, which were most often invisible to the naked eye, Grattan-Guinness aimed his camera in the same direction and filmed.

Later that evening at a party in my home, Mrs. Lansing showed some of her earlier films, including those of a purported UFO and its possible occupants,[190] several showing clocklike formations of UFOs,[194] and one film with a gliding ufonaut.

The uniqueness of her filmic material, needless to say, left its impact on the guests and indicated some of the countertransference-like difficulties one encounters in the study of Mrs. Lansing. Since the turmoil often accompanying production of her images might be necessary, a digression is in order.

An internist guest became upset, said everything was mechanical artifact, and left early in the evening, after laughing at what he had seen. A former Naval Air pilot and amateur photographer friend, who has been interested in UFOs for many years, became upset and at the end of the evening said to me that the images were due to defects in the camera and had nothing to do with UFOs. This was his impression despite the fact that, as far as I knew, he had not read any of the articles about Mrs. Lansing's alleged UFO experiences and numerous photographic accomplishments which could be objectively validated—whatever the interpretation might be. Two psychiatrist colleagues (perhaps not unlike Freud's opinion as expressed in a paper on medieval poltergeist phenomenon[79] in which he discoursed about the psychopathology of the people involved deftly avoiding coming to grips with the fascinating phenomenon itself), offered no comment on what they had seen but wondered if Mrs. Lansing had schizophrenia.[187] It should be evident, then, that the study of Mrs. Lansing's data, which is out of the mainstream of everyday experience or practice, poses methodological problems that are hardly less difficult than the investigation of the phenomenon itself.

2. LATER EXPERIMENT

Finally, between 1 and 2 A.M., on a clear, near-full-moon Thursday morning, September 5, 1974, Grattan-Guinness, Donald Selwyn who is an optical electronics inventor and Executive Director of NIRE, and I went out to my back yard to conduct some experiments with Mrs. Lansing. Grattan-Guinness again used the Eumig camera as he had earlier with the intention of filming in the same direction as Mrs. Lansing. For this occasion Mrs. Lansing used a contrivance engineered by Selwyn. The device is a bar to which two cameras are attached. By using cable releases simultaneously, it was hoped that in the hands of Mrs. Lansing the cameras (which could be set at different speeds) would film objects that could be measured for variations in speed. Both cameras belonged to Selwyn. One was an Argus/Cosina super-8. It was loaded with Kodachrome II film and adjusted to 24 frames per second. The other camera which was stereoscopically focused on the same test object with preliminary adjustment, was a Kodak Ektasound super-8 motion picture camera. It used Ektachrome 160 super-8 film with the speed adjusted to 24 frames per second.

In due course both Mrs. Lansing and Grattan-Guinness noticed a white object in the sky which made an erratic movement but which happened so quickly they couldn't film it. Grattan-Guinness wrote about his experiences:

'. . . at one moment, during our evening's filming, while Dr. Schwarz and Mr. Selwyn were in conversation a few feet away, both Mrs. Lansing and I saw a UFO. A light, which we had already filmed as a star, suddenly moved silently and rapidly in a shallowly descending path behind Dr. Schwarz's house. Unfortunately we have no record of the sighting, for Mrs. Lansing had no premonition of its occurrence. We both reacted simultaneously and spontaneously to it and described it in exactly the same detail afterwards. Although the motion was rapid, it was slow enough for me to notice its slight oscillatory character. It was nothing like the motion of a meteor, or a falling star, for the object neither left a trail, nor followed a conical path.

[Grattan-Guinness went on to summarize his reaction to Mrs. Lansing's films and the other experiments in which he participated as follows:]

"In themselves the film images and the sighting are of no particular significance, but the circumstances of the occurrence render them of considerable interest. I've never obtained unusual imagery on film or seen a strange light in the sky before, and I have no doubt that Stella's presence alongside me had something to do with them."

3. RESULTS

1. Trip to Dunninger's Home

Although scrutiny of Grattan-Guinness's film made on the afternoon trip to Dunninger's revealed nothing out of the ordinary, Mrs. Lansing's film, which was made simultaneously, showed several interesting effects. They were entirely similar to those she had obtained on many previous occasions, using a variety of cameras and films, both in the day and at night.

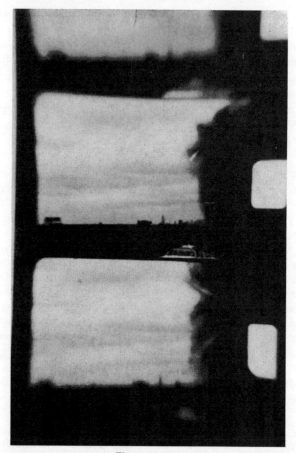

Figure 15–1A.

At two points she filmed typical clocklike formations of apparent UFO-like objects. Figure 15-1a shows this effect with Grattan-Guinness' hair in the background, and Figure 15-1b is the blowup of the objects. Figure 15-2a shows a second film series of similar clocklike formations with the side of Grattan-Guinness' face and camera in position in the background. Figure 15-2b is a blowup of some of the "craft."

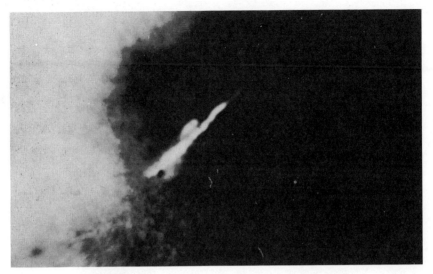

Figure 15–1B.

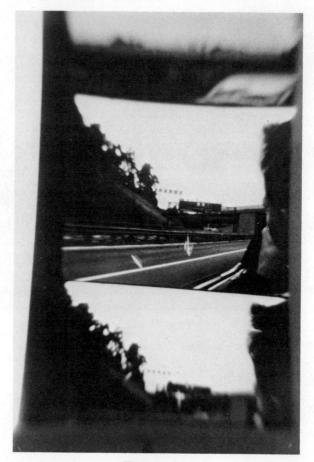

Figure 15–2A.

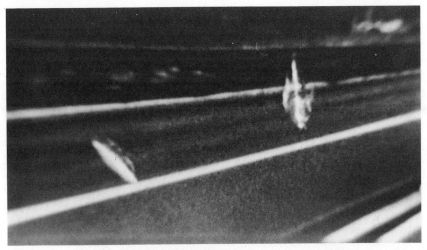

Figure 15–2B.

The next series on the same projected film showed a clearly discernible but transparent clocklike formation, with the George Washington Bridge and Mrs. Enid Grattan-Guinness's hand in the background. Unfortunately, it was difficult to make slides comparable to the projected images and suitable for publication.

All the films and slides were developed by Kodak (Photo-Cullen, a commercial lab in Montclair). The slides were made from the films using equipment specially constructed by NIRE.

Other artifacts than the clocklike patterns were noted in earlier segments of Mrs. Lansing's film. For example, when still in Massachusetts Mrs. Lansing had loaded her camera and filmed a huge, round, dark encysted-like object with a pitch-black night-sky background. While driving to New Jersey she photographed a large opaque object, low in the sky, a few feet above the ground between some high tension wire steel columns (see Figure 15–3).

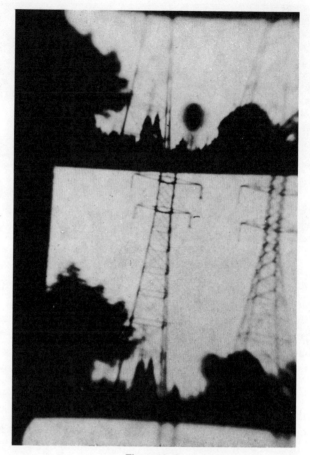

Figure 15–3.

2. Evening Films and Surprise: Selwyn's Mischief

The experimental evening films made by Mrs. Lansing with the cameras on the Selwyn bar, and by Grattan-Guinness with the Eumig, also had strange effects. Prior to filming the equipment was inspected and fresh film was inserted. Figure 15–4 shows Grattan-Guinness's sequence of the moon and just below it a luminous, blue gaseous-like rectilinear object surrounded by a brownish mass.

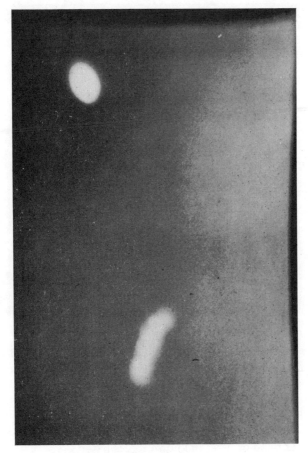

Figure 15–4.

Mrs. Lansing, perhaps because of the excitement of the evening, and the novelty of the Selwyn bar, did not release both cables simultaneously and as she looked alternately through the view finders of different cameras, she did not recall at what point she had either the zoom or wide-angle lens in focus. Unfortunately she only exposed a few feet of the sound motion picture film, which upon projection showed nothing extraordinary. However the projected Ektachrome film (Argus/Cosina camera) showed a huge, white object taking up much of the screen, and which at certain points seemed to simulate a white floating piece of paper with a shimmying effect (see Figure 15–5). This was noted on four separate occasions lasting a few seconds each, and extending over several frames.

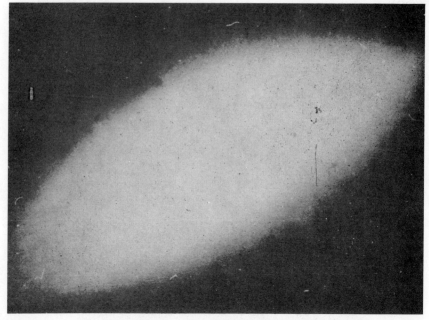

Figure 15–5.

The latter odd effect was provisionally attributed to an artifact-distortion of the moon. However, unknown to anyone at the time when Selwyn gave the bar-mounted cameras to Mrs. Lansing, he had secretly (and without my consent) screwed on to the Argus-Cosina camera a plus-10 dioptor lens, so that "it would be impossible for Mrs. Lansing to film anything in the sky with clear focus," and thereby "prove" if the images were in the sky [or projected from her mind or other unknown forces.].

At the conclusion of the outside part of the experiment Mrs. Lansing came into the house and Selwyn laughingly showed us how he had attached the extra lens. He removed the lens and Mrs. Lansing then took a few clearly focused control shots of an African violet plant. She later took a few feet of color television while Grattan-Guinness did the same. Although there was minimal exposure, it was hoped that as on numerous previous occasions, she might obtain more UFO-like objects (thoughtography?) while filming various TV shows of interest to her. However, later perusal of the developed film revealed this was not the case.

Because of the shimmying white rectilinear effect, I undertook controlled studies on two separate occasions when Mrs. Lansing was not present.* In

*Once, when I was with Mrs. Lansing while I was filming the "moon," the developed picture showed a clamshell-like object (Fig. 15–6a), and a more recent picture of her shows a blue globe and a ray above her hand (Fig. 15–6b).

Figure 15–6A.

100 feet of film, using Selwyn's Argus/Cosin camera with and without a plus-10 dioptor lens and filming such objects as a near-full moon, a street light, house lights, stars, and airplanes, nothing remotely similar was obtained to the rectilinear shimmying "moon"—if that was what Mrs. Lansing had. Although the shimmying effect is no more explainable than the clock-like and other images it does not seem to be the moon. Further experiments in reference to this effect were undertaken with the assistance of an opthalmologist colleague, Floyd Farrant. By using different lights from varying angles directed at the Argus/Cosina camera lens, it was impossible to simulate Mrs. Lansing's shimmying "moon." It is hard to see how a spherical aberration of the lens could make a round object like the moon rectilinear.

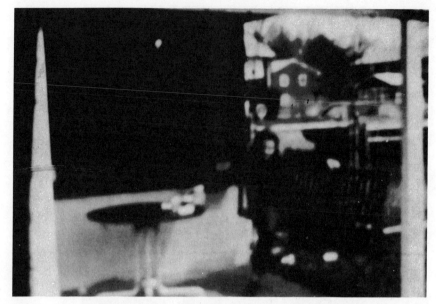

Figure 15–6B.

COMMENT

The facts indicate that Mrs. Lansing under *controlled* conditions can produce on motion picture film presumed UFO-like images that are not all artifacts. Thus, if there are approximately 4050 frames in a 50-foot film reel and
she obtained, as in her Canon camera film example, *seven* frames (including
over-lapping films) with unusual data (0.17% success), there must be an explanation. Previous experiments and also observations of her numerous
films taken either by and of herself[194] or in the company of others (i.e., the
author and his son have filmed similar things mostly when with Mrs. Lansing and rarely when not in her presence) support her claims. Joseph Dunninger, the late eminent telepathist and magician, studied Mrs. Lansing's
filmic images and felt that hoax, self-deception and technical flaws could not
account for her films.[194] He did not know what they were. Paul Sharits, expert in cinematography at the State University of New York at Buffalo, who
saw several of Mrs. Lansing's films, felt that some of her filmic images "con-
tradicted all time-space and filmic logic."

Just as it is erroneous to jump to the conclusion that Mrs. Lansing is actually filming UFOs, so it is presumptuous to state that what she frequently
photographs has no connection with UFOs. These problematic points, including the possible origin of the filmic images, are dealt with else-

where.[187,190,194,154] The major implication is that a human being can have a presumed molecular interaction upon a variety of films, either directly or through the mediation of other poorly understood forces: i.e., psi-induced, UFOs, or UFO-psi.

Psychiatrist Jule Eisenbud's researches on Ted Serios[51] spectacularly demonstrate thoughtographic (telekinetic) effects upon Polaroid film. Using his vast knowledge and experiences in parapsychology, Eisenbud has expatiated on the roles of the unconscious and psi[53] in thoughtography and thereby pointed the way to further investigations.

The physician might wonder at the attention to such an esoteric subject as thoughtography. Perhaps such presumed telekinetic events have a parallel with so-called psychic cures of various diseases. If paranormal effects can occur on film, it should be possible to accept psychic effects on organic systems. Understanding the modus operandi in one case might lead to an understanding of the other and possible practical clinical applications.

Although "psychic" cures of diseases are described in the popular press, little or nothing has been published in medical journals. This is not unusual when one considers the need for rigidly adhering to scientific criteria. Popular accounts give little recognition to the variability in the natural history and course of many diseases where spontaneous remissions frequently take place. In supposed psychic cures the conditions are often poorly controlled, inadequately described and documented.

Also, suitable clinical experiments employing a "psychic healer" often raise formidable medical-legal and ethical questions. Although claims for cures are legion, there is a dearth of solid evidence. The popular accounts are flawed with numerous technical shortcomings and gaping loopholes.

The problem of controlling such multiple variables as suggestion, placebo effect, and possible telesomatic influences, has retarded serious inquiry of psychic healing. It is no wonder that physicians are loath to heed claims for alleged "miraculous" psychic effects, UFO-mediated cures, or to participate in medically unsophisticated experiments.

Although there are all these shortcomings in evaluating possible psychic healings, physicians experience occasional cases where possibly psychically mediated (telesomatic) psychosomatic reactions might take place. Unlike near insoluble problems posed by psychic healing this method of studying telepathically precipitated physical disorders[180,191] lends itself to more precise, critical, clinical scrutiny.

Fortunately the "psychic healer" dilemma is partially resolved by such data, as Grad's[93,94] carefully controlled studies on the effects of a healer's treatment on wound healing in rats, and on the growth of barley seedlings. Related supportive studies might include mention of Jacques Romano[181] who had a "ray" that induced "cool breeze" paraesthesias that were appar-

ently not due solely to suggestion, and which, in a series of experiments retarded the growth of hybrid sunflower seedlings, whereas there was no
similar effect on a known genetic strain of hybrid corn.[175] (It was suggested
that paragnostic abilities (including possible telekinesis) were related to the
reported conflicting effects of so-called mitogenetic radiations). Mention
should also be made of Backster's report[2] of philodendron leaves allegedly
responding to various cognitive-affective states, and also several different intriguing accounts and references cited by Tompkins and Bird.[219] Careful experimentation should resolve some of the controversies about the data if not
the interpretations.

Andrija Puharich, the physician-parapsychologist, whose work on psychic
surgery has been described in the book *Arigo* by Fuller,[86] has recently
presented a variety of presumably telekinetic physical effects, including possible (paranormal?) induction of UFO film images by the Israeli Uri Geller.[147] The interpretation of Puharich's amazing studies is compounded and
controversial because of his allegations of UFO-associated events. However,
some of his work with Geller has been corroborated by controlled tests at
the Stanford Research Institute.[32]

Another neglected area of possible applied telekinesis might be the qualitative, apparent immunity of Holiness Saints to the ordeals by serpents, fire
and strychnine.[172]

CONCLUSION

Intensive study of the Stella Lansing effect on motion picture films, in addition to probing the fascinating mysteries of UFOs, might offer new investigative techniques and open up practical, clinically related areas of interest to
psychosomatic medicine.

16
Postscript: Possible "Impossibilities"

Where do we go from here?

My hope is that many others will explore psi in relation to psychopathology and psychophysiology. Psychiatry should know in more precise, preferably quantitative, terms how widespread psi ability is, and of course, all the details about how some people can develop psi, or have greater awareness for it than others, or how the various psi components (telepathy, clairvoyance, telekinesis, and precognition) differ in relation to psychodynamics and how they are similar.

Perhaps much of the current laboratory work may be premature, and what we need is a concerted approach embracing the natural history, qualitative, or psychodynamic approaches, as, for example, the researches on precognition, in the chair test developed by Professor Tenhaeff[214] in his pioneering work with Gerard Croiset. Why have so few investigators followed up on Professor Tenhaeff's "grab" or "chair test"? The psychodynamic approach to psi, beyond giving us a much deeper understanding of ourselves in relation to nature, might also uncover hitherto overlooked aspects of the phenomena: for example, better ways to dissolve resistance to psi, better ways to condition the psi ability, and ways to define and develop a more favorable permissive external and internal milieu. The computer should be able to digest the many clinical variables and might even uncover some hitherto overlooked clues. An excellent example of combined psychodynamic and quantitative laboratory technique is the well-controlled dream telepathy data of Ullman and Krippner.[225]

Many new clinical studies are necessary to define the borders of applicability of psi to creativity, invention, success in science, business, and the like. Much work remains to be done toward further sharpening the abilities of paragnosts and dowsers for solving crimes, finding missing persons, probing archeological mysteries, and so on. It is theoretically important, as well as

militarily practical to understand the psychic force that can account for telekinetic effects, clairvoyantly perceive distant installations or missile bases,
and telepathically eavesdrop on the minds of our adversaries.

Along this line Puharich[147] deserves credit for calling our attention to the
spectacular telekinetic results allegedly induced by Uri Geller. The facts are
one thing; interpretations are another. It behooves us to learn all we can
about the mind, unconscious processes, personality, and physiology of
someone like Uri Geller in order to obtain clues that might further the fundamental understanding of such abilities as bending spoons, starting broken
watches, jamming electronic switches, and the like. Unfortunately we have
as yet only a superficial glimpse into the dynamics of Geller's personality
and inner life. Undoubtedly there are many other persons with similar abilities. They must be discovered and studied.

One reason there is little information on the possible associated psychopathology of the Geller effect might concern clues obtained from personal examples of telekinesis and the psychotherapeutic situation. Although I have
collected bulging envelopes of such data, only a few examples have been included in these papers. Resistance to psi, and to telekinesis in particular, is
largely unconscious; however, there is also the mostly conscious, common
sense concern over the consequences of revealing all. Indeed, many of my
best telekinetic examples are so revealing that they cannot be published at
present. Since the possible underlying emotional factors for these examples
are similar between myself and a variety of patients, we can suppose that
there is a common mechanism and relevant state of consciousness and psychodynamic pattern. This data could reasonably be extrapolated to other
telekinetic situations and there might also be fundamental similarities to the
underlying psychological dynamite in poltergeist cases, for example, those
reported by Fodor and a few on which I am preparing reports.

On the negative side: if in a free society we do not understand the Geller
effect, totalitarian-state scientists who are actively engaged in psychotronics
may quite likely stumble upon discoveries which will be utilized to our dis-
advantage. In short, the hour might already be late. Our survival could be at
stake.

In one respect, however, the psi-psychodynamic techniques should give
open-society scientists an edge in this matter because their minds are not fet-
tered with political lysenkoism, and they are free to think in terms of the
unconscious and all that it means. Let us stress again that, as in much
psychic-psychodynamic research, the anonymity of the medium must be
protected. Unfortunately, when these abilities burst out, publicity frequently
follows. In the free world one can seldom discover a powerful physical medium with telekinesis without everyone knowing about it. Totalitarian states,
where censorship of the press is practiced, as well as other forms of thought

control, have a short-term advantage. We really don't know what they are doing.

I would emphasize that the ethical and religious aspects of psi are also completely suitable for scientific scrutiny. The valid data or "miracles" of the saints might still be happening today as in the past, the only difference being that now we have better methods and tools to study this data. No longer should there be any taboos that declare such study off limits. Furthermore, the often allied covert, erotic aspects should not be sacrosanct. Seeking the truth strengthens and should not weaken. Father Thurston[218] and other hagiologists have patiently recorded many of these strange events in the lives of religious figures and others from all of man's recorded history. This body of data would appear to be prime territory for psychiatric analysis: levitation, bilocation, astral traveling, teleportations, healings, stigmatisms, materializations, dematerializations, spirit photographs, direct voice, and paranormal audiotape voices. We would like to know how religious life and its accompanying mystical states of altered consciousness practiced by the different devotees or ascetics can seemingly account in some people for the development or enhancement of psi faculties. Also, on the other hand, we would be interested in how these apparent psi abilities can be directed toward destructive ends, as in some reported cases of alleged possession, poltergeists, so-called human spontaneous combustion, hauntings, or as perhaps in the political realm of a Rasputin or a Hitler. We still do not know what makes a genuine mystic—saint or devil—different from other people.

As an example of some of the underlying subtleties of ethical issues involving psi, let me cite what the late Dr. Seymour S. Wanderman, a friend of Jacques Romano, told me years ago. Dr. Wanderman recalled how Romano repeatedly gave spectacular psychic demonstrations at parties in the home of the well-known Wall Street broker, Julius Bache; but at no time did Bache ever offer, or did Romano ask for, any money, just his traveling expenses. Needless to say, Romano's extraordinary feats did not hurt Bache's business dealings. According to Wanderman, most of the guests thought that Romano was so ethical and honorable that it would be wrong for him to take any money, and it was because of this altruistic attitude that Romano succeeded in psi. However, matters are not that simple. The true reason was that if Romano took any money, his precarious prerequisite emotional equilibrium, or inner harmony, would be disturbed, and that would have impeded or suppressed his psychic demonstrations. For many people for whom experiments are devised and money is given as a reward for success, the experiments often might not be sufficiently sophisticated or individualized, since in fact they usually fail. Perhaps the reason for this is as it was with Jacques Romano: the rewards could motivate the desire to try too hard, and this intense conscious motivation might invoke hypothesized neocortical-cognitive mechanisms which shut out an awareness for psi. This awareness might be largely dependent on the unconscious mind and might originate from deep-lying limbic structures.

The disturbed conscious (neocortical)-unconscious (limbic) equilibrium shuts out awareness and the capacity to synthesize psychic (unconscious) impressions. A neurological analogy to this hypothesized mechanism is the clinical observation that a patient with Parkinson's disease might have a resting tremor of his hands, but when he is asked to write his name or concentrate on writing, the tremor is suppressed. In this way the patient invokes his undamaged cortex, which then effectively controls the tremor, which originates in the malfunctioning deeper neural structures: the basal ganglia and substantia nigra. Nevertheless, when the patient is again distracted or not concentrating on the specific task of suppressing the tremor, the deep-lying damaged structures again take over and reinduce the tremor. The process is similar to having the right dose of medicine—not too much and not too little.

These possible analogies obviously have greater ramifications than are presented here, but sufficient material exists to indicate how this principle might apply to many current laboratory experiments—some of which seem, from the interpersonal point of view, to be designed with a heavy hand.

With rare exceptions, study of the sexual lives of paragnosts in relation to their abilities is another neglected area for serious psi investigations. Despite the plethora of hints and clues about the significance of the sexual aspects of psi, as, for example, the penetrating studies of poltergeists and mediums by psychoanalyst-parapsychologist Nandor Fodor,[64,13] unfortunately little appears in the literature by those who are familiar with the clinical vagaries and the management of such problems. The establishment gives lip service to the study of man as he is and leaving nothing out; yet, when we come to sex we find, all too often, this curious omission.

Fodor's findings are indirectly supported by Professor Tenhaeff's[214-216] independent and thoroughly modern researches. There is need to follow up and expand on interview techniques as well as intensive psychometric projective testing of paragnosts. Probing unconscious sexual factors is a personal, sometimes traumatic, and revealing process for anyone. One cannot blame paragnosts, therefore, who, unlike experimental subjects in other fields, are asked to bare their souls completely and who suffer further because for both real and imagined reasons they are often suspected of fraud. Paradoxically those who for good psychodynamic reasons are masters of psychically invading the privacy of others frequently insist on their rights to personal privacy. Perhaps further studies of paragnosts and psi in the physician-patient relationship will tell us how instances of extreme repression of sexuality or hostility sometimes "select" psi as a final common pathway and at other times select various psychopathological and psychophysiological outlets.

Other ways of following up some of the neglected sexual aspects to psi may be mentioned. For example, it can be speculated that possibly the paragnosts, who often seem to have an unconscious androgynous makeup, can take in a wider range of experiential impulses and interpret them without having a wall of resistance and shut out material that would be otherwise biologically or culturally objectionable to most people without psi abilities. The paragnosts intuitively know through direct mechanisms. Perhaps these speculations are compatible with clinical observations of some gifted mediums or paragnosts who seem to have lively sexual drives, either in a natural heterosexual way or occasionally otherwise. In addition to many external psychodynamic variables, there might also exist the psychophysiological correlates. If psi is associated with limbic and reticular functions, the stirring up of unconscious processes, as seems to be the case during entrancement (or the ecstasy of mystics), may stimulate contiguous neuroanatomical areas which, when activated, cause a variety of autonomic psychosomatic effects, including bulimia, anorexia, desire for fasting (?), sexual excitement, etc. Although observed and gossiped about, for obvious reasons all too little is written about the sexual aspects with names attached; for in conjunction with some of the spectacular psychic feats, there are often background characterological factors of satyriasis, nymphomania, or the extreme opposites: possibly subliminated drives into highly intellectual, philosophical abstruseness or the converse: viz., instances of repressed or denied sexuality which are manifested in abstinence, asceticism, bizarre forms of behavior, as in possibly mortification of the flesh and in sexual deviations. Unfortunately, much of what is written on the sexual aspects pertains to people who have been dead for many years or even centuries, and the data is hearsay and often unreliable.

The earliest examples of the role of psi and sex can be traced back to episodes surrounding mating that occur when lovers share a communion, or sex in its broadest sense—the early, close parent-child (telepathic) nurturing relationships. Psychiatric studies have linked psi to a variety of states of consciousness, minus states, which happen after brain injury, during hypnosis, in body-image disturbances, etc. Careful case studies should now definitely expatiate on these interconnections; and then, hopefully, human and animal experiments can be devised that will bring this material into clear focus.

Aside from a series of possible telepathic dreams involving the death of Nandor Fodor and a few other examples, little has been mentioned in this book about one of the commonest examples of crisis telepathy. This omission is not unintentional, for I have envelopes stuffed with possible examples of this. However, when cases concerning presumed telepathic perception of death are analyzed, problems crop up similar to those already mentioned in the difficulties of preparing a report on clinical telekinesis. That is, when psychodynamically explored, some are too personal and the subject can become so painful, weighty, and solemn that it is burdensome to write up. However, there are some good studies on deathbed psi, for example, those reported by Osis[140] and more recently Osis and Haraldsson.[141] Although in no instances—excluding some haunting cases—does my personal material suggest communication with discarnate spirits as a likely possibility, there are good examples of this—most unfortunately in the literature of long ago. We need to re-examine the whole question of survival using new techniques.

In connection with survival, mention should be made of Ian Stevenson's[211] highly original researches on reincarnation. His well-documented studies and speculations about possible medical-psychiatric applications demand attention, for as in the case of psi, the possibly closely allied reincarnation hypothesis, if given careful consideration and found worthy, could hold much promise for improving our understanding of the human condition, various diseases, and possibly even offer new approaches to therapy.

Two particularly exciting areas that point to the future of parapsychiatric research involve thoughtography (paranormal or spirit photography) and paranormal audiotape recordings. Jule Eisenbud,[51,53] the psychiatrist who had already made monumental contributions to the psychoanalytic understanding of psi, has done some carefully controlled work with Ted Serios, who can produce pictures on Polaroid film which are related to thoughts in the unconscious mind. Dr. Eisenbud's scholarship, diligence, and genius are evident in his speculations on the possible methods of this unique talent. Although some magicians have disclaimed Serios's thoughtographic pictures as tricks, not one of them has ever accepted Eisenbud's challenge and duplicated the same results under identically controlled conditions. On the other hand, Eisenbud's work with Serios with selected controls has been replicated by others. Thoughtography is a practical, objective way of studying how the unconscious mind can influence these strange effects. Sadly, research and development laboratories in industry and academic science have almost ignored these revolutionary discoveries.

Psychic researcher Raymond Bayless[3] first published his work on paranormal audiotapes in 1959. That same year in Sweden, Jurgensen[112] began recording paranormal voices. His book was published in 1964, in Sweden. Four years later Raudive, [149] the psychologist, published his book in Germany. One wonders about the origin of these voices, the methods by which they presumably telekinetically affect the tapes, and the interpretation of the ideational content. Although there has been an enormous amount of alleged paranormal audiotape data produced by a few, it is shameful that this breakthrough has failed to cause a ripple among the parapsychological establishment, let alone elsewhere. I would be curious to know how a voiceprint from an alleged paranormal tape of a dead person would compare with a voiceprint made from that same person when he was alive.

Both paranormal photographic and audiotape techniques are germane to a third subject that dramatically points to the future. Ufology, or the study of unidentified flying objects (flying saucers), reveals that in many of the alleged close encounters with the entities of landed craft, in addition to various biological and psychophysiological effects, the witnesses often claim psychic effects, such as supposed telepathy, clairvoyance, precognition, telekinesis, teleportation, materialization, dematerialization of craft and creatures, apports, causation, relief of various illnesses, and the like. Many of these cases are well documented, and the witness (or other members of his family!) often experiences repetitions of close encounters. Also, the witnesses often recall family legends of ghosts, poltergeists, and hauntings going back for generations: or, again, these phenomena seem to develop shortly after or at the time of the encounters. More frequently however, these phenomena continue on and on, becoming part of their lives and posing problems for them. This wealth of data has largely been neglected by psychiatrists, parapsychologists, and to some extent by the ufologists themselves. It is begging for study and might offer clues that would rival or surpass the most spectacular psi discoveries of the last century, when for example, the famed scientist Sir William Crooks bravely studied materialization, fire immunity, and so on. Parapsychiatric study of the contactees and abductees—those who claim contact with the UFO entities—might be especially valuable since in great measure these persons have many similarities to gifted mediums or paragnosts. They are readily entranced, and experiments can be devised that seem to incite new UFO contacts and psychic phenomena, and, what is more important, conditions that lead to objective data—possible paranormal films of UFOs, paranormal audiotapes.

The subjective accounts of the contacts are often mind-boggling. The interpretations offered by the contactees and others are equally bewildering unless the psi hypothesis is utilized. Using it, in conjunction with a careful psychiatric work-up, gives—in most of the cases I have studied—an extremely complicated picture; but at least things seem to come together and some sense can be made out of otherwise contradictory data. The personal equation—the guts of the psychic and psychodynamics—might therefore be the key to much of the mystery. However, the failure to cope with this problem has retarded the researches, possibly because of ethical-technical reasons as well as such factors as unconscious resistance to probing the unknown and certain psychopathological (?) dangers. As in psychic research, the investigator is all too easily enmeshed in the phenomena, and his role can become part of the problem. For example, one psi clue that is frequently overlooked in many close-encounter cases is synchronicity: the same type of fortuitous events occurring over a period of time and involving the experients to the close encounter and later sometimes the investigators. It seems that the contactees, abductees, and possibly investigators are frequently led, as it were, to become part of the strange things that happen subsequently. As in clinical psi studies in general, the investigator's conscious and unconscious attitude and his latent psi abilities are relevant. Although purported injury from UFOs are, fortunately rare, psychosocial and psychic effects are another thing.

It might be desirable for the future investigator of psi and the psi aspects of ufology, like the psychiatrist, to possess considerable understanding of his own unconscious mind and reactions to often strange, unfamiliar data. Without heeding this caveat, any clinical investigation of psi and its presumed emotional and neurophysiological substrates would be incomplete. Possibly, as in some poltergeist or haunting cases, where the necessary measurements and description of the physical telekinetic events are recorded in their minutest detail while little or nothing, or lip service at best, is given to the underlying emotional conflicts, the study is also inadequate. Alas, to date all too few theoretically preferable psychic-psychodynamic studies have been undertaken. As, for example, in the case of the gifted physical medium with telekinesis, the problem is one of protecting the contactee's anonymity. There also exists the difficulty of finding a bona fide journal that would dare publish findings that often contain glaringly contradictory data, data frequently omitted in other articles, and data on psychodynamic-psi interfaces. It follows that parapsychology might have as much to learn from ufology as the reverse, and that both parapsychology and ufology might be dealing with the same underlying force.

Psi is not a question of belief or unbelief, but one of fact collecting, collation, critical study, analysis, and understanding. Psi is a science of possible "impossibilities." One does not have to ask the government for largess nor need one travel to the far corners of the earth to study psi, for the best examples are usually found in one's own backyard. By considering psi, man's horizons should be no less than those that confronted the early explorers when they first landed on the coast of North America or when the astronauts landed on the moon. In none of these instances did these individuals fully comprehend what they came upon, and today we are still trying to assimilate and fully examine the magnitude of their discoveries. Psi challenges man to discover and explore vast new worlds where there are no boundaries and time is a highly relative concept. Although Galen's writings at the time of his death (200 A.D.) became Holy Writ, they unwittingly ushered in a dark age of medicine that lasted for 500 years. New ideas and bold experiments were strangled by a rigid orthodoxy that claimed for itself the imprimatur of in-fallibility.

How little man changes! If he is to advance or to survive, he must consider subjects like psi with an open mind rather than rejecting the data out of hand, or refusing to probe arbitrarily proclaimed sacrosanct areas, because of spurious authorities, discredited knowledge, unconscious taboos, or text-books that tediously repeat errors and outworn doctrines of the past. How long can we afford such extravagances as not listening and paying attention (or not delegating the authority to other properly trained people) when some persons among us might tell about their strange, personal, psychic, UFO and Fortean experiences. How many gifted paragnosts, whether housewives, farmers, teachers, or what not, have we shamelessly turned away or discour-aged because of our fear of being contaminated by their farfetched tales, their possible psychosis, of our being tricked, or possibly on a deeper level, our fear of having our own frail sense of independence or reality questioned —a fear of being challenged anew to voyage into the great unknown!

References

1. Bagchi, B. K.: Mysticism and mist in India. *Journal of the American Society of Psychosomatic Dentistry and Medicine,* Vol. **16** (No. 3): 1–32, 1969.
2. Backster, C.: Evidence of a primary perception in plant life. *International Journal of Parapsychology,* Vol. **10** (No. 4):329–348, Winter, 1968.
3. Bayless, R.: A letter to the editor. *Journal of the American Society for Psychical Research,* Vol. **LII** (No. 1):35–38, January, 1959.
4. Beecher, H.: The powerful placebo. *J.A.M.A.,* **159:**1602, 1955.
5. Bendit, J. L.: ESP: a factor in human behavior. *Corrective Psychiatry and the Journal of Social Therapy,* **12** (No. 1):178–191, March, 1966.
6. Bergler, E.: *Laughter and the Sense of Humor.* Intercontinental Medical Book Corp., New York, 1956.
7. Bickford, R. C.: Sensory precipitation of seizures. *Journal of the Michigan State Medical Society,* Vol. **53:** 1018–1020, September, 1954.
8. Brill, A. A.: *Lectures on Psychoanalytic Psychiatry.* Vantage Books, New York, paperback, 1956, p. 140.
9. British Pharmacopocia, Pharmaceutical Press, London, 1953.
10. Burlingham, D. T.: Child analysis and the mother. *Psychoanalytic Quarterly,* **5:**69–92, 1935.
11. Cadoret, R. J.: Physiology and ESP. *Corrective Psychiatry and the Journal of Social Therapy,* **12:**164, March, 1966.
12. Carington, W.: *Thought Transference.* Creative Age Press, New York, 1946, p. 287.
13. Carrington, H., and Fodor, N.: *Haunted People.* Dutton, New York, 1952, pp. 175–212 (The Talking Mongoose).
14. Clark, E. T.: *The Small Sects in America.* Abingdon Press, Nashville, 1937.
15. Creighton, G.: Effects of UFOs on animals, birds, and smaller creatures. *Flying Saucer Review,* Parts 1–10, Vol. **16** (Nos. 1–6) 1970; Vol. **17** (Nos. 1–4) 1971.
16. Crookes, W.: Notes of seances with D. D. Home. *Proc. Soc. Psychical Res.,* **VI:**98, 1889–1890.
17. Davis, J. H., and Abbott, W. E.: The pathology of thermal burns—changing concepts, a review of the literature since 1945. *Surg.,* **40:**788, 1956.
18. Dean, E. D.: Personal communications to author.
19. ———Plethysmograph Results Over Distances and Through a Screen. Abstract, *Journal of Parapsychology,* **28:**285, February, 1964.

20. ———The Plethysmograph as an indicator for ESP. *Journal, Soc. Psychical Res.,* **41**:351, March 1962.

21. Devereaux, G., Editor: *Psychoanalysis and the Occult.* International Universities Press, Inc., New York, 1953.

22. Drill, V. A.: *Pharmacology in Medicine.* McGraw-Hill, Blakiston, New York, 1958.

23. Dunninger, J., as told to Gibson, W. B.: *Dunninger's Secrets,* Lyle Stuart, New York, 1974.

24. ———Personal communications to the author, Sept. 1, and 16, 1966, and Oct. 18, 1972.

25. Dunninger, J.: *What's On Your Mind?* World Publishing Co., Cleveland, New York, 1944.

26. *ibid.* pp. 51–61

27. *ibid.* p. 52

28. *ibid.* p. 52–54

29. *ibid.* p. 54

30. *ibid.* p. 77

31. *ibid.* pp. 102–103

32. Ebon, M., Editor: *The Amazing Uri Geller,* Signet Book (paperback), New American Library, New York, 1975.

33. ———*They Knew the Unknown,* World Publishing Co., New York, 1972, Chapter 6, pp. 77–78.

34. Edison-Reese Correspondence, Edison Laboratory Archives, Orange, N. J. 07050

35. Edwards, F.: *Stranger Than Science.* Ace Books, Inc., reprinted by Lyle Stuart, New York, 1959, pp. 184–187.

36. Ehrenwald, J.: *Telepathy and Medical Psychology.* W. W. Norton, New York, 1948.

37. ———*New Dimensions of Deep Analysis.* Grune & Stratton, New York, 1952, p. 316.

38. ———Telepathy and the child-parent relationship. *Journal of the American Society for Psychical Research,* **XLVIII**:43–55, April, 1956.

39. ———Telepathy: concepts, criteria and consequences. *Psychiatric Quarterly,* **30**:425–449, 1956.

40. Ehrenwald, J.: The telepathy hypothesis and doctrinal compliance in psychotherapy. *American Journal of Psychotherapy,* Vol. **XI** (No. 2):359–379, April 1957.

41. ———Hippocrates, Kairos, and the existential shift. *Amer. J. of Psychoanalysis,* Vol. **29**:89–93. 1967.

42. ———Mother-child symbiosis: cradle of ESP. *Psychoanalytic Review,* Vol. **58** (No. 3):455–466, 1971.

43. ———*The ESP Experience,* Basic Books, New York, 1978.

44. Eisenbud, J.: Telepathy and problems of psychoanalysis. *The Psycho-analytic Quarterly,* **15**:32–87, 1946.

45. ———The dreams of two patients in analysis interpreted as a telepathic rêve à deux. *Psychoanalytic Quarterly,* Vol. **16**:39–60, 1947.

46. ———Analysis of a presumptively telepathic dream. *Psychiatric Quarterly,* Vol. **22**:103–135, 1948.

47. ———Psychiatric contributions to parapsychology: a review. *J. of Parapsychology,* Vol. **13**:247–262, 1949.

48. *ibid.* pp. 251–252.

49. ———Book review of *Eleven Lourdes Miracles* by D. J. West. *J. of the Amer. Soc. for Psychical Research,* Vol. **LII** (No. 2):73–76, April 1958.

50. ———Psi and the nature of things. *International J. of Parapsychology,* Vol. **V** (No. 3):245–273, 1963.

51. ———*The World of Ted Serios.* William Morrow & Co., Inc., New York, 1967, p. 367.

52. ———Why Psi? *Psychoanalytic Review,* Vol. **53** (No. 4):647–663, 1966–1967.

53. Eisenbud, J.: *Psi and Psychoanalysis.* Grune & Stratton, New York, 1970.

54. ———Some notes on the psychology of the paranormal. *J. of the Amer. Soc. for Psychical Research,* Vol. **66**:27–41, 1972.

55. Elman, R., and Lisher, C.: The local skin lesion in experimental burns and its relation to systemic manifestations. *Surg., Gyn., and Obst.,* Vol. **78**:346, 1944.

56. Everson, T. C., and Cole, W. H.: Spontaneous regression of malignant diseases. *J.A.M.A.,* Vol. **169**:1737, 1958.

57. Feinberg, L.: Fire walking in Ceylon. *Atlantic Monthly,* V. 203:73, 1959.

58. Fisher, C.: Dreams and perception. *J. of the Amer. Psychoanal. Assoc.* Vol. **2**:389–445, 1954.

59. ———A study of the preliminary stages of the constructions of dreams and images. *J. of the Amer. Psychoanal. Assoc.,* Vol. **5**:5–60, 1957.

60. ———and Paul, I.H.: The effect of subliminal visual stimulation on images and dreams: a validation study. *J. of the Amer. Psychoanal.* Assoc., Vol. **7**:35–83, 1959.

61. ———Subliminal visual stimulation: a study of its influences on subsequent images and dreams. *J. of Nervous and Mental Diseases,* Vol. **129**:315–340, 1959.

62. ———Subliminal and supraliminal influences on dreams. *Amer. J. of Psychiatry,* Vol. **116**:1009–1017, 1960.

63. Fitzherbert, Joan: The nature of hypnosis and paranormal healing. *Journal of the Society for Psychical Research,* Vol. **46**:1, 1971.

64. Fodor, N.: The psychoanalytic approach to the problems of occultism. *J. of Clinical Psychopathology,* Vol. **7**:65–87, 1945.

65. ———*Mind Over Space.* Citadel Press, New York, 1952, p. 221.

66. ———Through the Gate of Horn: a clinical approach to precognitive dreams. *Amer. J. of Psychotherapy,* Vol. **IX**:283–294, April 1955.

67. ———*The Haunted Mind,* Helix Press, New York, 1959.

68. ———Telepathy–inhibitive, cathartic and malignant, *The Indian J. of Parapsychology,* Vol. **1** (No. 3):125–130, September, 1959.

69. ———*New Approaches to Dream Interpretation.* Citadel Press, New York, 1962, p. 368.

70. ———Cosmic winds, *Psychics International,* Vol. **1** (No. 3):1–42, November 1964.

71. Fodor, Amarya: Cosmic winds: does my husband communicate: FATE, Vol. **18** (No. 1):83–85, January 1965.

72. Fodor, N.: *Encyclopedia of Psychic Science.* University Books, Inc.,

73. *ibid.,* (Daniel Dunglas Home) pp. 171–175.

74. *ibid.,* (Mrs. Gladys Osborne Leonard) pp. 193–194.

75. *ibid.,* (William Stainton Moses) pp. 248–250.

76. *ibid.,* (Eusapia Paladino) pp. 271–275.

77. *ibid.,* (Mrs. Leonore E. Piper) pp. 283–287.

78. ———*The Unaccountable.* Award Books, New York, 1968, pp. 121–125.

79. ———*Freud, Jung, and Occultism.* University Books, Inc., New Hyde Park, N. Y., 1971, pp. 119–120.

80. *ibid.,* Chapter III, Freud and the Devil, pp. 16–19.

81. Freud, S.: *Dreams and Telepathy.* Collected Papers 4. Hogarth Press, London, 1925, pp. 408–435.

82. ———Dreams and the Occult. *Published in New Introductory Lectures on Psychoanalysis.* Hogarth Press, London, 1934.

83. ———*The Occult Significance of Dreams.* Collected Papers 5. Hogarth Press, London, 1950, pp. 158–162.

84. Friedman, S. M., and Fisher, C.: Further observations on primary modes of perception. *J. of the Amer. Psychoanalytic Assoc.,* Vol. **8**:100–129, 1960.

85. Fromm-Reichmann, F.: *Psychoanalysis and Psychotherapy.* Edited by Bullard, D.M., University of Chicago Press, 1959, p. 318.

86. Fuller, J. G.: *Arigo: Surgeon of the Rusty Knife.* Thomas Y. Crowell, New York, 1974.

87. Gaddis, V. and M.: *The Strange World of Animals and Pets.* Cowles Book Co., Inc., New York, 1970.

88. ———*The Curious World of Twins.* Hawthorn Books, Inc., New York, 1972.

89. Garrison, F. H.: *History of Medicine.* Saunders, Philadelphia, 1929.

90. Gerloff, H.: *The Crisis in Parapsychology: Stagnation or Progress?* Walter Pustet, 8261 Tittmoning Obb., Germany, 1965.

91. Gibson, E. P.: The American Indian and the fire walk. *J. Am. Soc. for Psychical Res.,* Vol. **XLVI**:149, 1952.

92. Gilmore, G. W.: Ordeal, in: *The New Schaff-Herzog Encyclopedia of Religious Knowledge.* Funk and Wagnalls, New York, Vol. **VIII**:249, 1910.

93. Grad, B., Cadoret, R. J., and Paul, G. I.: An unorthodox method of treatment of wound healing in mice. *International J. of Parachology, Vol.* **III** (No. 2):5–24, 1961.

94. Grad, B.: A telekinetic effect on plant growth, II, experiments involving treatment of saline in stoppered bottles. *International J. of Parapsychology,* Vol. **VI** (No. 4):473–498, Autumn 1964.

95. Greenbank, R. K.: A prophetic dream. *Corrective Psychiatry and the J. of Social Therapy,* Vol. **12**:213–218, March 1966.

96. Gregory, Anita: Important Russian telepathy findings. FATE, Vol. **24** (No. 7):45–51, 1971.

97. Gresham, W. L.: *Houdini: The Man Who Walked Through Walls.* Holt, Rinehart & Winston and Macfadden Books, 1959, p. 263.

98. Groethuysen, U.C., Robinson, D. B., Haylett, G. H., Estes, H. R., and Johnson, A. M.: Depth electrographic recording of a seizure during a structured interview. *Psychosom. Med.,* Vol. **XIX** (No. 5): 353–362, September-October 1957.

99. Hartwig, G.: *Aerial World.* D. Appleton & Col, New York, 1875, pp. 282–285.

100. Hastings, J. (editor): Ordeal, in: *Encyclopedia of Religion and Ethics.* Scribner's, New York, 1955, Vol. **IX**:507.

101. Hecoen, H., Penfield, W., Bertrand, C., and Malmo, R.: The syndrome of Apractognosia due to lesions of the minor cerebral hemisphere. *A.M.A. Archives of Neurology and Psychiatry,* Vol. **75**:400–434, 1956.

102. Henriques, F. C., Jr., and Moritz, A. R.: Studies of thermal injury, I, the conduction of heat to and through skin and the temperature therein. A theoretical and an experimental investigation. *Am. J. Pathol.,* Vol. **23**:531, 1947.

103. Home, Mme. D.: *D. D. Home, His Life and Mission.* Kegan, Paul, Trench, Trubner, London, 1921.

104. Johnson, A., and Szurek, S. A.: Etiology of antisocial behavior in delinquents and psychopaths. *J.A.M.A.,* Vol. **154**:814, March 1954.

105. Josephson, M.: *Edison: A Biography.* McGraw-Hill Book Co., Inc., New York, 1959, p. 98.

106. *ibid.,* p. 141.

107. *ibid.,* p. 284.

108. *ibid.,* p. 381.

109. Jung, C. G.: *Psychology and Religion: West and East.* Pantheon Books, New York, 1958, p. 592.

110. *ibid.,* pp. 596–597.

111.   ———*Man and His Symbols.* Aldus Books, London, 1964, pp. 149–157.
112.   Jurgensen, F.: Sprechfunk mit verstorbenen, cited in, Uphoff, W. and M. J., *New Psychic Frontiers, Your Key to New Worlds.* Colin Smythe, Ltd., 6 Staten Road, Gerrards Cross, Bucks, England, 1975, p. 63.
113.   Keel, J. A.: *Strange Creatures From Time and Space.* Fawcett Gold Medal Books, Greenwich, Conn., 1970.
114.   Kolb, L.: *The Painful Phantom.* Thomas, Springfield, Ill., 1954.
115.   Kretchmer, E.: *The Psychology of Men of Genius.* Harcourt, Brace & Co., New York 1931.
116.   LaBruyere, quoted by Lombroso, C.: *Man of Genius.* Charles Scribner's Sons, New York 1891.
117.   Lang, A.: The fire walk. *Proc. Soc. Psychical Res.,* Vol. **XV**, Part XXXVI:2, 1900.
118.   LeShan, L. L.: The vanished man: a psychometry experiment with Mrs. Eileen J. Garrett. *J. Am. Soc. Psychical Res.,* Vol. **62**:46–62, 1968.
119.   Lilly, J. C.: *Man and Dolphin.* Pyramid Publications (paperback), New York, 1962.
120.   MacLean, P. D.: Some psychiatric implications of physiological studies on the frontotemporal portion of the limbic system. *Electroencephalography and Clinical Neurophysiology,* Vol. **4**:407–418, 1952.
121.   ———The limbic system and its hippocampal formation; studies in animals and their possible application to man. *J. Neurosurgery,* Vol. **11**:29–44, 1954.
122.   McCreary, T., and Wurzel, H.: Poisonous snake bites. *J.A.M.A.,* Vol. **170**:268, 1959.
123.   Marden, L.: The island called Fiji. *Nat. Geo. Mag.,* Vol. **CXIV**:526, October 1958.
124.   Meerloo, J. A. M.: Telepathy as a form of archaic communication. *Psychiatric Quarterly,* Vol. **23**:691–704, 1949.
125.   Meerloo, J. A. M.: Archaic behavior and the communicative act. *Psychiatric Quarterly,* Vol. **29**:60–73, 1955.
126.   ———*Hidden Communion:* Studies in the Communication Theory of Telepathy. Garrett Publications, Helix, New York, 1964, p. 118.
127.   ———Unobtrusive and Unconscious Communication. *International J. of Parapsychology,* Vol. **VI** (No. 2):149–177, Spring, 1964.
128.   ———Sympathy and Telepathy: A Model for Psychodynamic Research in Parapsychology, *International J. of Parapsychology,* Vol. **10** (No. 1):57–83, 1968.
129.   ———*Along the Fourth Dimension.* John Day Co., New York, 1970, p. 144.
130.   Menard, W.: Firewalkers of the South Seas. *Tomorrow,* Vol. **6**:33, 1958.
131.   Miller, F. T.: *Thomas A. Edison, Benefactor of Mankind.* Edison Copyright, 1931, Francis T. Miller, pp. 268–272.
132.   *ibid.,* p. 295.
133.   Miller, R. De Witt, cited in *Impossible Yet It Happened.* New York, Ace Books, 1947, p. 80 (from Annales des Sciences Psychiques, 1915).
134.   Moritz, A. R., Henriques, F. C., Jr.: The reciprocal relationship of surface temperature and time in the production of hyperthermic cutaneous injury. Am. J. Pathol., Vol. **23**:897, 1947.
135.   ———Studies of thermal injury. II. The relative importance of time and surface temperature in the causation of cutaneous burns. *Am. J. Pathol.,* Vol. **23**:695, 1947.
136.   Moritz, A. R.: Studies of thermal injury. III. The pathology and pathogenesis of cutaneous burns; an experimental study. *Am. J. Pathol.,* Vol. **23**:915, 1947.
137.   Myers, F. W. H.: *Human Personality and Its Survival of Bodily Death.* Longmans, Green, London, 1903, Vol. 1, Chapter III, Genius, pp. 70–120.
138.   *ibid.,* pp. 598–634.
139.   National Formulary X. Lippincott, Philadelphia, 1955.

140. Osis, K.: *Deathbed Observations by Physicians and Nurses.* Parapsychology Foundation, Inc., New York, 1961, pp. 82–83.

141. Osis, K. and Haraldsson, E.: *What They Saw At the Hour Of Death.* Avon Books, New York, 1977.

142. Osmond, H.: A review of the clinical effects of psychotomimetic agents. *Annals of the New York Academy of Sciences,* Vol. **66**:418–434, 1957.

143. Parrish, H. M., and Pollard, C. B.: Effects of repeated poisonous snake bites in man. *Am. J. Med. Sci.,* Vol. **237**:277, 1959.

144. Pederson-Krag, G.: Telepathy and repression. *Psychoanalytic Quarterly,* Vol. **16**:61–68, 1947.

145. Poland, W. S.: The place of humor in psychotherapy. *Amer. J. Psychiatry,* Vol. **128**:5, 1971.

146. Pollack, J. H.: *Croiset the Clairvoyant.* Doubleday & Co., Garden City, New York, 1964.

147. Puharich, A.: *Uri: A Journal of the Mystery of Uri Geller.* Anchor Press, Doubleday & Co., Inc., Garden City, N. Y., 1974.

148. Puharich, H. K.: Transcript of the interdisciplinary symposium. The *Academy of Parapsychology and Medicine,* October 30, 1974, pp. 45–54.

149. Raudive, K.: *Breakthrough:* An Amazing Experiment in Electronic Communication With the Dead. Taplinger, New York, 1971.

150. Rhine, J. B.: (quoting F. A. Mesmer) Psi phenomena and psychiatry. *Proceedings of the Royal Society of Medicine,* Vol. **43**:804–814, 1950.

151. Rhine, J. B., and Pratt, J. G.: *Parapsychology, Frontier Science of the Mind.* Charles C. Thomas, Springfield, 1957, p. 220.

152. Richet, C.: *Thirty Years of Psychic Research.* Macmillan, New York, 1923.

153. *ibid.,* p. 506.

154. Roberts, A. C.: Tele-mystery. Commentary by B. E. Schwarz, M.D., *Flying Saucer Review,* Vol. **21** (No. 6):18–19, April 1976.

155. Robinson, D. B.: *Experiences, Affect and Behavior: Psychoanalytic Explorations of Dr. Adelaide McFadyen Johnson.* University of Chicago Press, Chicago, 1969.

156. Romano, J.: Personal communication to the author.

157. Ruggieri, B. A.: Pediatric telepathy. *Corrective Psychiatry and J. Soc., Therapy,* Vol. **13** (No. 4):187–195, July 1967.

158. Rumke, H.C.: Quoted by Tenhaeff, W. H. C., in *Tijdschrift voor Parapsychologie,* No. 1/2:42, 1966.

159. Runes, D. D. (editor): *The Diary and Sundry Observations of Thomas Alva Edison,* Philosophical Library, New York, 1948, p. 18.

160. *ibid.,* p. 20

161. *ibid.,* pp. 206–209, 224, 230, 235–238, 242–244

162. *ibid.,* pp. 224, 236

163. *ibid.,* pp. 207–216

164. *ibid.,* p. 215

165. *ibid.,* pp. 13, 44–55

166. *ibid.,* pp. 205, 209, 215, 233, 238–240, 244.

167. Ryzl, M.: *Parapsychology: A Scientific Approach.* Hawthorn Books, Inc., New York, 1970.

168. Sanderson, I. T.: *Investigating the Unexplained: A Compendium of Disquieting Mysteries of the Natural World.* Prentice Hall, Englewood Cliffs, N. J., 1972; personal communication March 10, 1972.

169. Sargent, W.: Some cultural group abreactive techniques and their relation to modern treatment. *Proc. Roy. Soc. Med.,* Vol. **42**:367, 1949.

170. ——*Battle For the Mind.* Doubleday, New York, 1957.

171. Schmidt, H.: PK experiments with animals as subjects. *J. of Parapsychology.* Vol. 34 (No. 4):255–261, 1970.

172. Schwarz, B. E.: Ordeals by serpents, fire and strychnine. *Psychiatric Quarterly,* Vol. 34 :405–429, July 1960.

173. ——Telepathic events in a child between 1 and 3-1/2 years of age. *Int. J. of Parapsychology,* Vol. III (No. 4):5–52, 1961.

174. ——Psychodynamic experiments in telepathy. *Corrective Psychiatry and the J. of Social Therapy,* Vol. 9:169–214, 1963.

175. ——Human presumed mitogenetic effect. *The Indian Journal of Parapsychology,* Vol. 5 (No. 3):113–137, 1963–64.

176. ——Psychic-Dynamics. Pageant Press, New York, 1965; *A Psychiatrist Looks at ESP.* New York, New American Library, 1968, paperback.

177. ——Built-in controls and postulates for the telepathic event. *Corrective Psychiatry and the J. of Social Therapy,* Vol. 12 (No. 2): 64–82, March 1966.

178. Schwarz, B. E.: The telepathic hypothesis and genius: a note on Thomas Alva Edison. *Corrective Psychiatry and the J. of Social Therapy,* Vol. 13(No. 1):7–19, January 1967.

179. Death of a parapsychologist: possible terminal telepathy with Nandor Fodor. *Samiksa* (Journal of the Indian Psycho-Analytical Society), Calcutta, India. Vol. 21 (No. 1):1–14, 1966–67.

180. ——Possible telesomatic reactions, *The J. of the Medical Soc. of New Jersey,* Vol. 64 (No. 11):600–603, November 1967.

181. ——*The Jacques Romano Story.* University Books, Inc., New Hyde Park, N. Y., 1968.

182. ——Telepathy and pseudotelekinesis in Psychotherapy. *J. of the Am. Soc. of Psychosomatic Dentistry and Med.,* Vol. 15 (No. 4):144–154, 1968.

183. ——Synchronicity and telepathy, *Psychoanalytic Review,* Vol. 56 (No. 1): 44–56, 1969.

184. ——*Parent-Child Telepathy: A Study of the Telepathy of Everyday Life.* Garrett Publications, New York, 1971.

185. ——Possible UFO-induced temporary paralysis, *Flying Saucer Review,* Vol. 17 (No. 2):4–9, March/April 1971.

186. ——Precognition and psychic nexus, *J. of the Amer. Soc. of Psychosomatic Dentistry and Med.,* Part I: Vol. 18 (No. 2):52–59, 1971; Part II: Vol. 18 (No. 3):83–93, 1971.

187. ——Stella Lansing's UFO motion pictures, *Flying Saucer Review,* Vol. 18 (No. 1):3–12 January/February 1972.

188. ——Possible geriatric telepathy. *J. of the Amer. Geriatrics Soc.,* Vol. XXI (No. 5):216–223, May 1973.

189. Schwarz, B. E.: Possible human-animal paranormal events, *J. Am. Soc. Psychosom. Dentistry and Med.,* Vol. 20 (No. 2):39–53, 1973.

190. ——Stella Lansing's movies: four entities and a possible UFO, *Flying Saucer Review,* Special Issue No. 5:2–10, November 1973.

191. ——Clinical studies on telesomatic reactions, *Medical Times,* Vol. 10 (No. 2):71–84, December 1973.

192. ——Saucers, psi and psychiatry, MUFON (Mutual UFO Network, Inc.) Symposium Proceedings, June 22, 1974, Akron, Ohio, pp. 81–95.

193. ——Telepathic humoresque. *Psychoanalytic Review,* Vol. 61 (No. 4):591–606, 1974–75.

194. ——Stella Lansing's clocklike UFO patterns, *Flying Saucer Review,* Part I: Vol. 20 (No. 4):3–9, January 1975; Part II: Vol. 20 (No. 5):20–27, March 1975; Part III: Vol. 20 (No. 6):18–22, April 1975; Part IV: Vol. 21 (No. 1):14–17, June 1975.

195. ——Talks with Betty Hill: aftermath of an encounter, *Flying Saucer Review,* Part I:

Vol. 23 (No. 2):16–19, 1977; Part II: The things that happen around her, Vol. 23 (No. 3):11–14, 31, 1977; Part III: Experiments and conclusions, Vol. 23(No. 4):28–31, 1977.

196. ———The man-in-black syndrome: follow-up on the Maine UFO encounter, *Flying Saucer Review.* Part I: Vol. 23 (No. 4):9–15, 1977 (published Jan. 1978). Part II: Vol. 23 (No. 5):22–25, February 1978; Part III: Vol. 23 (No. 6):26–29, April 1978.

197. ———Psychiatric and parapsychiatric aspects of UFOs, in Haines, R. F. (editor): *UFO Phenomena and the Behavioral Scientist* Scarecrow Press, Metuchen, New Jersey, 1979.

198. Schwarz, B. E., Bickford, R. G., Mulder, D. W., and Rome, H. P.: Mescaline and LSD-25 in activation of temporal lobe epilepsy. *Neurology,* Vol. 6:275, 1956.

199. Schwarz, B. E. and Bickford, R. G.: Electroencephalographic changes in animals under the influence of hypnosis, *J. of Nervous and Mental Diseases,* Vol. 124:433, 1956.

200. Schwarz, B. E., Bickford, R. G., Rasmussen, W. C.: Hypnotic phenomena, including hypnotically activated seizures, studied with the electroencephalogram, *J. of Nervous and Mental Diseases,* Vol. 22:564–574, 1955.

201. Schwarz, B. E. and Ruggieri, B. A.: *Parent-Child Tensions.* J. B. Lippincott Co., Philadelphia, 1958.

202. ———*You CAN Raise Decent Children.* Arlington House, New Rochelle, N. Y., 1971.

203. Servadio, E.: *Psychoanalysis and Telepathy,* pp. 210–220, translated by Devereux, G. (editor): Psychoanalysis and the Occult, op. at New York: International Universities Press, 1953.

204. Sevitt, S.: *Burns, Pathology and Therapeutic Applications.* Butterworth, London, 1957.

205. Sinclair, U.: *Mental Radio.* Albert and Charles Boni, New York, 1930, p. 239.

206. Soal, S. G., and Bateman, F.: *Modern Experiments in Telepathy.* Yale University Press, New Haven, Conn., 1954.

207. Sollmann, T.: *A Manual of Pharmacology and Its Applications to Therapeutics and Toxicology.* Saunders, Philadelphia, 1944.

208. Speiden, N. R.: Personal communication to the author, August 30, 1966.

209. Stekel, W., Eisenbud, J. (quoting Stekel): Psychiatric contributions to parapsychology: a review. *J. of Parapsychology,* Vol. 13:247–262, 1949.

210. Stevenson, I.: Telepathic impressions: a review and report of thirty-five cases. *Proceedings of the American Society for Psychical Research,* Vol. 29, June 1970.

211. ———The explanatory value of the idea of reincarnation. *The J. of Nervous and Mental Diseases,* Vol. 164 (No. 5):305–326, 1977.

212. Sullivan, H. S.: *Conceptions of Modern Psychiatry.* The William Alanson White Psychiatric Foundation, Washington, D. C., 1947.

213. Svorad, D.: "Animal hypnosis" (Totstellreflex) an experimental model for psychiatry. *Arch. Neurol. and Psychiat.,* Vol. 77:533, 1957.

214. Tenhaeff, W. H. C.: Proceedings of the Parapsychological Institute of the State University of Utrecht, Vol. 1, 1960.

215. ——— Vol. 2, 1962.

216. ——— Vol. 3, 1965.

217. ———*Telepathy and Clairvoyance.* Charles C. Thomas, Springfield, Ill., 1972.

218. Thurston, H., S. J.: *The Physical Phenomena of Mysticism.* Burns Oates, London, 1952.

219. Tompkins, P., and Bird, C.: *The Secret Life of Plants.* Harper & Row, New York, 1973.

220. Transcript of the Interdisciplinary Symposium, October 30, 1971, The Academy of Parapsychology and Medicine.

221. Tubby, G. O.: *James H. Hyslop—X, His Book, A Cross-Reference Record.* The York Printing Co., York, Pa., 1929.

222. Tylor, E. B. T.: Ordeal. *Encyclopedia Britannica,* Vol. 16:850, Chicago, 1957.

223. Ullman, M.: Herpes simplex and second degree burn induced under hypnosis. *Am. J. Psychiat.,* Vol. **103:**828, 1947.

224. ———On the occurrence of telepathic dreams. *J. of the Am. Soc., for Psychical Research,* Vol. **LII:**50–61, April 1959.

225. Ullman, M. and Krippner, S.: *Dream Studies and Telepathy: An Experimental Approach.* Parapsychology Foundation, Inc., New York, 1970.

226. Van Paassen, P.: *Days of Our Years.* Hillman-Curl, Inc., New York, 1936, pp. 248–251.

227. von Urban, R.: *Beyond Human Knowledge.* Pageant Press, New York, 1958, pp. 30–32.

228. *ibid.,* pp. 206–207.

229. Warcollier, R.: *Mind To Mind.* Creative Age Press, New York, 1948, p. 109.

230. Wilkins, Sir H., and Sherman, H. M.: *Thoughts Through Space.* Creative Age Press, New York, 1942, pp. 153–155.

231. Wolberg, L. R.: *Medical Hypnosis.* Two volumes. Grune & Stratton, New York, 1948.

232. Wuenschel, E. A.: *Self-Portrait of Christ, The Holy Shroud of Turin.* Holy Shroud Guild, Esopus, N. Y., 1957, p. 126.

INDEX

Telepathic discount, 232 n–233 n, 250
Telepathic displacement, 163
Telepathic dreams, 118, 133, 148–149, 217–218, 235, 246–247, 258–259
Telepathic "errors," 131, 166, 237
Telepathic hallucination, auditory, 108–110 visual, 132–139, 161
Telepathic-hyperesthesia, 91
Telepathic percipient, psychodynamics, 38, 41–42
Telepathic postulates, 129–143
Telepathic rapport, xxi, 106, 119, 236
Telepathic tracers, 80, 85, 94–95, 134–138, 150, 170, 186, 236–238, 253, 262
"Telepathology," 240
Telepathy, and abdominal pain, 114–115; and brain disturbance, 62, 105–106, 110–112, 140–141, 189, 250–256; and cartoons, 176, 213–215, 218–219; and crisis, 117–118, 169–170, 246–247, 285–287; and death, 41, 108–110, 148–149, 157–166, 169, 231, 234–235, 258–259, 263–266; fallacy of agent and percipient, 58, 61; and food, 96, 219–220, 257; foot-in-mouth, 217; and homeostasis, 224 (see also psychic equilibrium); and humor, 84, 174, 212–225; long distance, 208, 219, 221, 238–239, 250, 253, 256; Florida to New Jersey, 167–168, 240–241; Hawaii to New Jersey, 149–150; Sweden to New Jersey,132; and look-alikes, 242–243; and mental mechanisms, 96, 99; negative, 165; and occupation, age, sex and religion, 231; and oedipal conflict, 41, 98, 132–133; parent-child, 67–100, 115–116, 158–159, 171–172, 189–190, 213–215, 232, 235–238, 248 n, 262–263; with father, mother and grandmother, 93–94; and mental mechanisms, 99; with people and body image, 97; and surprise, 98; and sibling rivalry, 98; physician-patient, 230–231; and postulants for ministry, 231; and psychodynamic drawing experiments, 25–66; and red color, 39, 40, 44, 61, 65; remembering, 233; and sex, 38–40, 60, 214–215, 238–240, 260–261; and telephone, 125,146, n, 169, 206, 243, 247, 250, 252, 254–255, 258; a trois, 132, 207; and visual-auditory synesthesia and use of colloquialisms,63; and volley of drawing experiments, 42–50

(two persons), 51–52, 57–58 (four persons); wax and wane pattern, 92
Telepathy and Clairvoyance, 264
Telekinesis, possible, 102, 104, 108–110, 126, 145, 146 n, 149, 154, 163, 171–172, 179, 203, n, 208, 222, 231, 241, 259, 264 n, 265–266, 282, 287
Teleportation, 283, 287
Telesomatic reactions, 112–126, 231, 250–256, 280
Temperature and fire ordeal, 12
Temporal lobe, 64
Temporal lobe epilepsy, 116, 121, 252–253
Tenhaeff, W. H. C., xvi, xx, 102, 131, 151, 161, 165–166, 186, 200 n, 207, 229, 232, 264, 281, 284
Tetragrammaton, 189, 190
The Bible Unmasked, 183
The Curious World of Twins, 212, 237
The Return of Russell Colvin, 236
Thirty Years of Psychical Research, 89
Thompson, Stewart, 175
Thoughtography, 104, 144, 276, 279, 286
Thought transference, 101 n
Through the Gate of Horn, 191
Thurston, H., 283
Tompkins, P., 280
Tony, Dr., 120–121
Tooth, 41
Toothache and telepathy, 114
Totalitarian states, 282–283
Totstell-reflex, 10
Trance, 5, 18, 100
Transference, 132, 135, 148, 162, 174
Trauma, 151, 259
Traveling clairvoyance, 133, 136, 154–155
Trust, 171
Tubby, Gertrude O., xiii-xiv, 77, 79, 149, n–150 n, 154, 179
Tuxedo, 218
Twain, M., 212
Twins, 110, 121–122, 124

UFO (flying saucers), 210, 267–280, 287–288
Ulcerative colitis, 119
Ullman, M., 93, 102, 229, 281
Uncle, disliked, 148
Unconscious, xxii, 44, 60, 62, 68, 100, 119, 188, 235, 237; suggestion, 90
Urban, von, 199